ILLNESS IN THE HOME

A Study of 25,000 Illnesses in a Group of Cleveland Families

John H. Dingle, Sc.D., M.D.
*Elisabeth Severance Prentiss Professor
of Preventive Medicine and Associate
Professor of Medicine, The School of
Medicine, Western Reserve University*

George F. Badger, M.P.H., M.D.
*Professor of Biostatistics, Division of
Biometry, The School of Medicine,
Western Reserve University*

William S. Jordan, Jr., M.D.
*Professor of Preventive Medicine and
Professor of Internal Medicine,
University of Virginia School of Medicine*

The Press of Western Reserve University
Cleveland — 1964

PREFACE

The study described in this book is an attempt to determine and define the behavior of illness and health in a selected and stable group of families over a period of years. Our concept of studying illnesses in a stable civilian population to a large extent grew out of the wartime experiences of the Commission on Acute Respiratory Diseases of the Army Epidemiological Board in observing disease at a recruit training camp where of necessity the population was regimented. The question naturally arose "Would it not be possible to obtain more reliable information on the fundamental problems of the occurrence of disease and departure from a state of health by a long-term study of a stable civilian population with a broader age span?"

After much planning and a preliminary trial in 1946 and 1947, the full-scale study began on January 1, 1948, and continued until May 31, 1957. In anticipation of the first epidemic of Asian influenza the study was reactivated for the period from September 22 through November 30, 1957. Long-term studies of this sort require not only the cooperation of the families, but also adequate professional staff and financial support. The work has been a major activity of the Department of Preventive Medicine, School of Medicine, Western Reserve University. The planning in the early years of the study was carried out by Drs. G. F. Badger, J. H. Dingle, A. E. Feller, R. G. Hodges, W. S. Jordan, Jr. and C. H. Rammelkamp, Jr. Other persons who have participated in some phase of the study are as follows:

Professional staff.—Drs. William C. Boake, Constance Curtiss, Floyd W. Denny, Jr., Harold S. Ginsberg, Eli Gold, William E. S. James, Sidney Katz, Arthur S. Littell, Lois P. McCorkle, Irving Miller, Vaun A. Newill, Robert Oseasohn, Herbert Rosenbaum, and I. G. Tillotson, and Mr. David A. Stevens. The reports based on the study (1-26)* which are quoted extensively in this book reflect both in their authorship and acknowledgements the roles played by these staff members.

Home visitors.—Grace S. Achtermann, Mary Clare Harmon, Harlene Jones, Grace E. Lindsay, Marilyn E. Linn, Dorothy H. Sanderson, Joan L. Schlobohm, Mary G. Stokes, Patricia A. Watts and Anne H. Wolf.

---

*See list of numbered references, pg. 388.

Technical and laboratory staff.—Esther Bach, Ruth Banfield, Cornelia Bates, Naomi A. Buehler, Virginia Colville, Mary K. Dixon, Alice T. Dow, Julia Foster, Doris Garvin, Ruth Genutis, Joyce L. Greene, Agnes G. Haff, David Heard, Mary C. Heard, Marjorie N. Kodis, James J. Lamberti, Nancy C. McGraw, Mary H. McParland, Bernice Miraldi, Helen Mohnacki, Jeannette Rathfelder, Sylvia R. Rodriquez, Juanita M. Ruffier, Nancy C. Steiner, Ernest I. Stewart and Phyllis Todd.

Secretarial and clerical staff.—Barbara Barnard, Margaret L. Barriball, Laura M. Birnbaum, Edith K. Brown, Alice A. Burke, Corinne S. Cotharin, Rebecca Danon, Nancy S. Gilbert, Marlene Gustafson, Patricia C. Hecht, Jean P. Hinson, Dorothy R. Hollis, Esther Johnson, Ruth Labovitz, Josephine M. Morris, Margaret H. Sawyer, Joan M. Sokolik, Esther C. Taylor and Joan A. Venetta.

The climate of Cleveland was particularly favorable for a study of this sort because of the interest of the Brush Foundation and the previous studies of Professor T. Wingate Todd on child growth and development which that Foundation had supported. A number of the parents in the present study had previously been children in Professor Todd's study. The investigation was conducted under the sponsorship of the Commission on Acute Respiratory Diseases, Armed Forces Epidemiological Board, and was supported in part by the Office of The Surgeon General, Department of the Army, and by grants from the Brush Foundation, the Cleveland Foundation, the S. P. Fenn Trust, the Robert Hamilton Bishop, Jr., Endowment Fund, Mr. Philip R. Mather, and the Republic Steel Corporation. In the final editorial phase of preparation partial support was obtained through NIH grant GM 09310. In addition the study had the approval and support of the officers and Board of Directors of the Cleveland Academy of Medicine and of many family physicians and pediatricians in Cleveland. We are particularly indebted to Dr. Hymer L. Friedell and his staff for their careful study of the x-ray films, and to the New York State Department of Health Laboratory, Lederle Laboratories Division of the American Cyanamid Company, and the laboratories of the Communicable Disease Center, United States Public Health Service, for supplying pneumococcal and streptococcal grouping and typing sera. We also wish to acknowledge the interest and advice of Dr. Lowell J. Reed, particularly during the planning period, and the continued support of Dr. Joseph T. Wearn. We are indebted to Dr. A. E. Feller for reading the final manuscript.

This book presents, insofar as possible, the total experience of the families during the 10-year period of the study. A number of publications (1-26) have appeared in the literature dealing particularly with the results obtained during the first three to five years of the study. We are indebted to the various journals in which these publications appeared, and which therefore are the copyright owners, for permission to reproduce material pertinent to this book. These journals are the American Journal of Public Health (23), copyright by the American Public Health Association, Inc., 1955, the American Journal of Hygiene (1-5, 10-14, 16, 17, 20, and 21), the Journal of Experimental Medicine (7), the AMA Archives of Internal Medicine (25), and the New England Journal of Medicine (6, 8, 9, 15, 18, 19, and 22). We are also indebted to the Academic Press, Inc., for permission to quote from the Harvey Lectures (26).

Finally, we are most indebted to the families whose interest and cooperation made the study possible, and in particular to the mothers who tolerated the weekly invasion of their homes, who controlled the children at the time of the semiannual blood-lettings, and who became observant recorders of the daily symptoms at the times of illness in members of their families.

TABLE OF CONTENTS

TABLE OF CONTENTS

Chapter I
INTRODUCTION

This volume presents the results of a 10-year study of a defined population of civilian families in Cleveland. The primary objectives of the study were twofold: first, to obtain answers to some rather obvious questions for which only limited data were available, such as: How much illness actually occurs? What is the etiology of the illnesses? How important is the family unit in the spread of illness? Do individuals and families vary in susceptibility to illness, and, if so, to what extent? Do families have a characteristic pattern of illness?; second, to study specific disease entities, following leads obtained from clinical, epidemiological and laboratory aspects of the investigation. The literature contains surprisingly little accurate information dealing with the true occurrence of illnesses, especially minor illnesses, in civilian populations. A number of investigations and surveys of various types have been carried out in the past in Great Britain, Holland, the United States, and other countries, the majority being cross-sectional surveys, usually of different individuals at different time periods. Often such studies have been based on data derived from questionnaires or interviews with individual lay members of the population studied, without medical examinations or medical diagnoses, and thus have been subject to considerable inaccuracy. Such surveys, however, have been of value in providing rough estimates of illness problems on a broad basis.

Few attempts have been made to observe a defined population for a period of years in order to obtain reliable and detailed data regarding both specific and total illnesses. Excellent studies have been carried out or are in progress, however, on segments of a population. Sir James Spence and his associates, for example, are studying approximately a thousand children born into families in Newcastle upon Tyne, and plan to continue their observations until the children reach 15 years of age (100, 125); here the emphasis is being placed on children. Other studies of families have been carried on for variable periods of time (36, 40, 43, 55). It was our desire to study the occurrence and behavior of illnesses over a period of years in a population composed of families, since the basic social unit of our population is the family and this unit may well be the basic epidemiological unit having a major influence on health and disease. The accumulation of data, however, was not the only purpose of this study. It was hoped that the experience gained would provide a knowledge of methods and techniques for dealing with and obsering larger populations, as for example, those required to study long-term or chronic illnesses, as well as to provide information that might be of value for educational purposes.

Our interest in a study of this type arose from work in the Armed Forces which demonstrated that detailed basic data could be obtained with respect to the behavior of various specific diseases, since the military organization and facilities permitted the establishment of criteria for case finding at several levels of severity, such as hospital admissions, dispensary visits, sick call reports, and field surveys. Incidence rates could be calculated with a high degree of accuracy, since numerators could be determined for inapparent as well as overt illnesses and the total population concerned, or the denominator, was known. Such data provided the basis for reliable clinical and epidemiological descriptions.

It is apparent, however, that a military population has obvious deficiencies for the study of disease, since the age and sex composition of the personnel is arbitrarily limited, the period of observation of any individual or group is short, and the living conditions, peculiar to the needs of the services, are strictly regimented. It seemed possible that the advantages inherent in the military forces for the investigation of the behavior of illness might be achieved, and the disadvantages overcome, by the selection and study of a stable group of civilian families. Such has been the concept underlying the work presented here.

Initially it was hoped that two populations of families might be observed, one in the middle and upper economic level and the other in the lower economic level, so that the occurrence of illness could be compared in the two groups. After a preliminary study of population migrations in the city of Cleveland, however, it became apparent that the migration of the lower income families, both in and out of the city proper, was such that it would be impossible to follow adequately such a group over a period of years. For this reason the families observed had to be selected from the middle and upper economic groups. There was no population for direct comparison and the only comparisons that could be made were those within the family population itself. This population does not represent a random sample of the community and the data obtained cannot be applied to the population at large except, perhaps, in a very general way.

The general plan of study consisted of four parts: 1) the observation and recording of the illnesses or events occurring in each individual and family; 2) the differentiation of known entities such as streptococcal infections, influenza, or noninfectious diseases, and the study of their behavior; 3) the investigation of possible entities of unknown etiology based on individual and distinct patterns of clinical or epidemiological behavior; and 4) the study of specific problems such as the spread of an infectious agent in the population, the evaluation of therapeutic or prophylactic agents, and the occurrence of noninfectious processes. The methods and results for the most part are summarized in the body of the report and are augmented in the appendices.

Chapter II
METHODS OF OBSERVATION

After more than a year of planning and consultations with colleagues, a "pilot study" of five families was instituted in July 1947 to determine the feasibility of the approach and the procedures employed. After a period of 4 months it was apparent that the desired observations could be made and the population was accordingly enlarged. The data obtained prior to January 1, 1948, have not been included in tabulations and analyses because of the small number of families under observation during this period.

The recruitment of families for the study began with the help of Dr. C. W. Wyckoff, a pediatrician and president of the Academy of Medicine at the time. His interest and active support led to the enlistment of five families from his private practice for the "pilot study." News of the study spread from parents already enrolled to their friends, who became interested and contacted their physicians or the Department of Preventive Medicine for further information. Subsequent families were accepted into the study on the recommendation or with the approval of their family physicians or pediatricians. As mentioned before, the families constituted a highly selected population chosen for stability in the community and for intelligent cooperation. The purposes and nature of the study were presented in detail to prospective participants who were urged to consider all aspects carefully before deciding to enroll. The families were presumably normal and were not selected because of illness in any member or because of either unusual frequency or absence of illness in the family unit. The parents of the families were young adults who had at least one child.

From the time of admission until the end of the study, objectivity and uniformity were sought by the use of records devised for these purposes (Appendices 1 and 2). On admission of a family to the study, the medical status of each member was determined by history, physical examination, roentgenogram of the chest and examination of the blood and urine. Other types of examination, such as electrocardiograms or blood chemistry, were performed as indicated. A specimen of blood was obtained as a basis of reference for later serological studies. Interval histories, physical examinations, routine laboratory examinations, and roentgenograms of the chest were repeated at 6-month intervals for children and annually for adults until the last 2 years of the study. At that time the frequency of the examination of children was reduced to once a year. Blood specimens for serological studies were obtained twice a year, in the spring and the fall. Roentgenograms of the chest were taken additionally in connection with certain respiratory illnesses, and blood was also collected in relation to special illnesses and at the end of each trimester of pregnancy. Cord blood was obtained at the time of delivery and each infant was examined in the neonatal period.

Procedures for special studies were designed for the particular purpose of those investigations and will be given where pertinent in the subsequent chapters or are included in the Appendices. Bacteriological, virological and serological methods used were standardized procedures that either were in common usage or are described in Appendix 3.

Most of the data used in the analyses of illnesses came from records made as the illnesses appeared in each family. The maintenance of a constant flow of information involved the efforts of three key people: the mother, the field worker and the staff physician. The mother was instructed in detail regarding notification of the Department at the time of illness, however minor, in any individual in the household (Appendix 2). At the beginning of each month, the mother was given a new record sheet for each member of the family on which to note symptoms as they appeared on any day. The family physician was called by the mother if the illness was one for which he would ordinarily be notified. The study records and any data regarding illnesses were available to physicians of the families at all times. The members of the professional staff of the Department acted as observers only, but it was inevitable that at times they felt it necessary to urge the parents to call their family physician. Needless to say, the study was dependent in considerable measure on the mother as an observer, as an efficient recorder, and as a cooperative and intelligent person in general.

Each family was visited weekly by a field worker who reviewed the health status for the preceding week, made notes on her own records, discussed the mother's records with her and obtained a throat culture from each member of the household. This visit was important because the mother was a busy person and needed friendly prodding from time to time.

At times of illness during the early years of the study, the patient was examined by a staff physician who evaluated the illness clinically and epidemiologically and obtained cultures, blood and other specimens as indicated for etiological studies. During the later years of the study, patients with mild, afebrile minor illnesses were not routinely examined. The physician's observations were entered on records designed for this purpose. The frequency of follow-up visits varied with the severity and duration of the illness. Patients who were hospitalized were seen in the hospital during the period of acute illness.

When special studies were undertaken requiring changes in procedures, as for example, the collection of stool specimens during the epidemic of poliomyelitis in 1952 and the attempt to evaluate treatment of common respiratory diseases with antihistaminic drugs, a letter was written to the parents explaining the nature of the proposed study. The professional staff and field workers then discussed the proposal with the parents in order to give them as complete an understanding as possible. These parents were keenly aware of health matters and were knowledgeable about medical issues in the public eye. The professional staff was continuously challenged to provide evidence concerning progress of the study. Once a year, a general meeting of the parents was held to acquaint them with different aspects of the work being done and of the results obtained.

The records of the mothers, the field workers and the staff physicians were reviewed regularly by members of the professional staff and a diagnosis was made for each illness. The assignment of a diagnosis to each illness was obviously attended by varying degrees of difficulty, some illnesses, such as chickenpox, being recognized with a higher degree of reliability than others. The details concerning the appraisal of an illness itself, or periods of ill-health, are dealt with elsewhere.

Chapter III

DESCRIPTION OF THE FAMILIES AND THEIR REACTIONS TO THE STUDY

During the 10-year period from January 1, 1948, through May 31, 1957, a total of 86 families* and 443 individuals were in the study at one time or another for a combined total of 977,036 person-days, 2692 person-years and 556 family-years, of observation. The population consisted of 172 parents, 138 male children and 133 female children. One individual was in the study for only 35 days, while 17 individuals were observed for the entire period of 3439 days; the median period of observation was 2100 days.

The numbers of families and individuals admitted to and dropped from the study are shown in table 1. Most of the families entered in 1948 and 1951 and the last family was admitted in 1953. The latter family was one which had earlier moved out of town, but re-entered on its return to the city. Prior to that time the last new family entered in 1951.

Eighty-four children, including one set of twins, were born into the study. These births occurred in 56 of the 86 families. Two babies were born to each of 20 families, 3 to each of 4 families, and 1 child was born to each of 32 other families.

Twenty-six families were lost or withdrew from the study prior to its termination. Three of these were families of staff members who participated as subjects only to gain first-hand information regarding such problems as the observing, reporting and recording of symptoms and illnesses in members of their own families. The actual loss was thus 23 of 83 families, or 28%, throughout the entire period of study. The reasons for leaving were varied. Thirteen families moved out of town; divorce occurred in six families; three families were dropped at their own request. Only one family was lost because of lack of cooperation. Two of the six divorced families remained in the study after the father was separated from the family; in one family five members remained for 304 days each and in the other family four members remained for 488 days each. Hence a total of 3472 person-days was devoted to these two families. Eight additional persons were lost from the study: the two fathers of the divorced families mentioned above; three children who died; and three children who left for college.

---

*One family of four individuals has been counted twice because it left the study and later re-entered; there were actually 85 different families and 439 different individuals included.

TABLE 1

Number of families and individuals in the study by calendar year*

Year	In study January 1		Added during year		Dropped during year	
	Families	Individuals	Families	Individuals	Families	Individuals
1948	12	46	45	208	1	4
1949	56	250	6	33	6	26
1950	56	257	0	9	3	16
1951	53	250	22	95	3	14
1952	72	331	0	17	4	23
1953	68	325	1	16	4	23
1954	65	318	0	10	1	5
1955	64	323	0	3	3	13
1956	61	313	0	3	1	7
1957	60	309				

*Family 35 entered on May 1, 1948, and left (moved away) on October 30, 1948. The family moved back to the area and was readmitted on September 1, 1953. This family has been included twice in the above table, as have the four individuals in the family.

The size of the families ranged from three through eight members, with the most common size being five. In terms of maximum size, there were 3 families with 8 members, 5 with 7, 19 with 6, 37 with 5, 19 with 4, and 3 with 3 members each. Since family size changed during the study, due principally to birth, the actual periods of observation of families were best expressed as family-days of experience for each family size (Appendix 4, table 1). Families of sizes four, five, and six contributed approximately 90% of the total family-days of observation.

The median age of the parents in the 86 families at the time of entering the study was 30 years for the mothers and 33 years for the fathers. The age of the youngest parent at the time of entry was 22 years. At the end of the study, the oldest parent was 51 years of age. The median age of the parents at the time of departure from the study was 39 years for the fathers and 36 years for the mothers. The median age at entry for a child was 1.7 years, with the oldest child at the time of entry being 12 years of age (the youngest having been born into the study). The median age of children at time of departure from the study was 8.4 years, the oldest child being 18 years old.

The educational level of the parents was high (Appendix 4, table 2). Seventy-nine of the fathers and 58 of the mothers had attended college, while 23 of the fathers and 10 of the mothers had post-graduate or professional training after graduation from college. In line with their educational attainments, occupations of the fathers were those of responsibility in business or a profession as classified by the Bureau of Census (134) (Appendix 4, table 3). Most of them worked as members of business organizations, for example as partners in large law firms and executives of companies. None of the mothers was employed. Upon entry the families were in the middle or upper economic groups (Appendix 4, table 4), and 73 of them owned their own homes (Appendix 4, table 5). Except for short periods early in the study, each family lived by itself in a single house and was looked upon as an epidemiological unit.

These families living in a suburban area approached as nearly as possible a state of healthful living according to current standards (46). Although it was taken for granted by the families, it should be emphasized that there was no want of food, clothing, shelter, or cleanliness. Each home had central heating. Each child had a bed of his own and usually there were no more than two people in a bedroom; no one slept in the living room, dining room or kitchen. In every home there were flush toilets, efficient disposal of garbage, hot and cold running water, soap, and washing machines. The majority had dishwashers as well.

Despite the trend in these times toward identification with business organizations and recreational groups, the concept of the "family unit" in the United States today is a very firm one and in general is well-typified by the families in this study. Definite impressions of the general characteristics of the families were gained and formed the basis of much of the description presented here. The mothers were devoted to the efficient management of their households and cared deeply that their husbands were happy and successful in their work and that their children were making a good adjustment in school and in play. Suburban living and a social conscience promoted strong community feelings and most of the parents participated in civic organizations such as the Parent-Teacher Association and other voluntary welfare activities. They enjoyed friendships with others, and entertainment in the home and recreation in clubs were common to their way of living. Unlike other areas of society where work and exercise are often combined, they commonly thought of physical activity as a form of recreation, an emotional outlet, or an important way of maintaining health.

Anxieties in this population were numerous, but the parents

mostly worried about finances, business problems, the family budget, and responsibilities. Planning for old age, for security of the family in case of death of the father, for periods of ill-health and for protection against accidents was part of their philosophy.

The parents took steps for the maintenance of good health in their families, were wont to consult a physician for a "check-up" as well as an illness, and sought new knowledge of medical matters. Problems of mental health, radiological hazards, cancer, heart disease, and accident prevention were subjects of discussion, while the problem of infectious diseases seemed to be of less importance.

On the basis of the routine histories and physical examinations at the time of admission to the study, the general medical status of the population was considered to be excellent, and no one at this time had an incapacitating chronic disorder. Even one child, who had been blind since birth, attended school and proved to be a bright and energetic boy. As time went on, various individuals developed abnormalities such as diabetes mellitus, multiple sclerosis, gout, and otosclerosis, and certain other entities such as essential hypertension and chronic rheumatic heart disease became more evident in a small number of adults. No child developed rheumatic fever and no one had frank rheumatoid arthritis. Furthermore, no one experienced a myocardial infarction or angina pectoris. Malignancy was found only in one little girl who died of acute leukemia. Although acute respiratory infections proved to be the most common ailments in this population, chronic pulmonary disease was not a problem. A few individuals experienced asthma and acute bronchitis with respiratory infections or during the hay fever season, but chronic bronchitis or bronchietasis was not observed. Most of the medical problems were illnesses of short duration or localized pathologic processes that received medical care when needed. In fact, in this population, any discernible abnormality was brought promptly to the attention of the family physician.

During the first years of the study, an attempt was made to visit every infectious illness, if manifest only by sniffles. When illness rates were high, the physicians became frequent visitors to the homes. For example, a family of six experiencing an episode of respiratory disease or gastroenteritis might be visited three or four times during a single week. The illnesses were seldom severe, so there was usually no anxiety. The study physician's bag contained throat swabs and culture tubes, not needles and syringes. The children learned that this doctor just looked, and that the tongue blades he carried made good aeroplanes which could be marked with the big red wax pencil he used on the tubes. What's more, he sometimes arrived with a white mouse or guinea pig—once, even, with a goat.

When the study first started, the mothers were neatly dressed with every hair in place when they opened the door for the physicians making morning calls. When he kept returning every week, and even every day, realism returned along with slacks and pin curls. Sometimes, the mother was shopping or at a meeting and wasn't there to open the door. With or without the help of the maid, the physician found his "patient" playing in the sunroom or in bed upstairs. The field workers and the physicians became part of the routine of living. One field worker's schedule was such that the timing of the weekly visit coincided with an important daily household routine—the door was opened for both the worker and the cat.

The older children soon came to know what was expected of them, but such knowledge didn't always mean cooperation. For about 2 years, one little girl always ran to hide under her bed when the study doctor called, only to be dragged out screaming by her embarrassed mother. Today, this little girl is a friendly, poised young lady. Then there was the little boy who didn't want to be examined until he had finished reading a comic book. In this instance, it was difficult to know whether this reaction represented defiance or simply boredom with the study.

Most of the children became quite nonchalant about the home visits and examinations. Many even became nonchalant about the periodic venapunctures. In this regard, they did almost as well as their parents; indeed, there seemed to be a fair correlation between the attitude of the mother and the reaction of her children. The mother who kept putting off her own venapuncture by submitting numerous excuses had two daughters who became increasingly difficult to bleed. The tense parents usually had tense children, and such parents became very upset because of the behavior of their children. The relaxed, more stable families usually had children who would submit to venapuncture, albeit sometimes with tears, without difficulty. Of course, there was considerable variation, and no data were collected to test the validity of these impressions. Special mention is due one father who willingly reported to the medical school or hospital to be bled although he was susceptible to syncope. The total record is a fine tribute to the cooperation of parents and children alike.

Only one family withdrew from the study because of their concern that hypochondriasis might be produced in their children. The possibility that constant questioning about symptoms and repeated examinations might transform the children into hypochondriacs was seriously considered at the beginning of the study, but there was no evidence that this happened. It is possible that participation in the study may have had the opposite effect, for many of the children became rather knowledgeable about minor illness, some submitting school themes describing their roles as "guinea pigs" and presenting data obtained by the investigation. Observation did not appear to alter the pattern of reaction to illness already established for the family, a pattern which in general reflected the mother's attitude toward illness. Some mothers were overprotective. Needless to say, all mothers were annoyed by the occurrence of illness; some accepted it with philosophical resignation; others reacted with irritation and resentment. Some easily fitted nose drops and vaporizers into their daily routine; others busied themselves so with the sick that they had little time for the routine.

Of necessity, the accuracy of much of the data depended on the degree to which the mothers were conscientious recorders. It soon became obvious that some variations in degree were related as much to personality as to willingness to cooperate. The telephone message from one mother usually indicated a severity of illness not found to exist. Another played at being a physician and diagnosed all of the illnesses instead of reporting symptoms. A third might let her willingness to cooperate come before her willingness to be accurate, for it seemed that she felt obligated to report illnesses and was rather disappointed when she couldn't.

Knowledge of the personalities of the members of the families also influenced interpretation of the symptoms recorded. In a number of instances, as observations continued over the years, recurrent somatic complaints could be related to periods of tension and stress. In a few cases, symptoms were so constantly present that the individual had to be counted as a hypochondriac. One mother had such frequent headaches and neckaches, that in terms of counting new illnesses, headaches were hardly abnormal for her. The presence or absence of a true illness was sometimes difficult to establish in children prone to feign somatic complaints to avoid school. One child, whose father had recurrent episodes of abdominal pain and vomiting diagnosed as pylorospasms, complained of abdominal pains. Other children complained of sore throats or a variety of other aches in the hope of missing some quiz or book report.

As shown by the longitudinal analysis of illness rates, there was considerable spread between the highest rates in families and individuals and the lowest rates. A constant source of concern was how much these rates were influenced by the conscientiousness of the recorder, i.e., the mother. For several years, one family was discussed in conference from time to time because almost no illnesses were reported. No symptoms were recorded for the parents; the children had chickenpox and an occasional coryzal illness. It seemed unlikely that any family could be so "healthy" and after a particularly long period of "freedom" from illness, it was decided to face the parents with the problem and find some way to drop them from the study for the sake of accuracy. The mother and father had manifested interest by attending the annual meetings, but it was known that both were busy with many activities. Perhaps they would be happy to be relieved of the added burden imposed by the study. Accordingly, a study physician made an appointment to visit the parents one evening. He was received graciously, and his hosts expressed a sincere interest in the progress of the study. When the matter of reporting illnesses was raised, both wife and husband agreed, indeed insisted, that few illnesses had been reported because they and their children were rarely ill. They volunteered to drop out of the study to make a place for a family with more illnesses, but questioned whether this might not bias the results. These were people of integrity; the physician thanked them for their cooperation and assured them that their family was wanted in the study. The illness rate in the family remained low, until three of the four members had typical influenza and Asian virus was isolated from each.

Chapter IV

CERTAIN PROBLEMS IN THE DEFINITION AND ENUMERATION OF ILLNESS

In describing the amount of illness experienced by a population, illnesses must be defined in units which can be counted. This is not a simple matter and has been a source of difficulty in most morbidity studies. Dorn (52) summarized a number of the definitions which have been used by various investigators and this excellent summary will be quoted throughout the present discussion, for many of his statements have real pertinence to the problems recognized by us.

The present study was conceived primarily as an instrument for gathering data which would lend themselves to epidemiological interpretations. For this reason illnesses, diagnosed as specifically as possible, rather than periods of ill health, seemed to be the most appropriate units for enumeration. The basic problem with respect to either of these units of enumeration is defining when a departure from a state of good health occurs. When that has been defined, it is possible to determine the onset of either an "illness" or a "state of ill health." Then attempts can be made to determine the diagnosis or cause of the illness and the duration of the "state of ill-health." We have arbitrarily defined an illness or departure from a state of good health as the occurrence of one or more symptoms abnormal for the individual concerned.

In a comparable fashion, Dorn defined a "period of ill health" as a "continuous interval of time during which a person experiences a departure from a state of good health." During this period of ill health, "one or more separate diagnostic entities or causes of ill health may exist;" these are "called illnesses or diagnoses with the understanding that illness includes conditions resulting from disease, poisoning, and injury."

In actual experience, of course, it is not always easy or even possible to distinguish between illnesses and periods of ill health. Dorn touched on this problem when he stated: "Illnesses from which a complete recovery is possible may be counted the first time they occur in each period of ill health ... A second attack of the same illness during a single period of ill health creates a more difficult problem, for it is necessary to decide whether a second attack is merely a prolongation of the first or is a new attack of the same disease."

We have referred to this difficulty in several publications. In one of these (2) we stated:

"Another problem exists in the application of a definition of respiratory 'illness' for purposes of delineating new infections. The question is frequently encountered as to whether an exacerbation of previously existing symptoms, or the appearance of new symptoms superimposed upon those already present, is a new illness or the progression of an old one. Our attitude in interpreting such situations is quite different from that of other investigators. Sydenstricker (130), for example, considered an illness to continue until there was a period of freedom from symptoms; using this criterion 'all respiratory illnesses were carefully edited to see that the same continuous sickness was not counted as two illnesses when due to what seemed to be successive or progressive conditions.' Other studies have used the same or similar criteria. According to our interpretation, it is quite possible to have a new illness superimposed on the remnants of a preceding one and the situation is best decided on the basis of clinical judgment. Similarly, it is possible that a period of freedom of symptoms does not necessarily mean that new symptoms appearing after a few days are the result of a new infection. Neither set of criteria is subject to evaluation, and both undoubtedly lead to some misinterpretation of the facts, the extent of which must remain unknown."

The degree to which we have been successful in distinguishing the number of illnesses is thus unknown, and we certainly do not entertain the idea that we were entirely successful. In an attempt to achieve as much reliability as possible, however, many of the illnesses (even the minor ones) were seen by clinicians attached to the study and all diagnoses (i.e., identification and labeling of illnesses) were made by them. In spite of this, it was not an infrequent occurrence for the clinician to express bewilderment as to whether one or several successive or even superimposed illnesses were present.

This confusion was especially pronounced when both respiratory and gastrointestinal symptoms were present during a given period of ill health. A special statistical study of this problem was made (Chapter XI) and the conclusion was reached that many of these instances represented a single infection, but that some represented two simultaneous illnesses. A statistical measure of the relative frequency of each type was derived, but this was useless as an aid to diagnosis in specific periods of ill health.

In summary, then, it is quite possible that periods of ill health may be counted more accurately than is possible with illnesses. For epidemiological purposes the illness is a more useful unit of measurement and we have used it in discussions of acute illnesses from which eventual recovery is apparent. Except in the study mentioned (relating to the simultaneous occurrence of respiratory and gastrointestinal symptoms) the concept of "period of illness" has not been employed. The problem of distinguishing between an exacerbation of the initial illness and a new attack of the same disease might well be expanded to include the difficulty in distinguishing between multiple illnesses which occur simultaneously and multiple manifestations of the same illness (Appendix 5).

The preceding discussion assumes that even though separate or independent illnesses may not always be distinguishable, there are such illnesses and if knowledge were adequate, they could be identified and counted individually. We believe that identification of the acute and presumably self-limited diseases as separate illnesses was in general successful.

A most difficult problem is to decide how to enumerate those diseases which are characterized by recurring attacks or exacerbations of what may be a single disease, such as hay fever, asthma, herpes simplex, and furunculosis. They may be counted as single illnesses or in terms of the number of recurring attacks.* Actually, an attempt was made to identify each attack of such illnesses and to classify them as exacerbations, recurrences, or new illnesses. No arbitrary rules were made for this purpose but reliance was placed on the judgment of the clinicians.

As an example of this problem, furunculosis tends to reappear repeatedly in the same individual (see Appendix 5, table 1). Two persons each recorded furunculosis as appearing eight times while enrolled in the study. In the total experience, furunculosis was recorded 136 times, but involved only 76 individuals. If one is interested in the total times the condition was experienced, 136 is the number. Quite another type of information is provided by knowing that 76 individuals were involved; possibly this figure indicates the frequency with which some type of constitutional abnormality was present.

It was, then, possible to count: a) the number of individuals who at some time in the study recorded an acute manifestation of a recurrent disease; b) the number of attacks each person suffered; and c) the total number of attacks. If such counts of illnesses are

---

*Similar problems exist with the chronic degenerative diseases but are not of concern here because of the age and small size of the population.

of value, there still remain difficulties in applying the principles listed above. One of these refers to difficulties in deciding just what are manifestations of a given abnormality. For example, should allergies as expressed by hay fever and eczema be counted as one disease, and the number of times one or both manifestations occurs be used as the number of attacks of that disease, or should they be considered as separate diseases? Such decisions must frequently be quite arbitrary, especially if the purpose of the count is no more than to present a list of illnesses encountered. Another difficulty is in deciding just what entities should be included as chronically recurring diseases. For example, are such things as headache, stiff neck, "sick stomach," and even the common cold, which tend to recur in the same individuals, of the nature of chronic conditions with repeated attacks, or should each attack be considered as an individual acute illness? Depending upon the answers to these questions, which are largely a matter of opinion or of interpretation of known facts, an exceedingly large variation can be obtained as to the number of illnesses which occurred in the study. For example, if allergies are considered as a group, 166 individuals recorded 529 attacks of one kind or another. If the allergic manifestations are subdivided into nine groups (e.g., allergic conjunctivitis, hay fever, asthma, etc.), the number of attacks remains the same, but the sum of the number of persons assigned to the categories is 238. Thus, if we were considering the number of possible diagnoses, allergy would account for 166 or 238 (or some other number) depending on the groupings made in the diagnostic classification. The same, of course, is true for many other classes of illness.

Another source of possible confusion in counting illnesses is concerned with surgical procedures. Presumably, a surgical procedure is carried out in order to correct some pathological process or abnormality. A tonsillectomy may be performed and that tonsillectomy is the only recorded recognition that the abnormality exists. Theoretically, at least, the reason for the tonsillectomy is just as real a condition as is some well-defined disease for which no surgical correction is applicable. In other situations, such as in appendectomies, the surgery may be preceded by a well described acute episode to which a name, appendicitis, may be attached. In early tabulations it was our practice to identify and count each diagnosis when it was possible to state it, and each surgical procedure as an illness. This led both to inconsistencies and to a certain amount of double counting, in that a tonsillectomy for an unstated reason was counted once, but appendicitis with an appendectomy was counted as two events. In attempts to summarize the total morbidity experience, a more consistent pattern was followed. If a condition was diagnosed specifically (such as appendicitis), it was counted once as "appendicitis followed by appendectomy," while with most tonsillectomies the diagnosis was "unspecified condition leading to tonsillectomy and adenoidectomy." The many other types of situations leading to surgery were handled in a similar manner.

Data regarding the total occurrence of illness, then, can be quite misleading unless one is acquainted with the "rules" of counting which were followed; these data can be employed to advantage only if the rules which were used are consistent with the purpose for which the data have been gathered. In the following chapters, when the data are put to a specific use, the special rules of counting involved will be explained. Unless otherwise stated, the general rules were: that clinical judgment was widely used; that in dealing with what might have been recurring manifestations of one condition, each occurrence was counted; and that a condition leading to surgery was counted even though a specific diagnosis had not been assigned to that condition. The various diagnostic classes that were used are shown in Appendix 5, tables 1 and 2, together with the total number of times each diagnosis was made and the number of individuals concerned. A frequency distribution of the latter according to the number of times the diagnosis was made is also included in these tables. Finally, the number of operative procedures and the number of persons on whom these procedures were performed are also shown. The analyses presented in the next chapter are based on the illnesses enumerated and classified in Appendix 5, table 1.

Chapter V

PATTERNS OF ILLNESS

A total of 25,155 diagnoses was made—a rate of 9.40 illnesses per person-year. The number of illnesses and average incidence rates for several broad diagnostic categories are shown in table 2.

TABLE 2

Incidence of major classes of illness

Class of illness	Number of illnesses	Illnesses per person-year	% of all illnesses
Total illnesses	25,155	9.4	100
Common respiratory diseases	14,990	5.6	60
Specific respiratory diseases	793	0.3	3
Infectious gastroenteritis	4,057	1.5	16
Other infections	1,931	0.7	8
Other illnesses	3,384	1.3	13

The term "common respiratory diseases," which was used to describe 60% of all diagnoses, includes the common cold, rhinitis, laryngitis, bronchitis, and other acute respiratory illnesses of undifferentiated types. "Specific respiratory diseases" includes streptococcal tonsillitis and pharyngitis, nonbacterial tonsillitis and pharyngitis, primary atypical pneumonia, pneumococcal pneumonia and influenza.

There was some inconsistency in the rules for distinguishing between "specific respiratory diseases" and "common respiratory diseases." An influenza-like illness was classified as a common respiratory disease unless laboratory evidence was available to identify it as true influenza. Similarly, laboratory evidence was required before an illness was classified as streptococcal in origin. On the other hand, nonbacterial tonsillitis and pharyngitis was diagnosed clinically, as were the pneumonias. These rules were set up in 1948 after considerable debate as to what rules of classification would lead to the most meaningful description; they would be different if arrived at today in the light of the considerable progress which has been made in etiological studies of acute respiratory infections. These inconsistent rules, however, applied to a relatively small number (about 5%) of all acute respiratory illnesses (table 3).

TABLE 3

Number and percentage of respiratory illnesses by diagnosis

Diagnosis	Number of illnesses	Percentage of total
Common respiratory diseases	14,990	94.98
Streptococcal tonsillitis and pharyngitis	437	2.77
Nonbacterial tonsillitis and pharyngitis	219	1.39
Primary atypical pneumonia	42	0.27
Pneumococcal pneumonia	6	0.04
Other or undiagnosed pneumonia	15	0.10
Influenza	74	0.47
Total	15,783	100.00

The category of infectious gastroenteritis enumerated in table 2 excludes those instances in which the gastrointestinal symptoms were thought not to be primary symptoms. Approximately one-half (2,139) were considered to be acute infectious gastroenteritis and most of the remaining (1,918) were thought to be the same, although the evidence was less convincing (i.e., either they were diagnosed because of an epidemiological association with other cases or they had too few symptoms to warrant a diagnosis of gastroenteritis). The gastrointestinal illnesses described here constituted the second most frequent group of illnesses encountered in this study.

"Other" infections include the usual diseases of childhood, otitis media, herpes, and a miscellany listed in Appendix 5, table 1. A large number (259) were instances of unexplained fever without respiratory or enteric symptoms or other evidence of localization. The category "other illnesses" is made up of a variety of events, chiefly noninfectious in nature (Appendix 5, table 1).

The incidence rates for each of these groups of illnesses over the whole period of the study are shown in table 2; in addition, the percentage distribution of illnesses according to this gross clinical grouping is shown. On the average, each person suffered 5.6 illnesses from the common respiratory diseases each year. The gastrointestinal illnesses made up one-sixth of all illnesses, the average incidence rate being 1.5 cases per person-year.

Table 3 is presented to show the relative frequency of the various classes of acute respiratory disease. Common respiratory diseases comprised 95% of all acute respiratory disease. About one-half of the remainder were of streptococcal etiology. The relatively low incidence of influenza is somewhat artificial, since laboratory evidence of this infection was not sought routinely in all respiratory illnesses.

The illnesses termed "nonbacterial tonsillitis and pharyngitis" were classified as a group for two reasons: 1) an illness characterized by exudate was encountered rather frequently in studies which had been carried out in the Army by several of the individuals concerned with the present study and they were therefore interested in this feature of respiratory disease; and 2) an outbreak of illnesses in which exudate was noted occurred among the families during the summer of 1948. However, interest in this disease, or group of diseases, was not maintained uniformly throughout the study, and it is doubtful that the figures in table 3 accurately represent the frequency with which nonbacterial tonsillitis and pharyngitis was encountered. (See Appendix 6, table 1)

TABLE 4

Incidence of illnesses by year

Year	Common respiratory diseases	Infectious gastroenteritis	All other illnesses	Total illnesses
1948	6.31	1.52	1.88	9.71
1949	6.27	1.62	2.02	9.91
1950	6.15	1.50	2.38	10.03
1951	6.00	1.66	2.54	10.20
1952	6.15	1.73	2.69	10.57
1953	5.28	1.28	2.00	8.56
1954	5.09	1.28	1.80	8.17
1955	5.17	1.40	2.53	9.09
1956	4.86	1.71	2.44	9.01
1957	4.95	1.49	2.46	8.90
Total	5.60	1.52	2.28	9.40

As shown in table 4, the incidence of the common respiratory diseases as recorded declined throughout the study, being 6.31 cases per person-year during 1948 and 4.95 during the first 5 months of 1957. This decrease apparently was due to both an aging population and either a real decrease in the occurrence of the common respiratory diseases or a decrease in the completeness with which illnesses were recorded. The incidence of infectious gastroenteritis and miscellaneous diseases (all others combined, including specific respiratory diseases, other infections and "other illnesses" of table 2) fluctuated considerably, but no trend, either up or down, was noted.

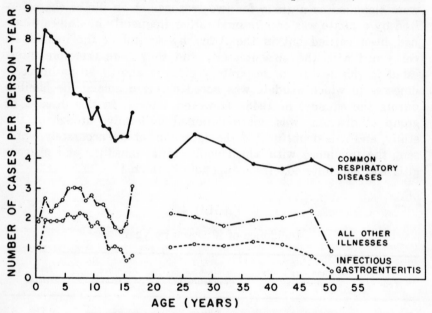

Fig. 1   Incidence of illness by diagnosis and age

The incidence and comparative frequency of these three groups of illnesses by age are shown in figures 1 and 2 and in Appendix 6, tables 2 and 3. The variation of incidence of the common respiratory diseases with age will be discussed at some length in Chapter VI. All three groups of illnesses showed an increased incidence between the first and second years of life. The common respiratory diseases decreased in incidence from then on; even in adults there was a slight decrease with increasing age. Infectious gastroenteritis remained at a fairly constant level up to about 12 years of age, then dropped slightly to a lower level which persisted throughout adulthood. The incidence of all other illnesses more or less paralleled that of infectious gastroenteritis, except for a slight rise and

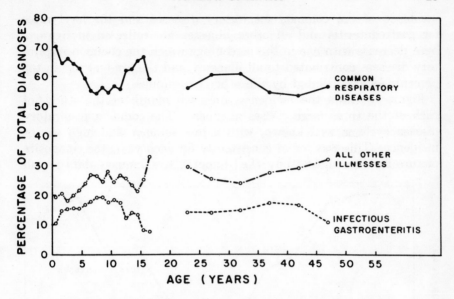

Fig. 2   *Percentage distribution of cases by diagnosis and age*

fall in childhood with a peak at 6 and 7 years of age. This rise and
fall reflects, primarily, the incidence of the acute infectious diseases.

The percentage curves of figure 2 are somewhat more complex,
but the relative positions—highest for common respiratory diseases,
lowest for gastroenteritis, and central for all other diseases—were
maintained throughout the age scale. The general decrease in the

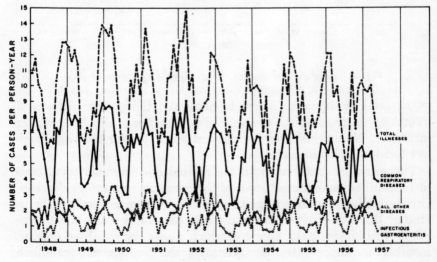

Fig. 3   *Incidence of illnesses by month and year*

incidence of the common respiratory diseases and the level rates
for gastroenteritis and all other illnesses are reflected in figure 2
by a decrease with age in the percentage which the common respiratory diseases contributed to all illnesses, and the gradual rise in the
percentages contributed by the other two groups.

Figure 3 shows the incidence, for each month of the study, of
each of the three large classes of illness. The common respiratory
disease cycle is well known, with a low summer and high winter
incidence. This was found consistently for each year; the composite
picture for the whole study (i.e., lumping the January data for all

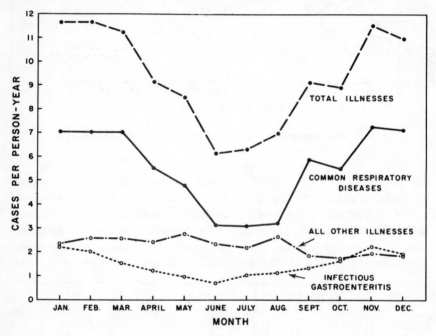

Fig. 4   *Incidence of illnesses by diagnosis by month of year*

years, etc.) is shown in figure 4. Similarly, the general pattern of
infectious gastroenteritis was one of low summer and high winter
incidence. No marked seasonal pattern was noted for the miscellaneous residue of illnesses.

The principal factor in both the annual and seasonal occurrence
of total illness was the behavior of the common respiratory diseases.
Other surveys of minor respiratory illnesses have generally demonstrated three or four winter peaks between the months of September and May (54, 63). Figure 4, which shows the weighted average
monthly incidence rates, demonstrates the September rise which
occurred in each of the years (see figure 3) but after a slight drop

in October the average rates for the 5 months November through March were remarkably constant.

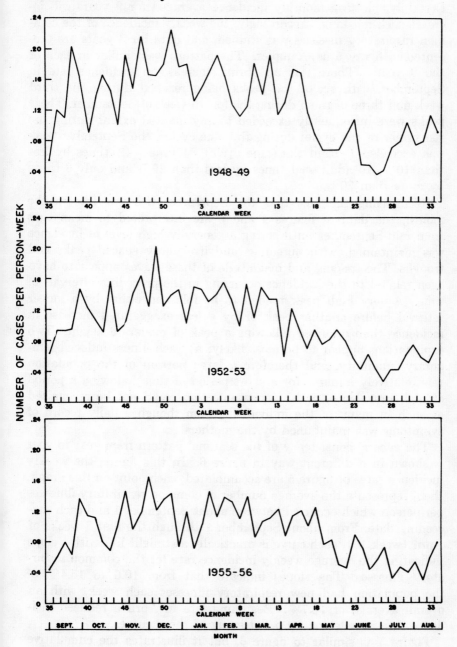

Fig. 5   Incidence of the common respiratory diseases by week for each of 3 selected years beginning about September 1, 1948, 1952, and 1955

The study of Frost and Gover (63) showed that plotting the occurrence by month may mask significant fluctuations in incidence. Certainly, plotting monthly incidence averaged for 9 years will increase such masking. Accordingly, the weekly incidence of the common respiratory diseases was studied, and data for 3 years are presented in figure 5 as examples. The pattern was similar in each of the 9 years. There was an abrupt increase in incidence late in September, with six of the peaks being reached during the third week and three of them during the fourth week of September. These peaks were infrequently exceeded to any marked extent during the remainder of the cycle; during the nine cycles, the September peak was exceeded (within the same cycle) 34 times—21 times by less than 10%, 10 additional times by less than 20% and only 3 times by more than 20%.

Recognizing the fact that the September rise was late in the month, the data of figures 4 and 5 are interpreted to mean that from mid-September until spring a generally high level of incidence was maintained, with numerous and irregularly spaced peaks and troughs. The spacing and magnitude of these waves appear to have been related to the incidence occurring in the preceding intervals of time. A very high peak tended to be followed either by a longer interval before another peak or by a less exaggerated increase in incidence than occurred following a peak of moderate height. Two explanations appear to be most likely: a) each illness induced temporary immunity, and therefore a large portion of the population was relatively immune for a short period of time following a period of high prevalence, or b) a new infection could not be recognized as such in many of the individuals, even though a daily record of symptoms was maintained by the mothers.

The general consistency of the seasonal pattern from year to year is shown in a different way in figure 6. In this figure, the weekly incidence rates of figure 5 are accumulated; each point on this graph, then, represents the average number of common respiratory illnesses per person which occurred between about September 1 and each succeeding date. From about September 1 through the first 3 weeks of April (week 16), each curve is practically a straight line with a slope indicating the average weekly incidence rate for the common respiratory illnesses. The slopes indicate that from 10.6 to 15.4% of the population had new respiratory illnesses each week, with an overall average of 12.7%. Beginning late in April a reduced incidence rate is reflected by a flattening of these curves.

Figure 7 is similar to figure 6, but it illustrates the cumulative incidence for all infectious illnesses. Except for the common respiratory diseases, these illnesses consisted mostly of those designated

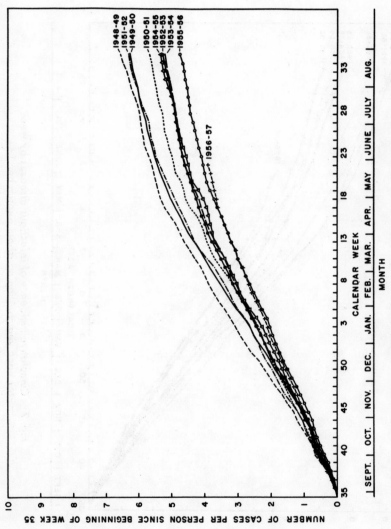

Fig. 6 Cumulative incidence of the common respiratory diseases by week, for each year beginning about September 1

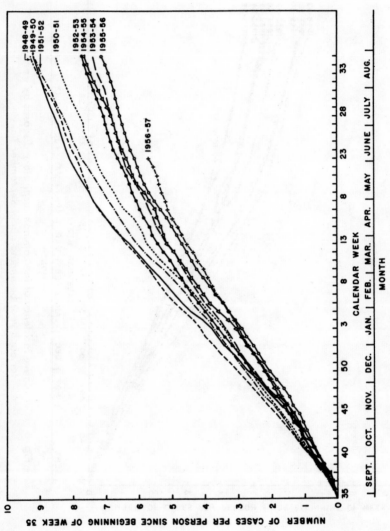

Fig. 7   Cumulative incidence of infectious diseases by week,
for each year beginning about September 1

as infectious gastroenteritis, but also included the specific respiratory diseases, the communicable diseases of childhood, and any other illness thought to be of infectious origin. These incidence curves are very similar to those for the common respiratory diseases, except that they reach higher levels.

ILLNESSES DURING THE FIRST YEAR OF LIFE

Infants in their first year of life were of special interest because of the opportunity to observe and record reactions that were largely determined by factors operating in a family environment (Appendix 7). Except for two babies (one with severe eczema and another with a meningo-myelocele), they grew and developed normally. There were 869 illnesses in 107 infants, a rate of 9.6 illnesses per

TABLE 5

Incidence of major categories of illness during the first year of life of 107 infants*

Category of illness	Number of illnesses	Illnesses per person-year	% of all illnesses
Total illness	869	9.6	100
Common respiratory diseases	613	6.8	71
All other illnesses	256	2.8	29

*There were 84 newborn infants and 24 other infants who were less than one year of age when their families joined the study. However, one newborn baby had severe eczema and was away from home during most of his first year of life and was excluded from the count of illnesses.

person-year during the first year of life. Common respiratory infections accounted for about 70% of all disease during the first year (table 5) and thus mainly determined the level of total illness during each month of age (figures 8 and 9). There was a progressive rise in the occurrence of total illness from birth to a maximum incidence of 12 cases per person-year during the sixth month of age. The rates of total illness during each month of age continued close to this level throughout the remainder of the year. Diseases other than common respiratory infections accounted for about 30% of the total illnesses. Among these, two-thirds were frank infections and one-third were due to other diseases such as noninfectious dermatitis, reactions to immunizations, fevers of unknown origin, miscellaneous diseases and accidents (Appendix 7, table 3). It is

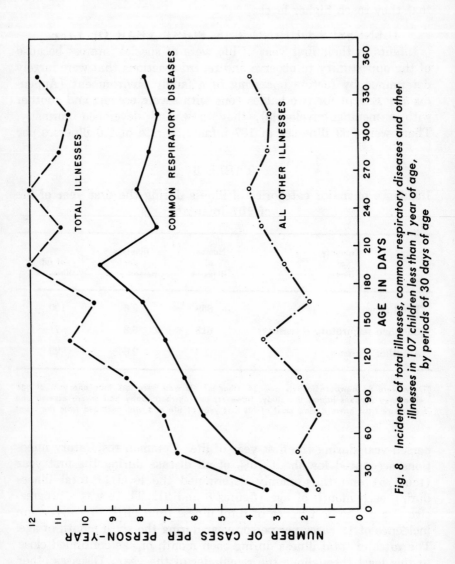

Fig. 8 Incidence of total illnesses, common respiratory diseases and other illnesses in 107 children less than 1 year of age, by periods of 30 days of age

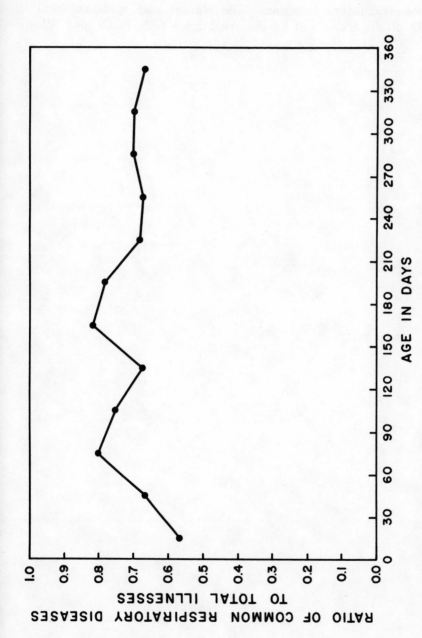

Fig. 9 Ratio of common respiratory diseases to total illnesses in 107 children less than 1 year of age, by periods of 30 days of age

readily apparent that the major experience of the newborn infant in the shelter of his home was infectious disease, particularly common respiratory infections. The clinical and epidemiological aspects of the latter will be discussed more fully in Chapter VI.

Chapter VI

COMMON RESPIRATORY DISEASES

Respiratory diseases constituted the major illness problem in the present study. About 63% of all new illnesses recorded were of this type and of these, approximately 95% were classified as the "common respiratory diseases." This category includes illnesses commonly diagnosed as the common cold, rhinitis, laryngitis, bronchitis and other acute respiratory illnesses of undifferentiated type.

INCIDENCE

The total incidence of the common respiratory diseases and variations by age and season were shown in the preceding chapter, as was the long-term trend in incidence rates. Table 4 shows that the recorded incidence of the common respiratory diseases decreased with the passage of time. This decrease was the subject of some study in order to learn whether or not it was real. Details are given in Appendix 8. In brief, the evidence is quite clear that there was a decreased incidence of the common respiratory diseases recorded as the study progressed, that this decrease was most evident in the months of high incidence (September through April), and that it occurred consistently in each age group. Part of this decrease was due to a shift in the age distribution of the childhood population; for example, during 1948-49, 60% of the individuals in the study were under 5 years of age and therefore subject to high incidence rates, while in 1956-57 only 20% were in this age group. This fact alone would lead to a decreased total incidence rate. The exact proportion of the decrease which was due to aging is impossible to determine, but an estimate showed that about one-fourth of the decrease in reported incidence was due to aging of the population, while about three-fourths was due to some other factor or factors which could not be identified. There was no significant decrease in the incidence rates during the summer months (May-August).

INCIDENCE BY AGE

It is common knowledge that children have more respiratory illnesses than do their parents, and that persons of all ages tend to have several such illnesses each year. Figure 1 shows the average incidence of the common respiratory diseases by age (see also Appendix 9, table 1).

Children under 1 year of age had about seven respiratory illnesses per year on the average which is lower than the rates during the next few years of life. The highest incidence occurred among

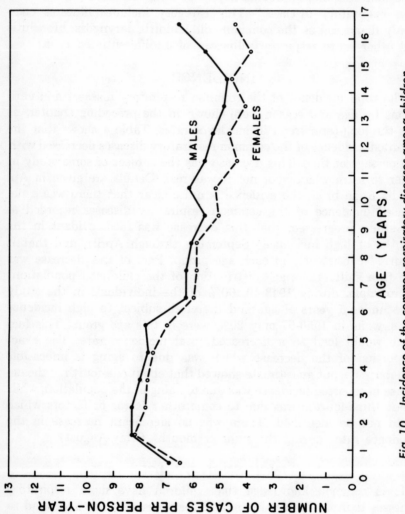

Fig. 10   Incidence of the common respiratory diseases among children by age and sex

1-year-old children (8.3 cases per year) and the rate remained quite high through age five (7.4 cases per year). Beginning at age six, there was a progressive decrease in the frequency of respiratory illnesses. Adults had relatively fewer illnesses than did children — slightly over four per year.

INCIDENCE BY SEX

During childhood the average incidence of the common respiratory diseases was slightly higher for boys than for girls. This was true consistently at every year of age, as shown in figure 10 (see also Appendix 9, tables 2 and 3). The reverse was found among adults: mothers had higher rates than did fathers. Fathers had about the same incidence rate in each age group; mothers, on the other hand, showed a decline in average incidence of respiratory illness as age increased (Appendix 9, table 4).

INCIDENCE IN RELATIONSHIP TO SCHOOL ATTENDANCE

The frequency and intimacy of contacts with other individuals is generally thought to be a major factor in determining whether a given individual has few or many respiratory illnesses. It is, of course, impossible to classify individuals on any quantitative scale of adequate contact, but persons in the present study have been classified in two respects which certainly are related to this variable. One of these is concerned with attendance at school, the other with size of family.

In studying the relation of school attendance to the incidence of common respiratory disease, each child was classified as: a) a school child, b) a preschool child with a sibling attending school, or c) a preschool child with no sibling attending school. Figure 11 shows the age-specific incidence rates for each of the three classes of children. For every year of age, the rates for children attending school were higher than those for preschool children.

The high incidence among school children, who had many contacts outside the home, indicates that those contacts directly influenced the incidence of respiratory illness. The influence of school children on the incidence of respiratory illness among their siblings is shown by comparing the rates for the two groups of preschool children. The preschool siblings of school children had a higher rate of illness than did the other preschool children. The data for preschool children aged 5 years are small and therefore the absolute values of the incidence rates are poorly established.

Presumably the majority of infections in the preschool age group are acquired in the home, and thus this rate may be an indication of a basic home risk. The rate of the preschool children in families with school children is at an intermediate level and may be con-

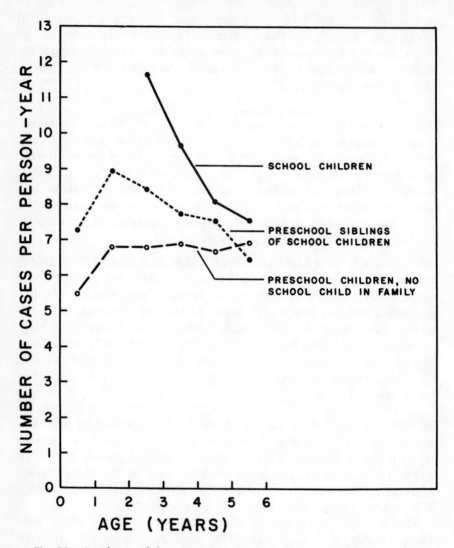

Fig. 11   Incidence of the common respiratory diseases in children under
6 years of age, according to school status

sidered to represent this basic risk plus the added risk of acquiring infections from siblings who are attending school. The curves for school children represent the basic risk plus the risk of acquiring infection in school. Thus the difference between the lowest and the highest groups may be a measure of the community risk for these children. The basic home risk, however, contributes to all three groups, and it would thus appear that the home is the most important place of spread of these infections.

This interpretation was strengthened by examining the incidence rates separately for that period of the year when school is in session (September - May) and the summer vacation period (June - August) (see figure 12). In general, the variation in incidence rates by class of child was found during the school period and was not present in the summer. Behavior during the school period thus determined the differences shown in figure 11.

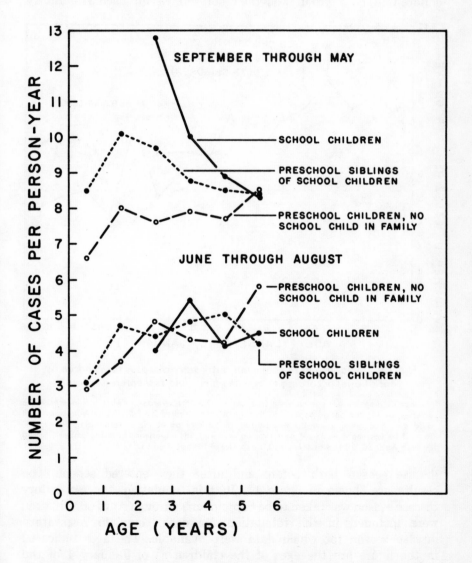

Fig. 12 *Incidence of the common respiratory diseases in children under 6 years of age by year of age, according to school status and season*

INCIDENCE ACCORDING TO AGE AT WHICH CHILD FIRST ATTENDED SCHOOL

To study the effect of early attendance at school on the subsequent incidence of the common respiratory diseases, individuals were divided into three groups according to the age at which they first entered school. The incidence of respiratory diseases for the children in each group was then determined for each respiratory

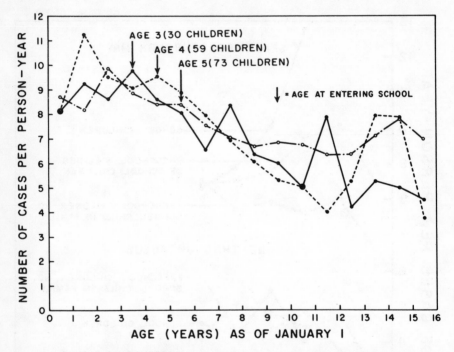

Fig. 13   Incidence of the common respiratory diseases for children by year of age, according to age at which child first entered school*

*Number of illnesses per person-year (the ordinate) is the average number of illnesses which occurred during the period September through April multiplied by 1.5. The experience of each child during a given 8 months was related to his age as of the corresponding January 1. Thus, if he became 4 years old on November 1, 1950, his experience from September 1, 1950 through April 30, 1951 was taken as his experience for age 4 years.

disease season both before and after they entered school. The results are shown in figure 13. In this tabulation, the respiratory disease season was taken to be September 1 through April 30. Children were included in the tabulation for each complete respiratory disease season for which data were available. The ages indicated in the figure are the ages of the children as of January 1 of the respiratory disease season in question. A few children who entered school, withdrew, and later reentered, were eliminated from the present analysis. Early attendance at school had no apparent effect on a child's ability to build up immunity to the common respiratory diseases, nor was any relationship found between early attendance at school and subsequent incidence of respiratory disease.

INCIDENCE BY SIZE OF FAMILY

The other factor studied was size of family. One might expect that larger families would experience more illnesses per year than would smaller families, merely because of the presence of more persons to have illnesses. That this was observed is shown in

TABLE 6

Incidence of the common respiratory diseases by size of family

Family size	Person-days	Family-days	Number of illnesses	Illnesses per family-year	Illnesses per person-year
3	38,991	12,997	483	13.6	4.5
4	269,604	67,401	3,846	20.8	5.2
5	399,450	79,890	6,043	27.6	5.5
6	201,396	33,566	3,472	37.8	6.3
7	36,491	5,213	666	46.6	6.7
8	31,104	3,888	480	45.1	5.6*
Totals	977,036	202,955	14,990	27.0	5.6

*Based on three families

table 6. Further, it might be expected that each individual in the larger families would have more illnesses per year than individuals in the smaller families: since there are more people to introduce illness, the individual members of larger families would be exposed more frequently within the home than would those of smaller families. Table 6 shows an increasing over-all average frequency of illness as family size increased from three to seven members. The experience with families of eight members was too small for use in establishing meaningful values.

The incidence of respiratory illness according to family size was studied for various age groups of individuals, and among young children, by school status. No clear-cut patterns were discernible relating incidence of respiratory disease to the various combinations of age of child and school status, according to family size. Therefore, data bearing on these points are not included.

TABLE 7

Incidence of the common respiratory diseases in parents by
size of family

Family size	Fathers			Mothers		
	Person-days	No. of illnesses	Illnesses per person-year	Person-days	No. of illnesses	Illnesses per person-year
3	12,997	109	3.1	12,997	159	4.5
4	66,913	549	3.0	67,401	813	4.4
5	79,586	793	3.6	79,890	1094	5.0
6	33,566	366	4.0	33,566	475	5.2
7	5,213	58	4.1	5,213	87	6.1
8	3,888	37	3.5	3,888	49	4.6

Among parents (table 7) the incidence increased for both mothers
and fathers as size of family increased from four to seven.

INTRODUCTION AND SPREAD OF THE COMMON RESPIRATORY DISEASES IN THE FAMILY

It is generally accepted that the common respiratory diseases
are infectious and that they spread from person to person. If this
is true, then the present study should provide information concerning the role of family members in bringing these infections
home and in spreading and acquiring infections once introduced.

Because these diseases are highly prevalent in the community
at all times, it is not possible to state with any certainty where
specific infections were acquired. Apparent spread within the family
may actually have resulted from multiple independent exposures
outside of the family. Also, since these diseases occur in extremely
mild forms, an apparent introduction into the family may actually
have been an acquisition from an inapparent case within the home.
In addition, and most importantly, there were many instances where
events were just too confused to warrant any attempt to label cases
as to whether they were acquired from without or within the family.
For these reasons, the present data will at most provide measures
of relative frequency; the absolute numbers should not be interpreted
literally.

The following analyses are based on selected instances of what
were apparently family outbreaks or episodes. The purpose of the
selection was to eliminate instances which appeared confusing, hop-
ing that the residue represented a reasonable sample, obviously

not random, upon which to base a description of the introduction and spread of the common respiratory diseases within the family.

The criteria for inclusion in the episode analyses were, of course, arbitrary. The episode started with an index case, defined as a case of common respiratory disease which appeared in a family 10 or more days after the onset of the last respiratory disease of any nature. For example, if a respiratory illness started on April 1, the next illness in the family could be classified as an index case only if its onset was on April 11 or later. If two or more cases developed on the same day and they met the criteria for an index case, both were considered as index cases. The period of an episode continued for 10 calendar days and all respiratory illnesses that started within that period constituted illnesses of the episode. The cases which developed in the nine calendar days following that on which the index case or cases appeared were designated as secondary cases.

Temporary absences from home by a member of the family were ignored in spite of the fact that such a procedure undoubtedly led to some inaccuracies. Exclusion of such persons might have led to an assessment of the suituation as incorrect as that which resulted from their inclusion. For example, a father might have been in an infectious, though preclinical, phase of an illness before he left on a trip. To have eliminated him from the study when he left the family would have charged the next member who became ill with the responsibility of having introduced the infection into the home.

After selecting episodes according to the above criteria, certain episodes were then excluded. These were the ones during which: (a) some person became ill more than once during the period of the episode; (b) an illness diagnosed as a specific infectious disease, such as streptococcal tonsillitis or primary atypical pneumonia, occurred in one or more members of the family during the period of the episode; and (c) the exact date of the onset of some case was in doubt.*

INTRODUCTION OF THE COMMON RESPIRATORY DISEASES INTO FAMILIES

It is obvious from the above discussion that no attempt was made to identify each infection which was acquired outside the home and thus to establish the rate at which persons became infected from the community. Rather, analyses were limited to attempts to measure the relative risk that various classes of individuals carried of introducing infections into the home, so that a statement could be made, for example, that the mothers brought home X times as many infections as did the fathers.

The relative frequency with which various classes of individuals introduced infections into the home is shown in table 8. Detailed analyses which led to this table are presented in Appendix 10. Fathers brought home the fewest infections. Mothers were infected outside the home somewhat more often than the fathers. Preschool

---

*In the analysis of the 1948-1950 episodes, previously published (3, 4), the criteria a, b, and c for excluding episodes were applied to analyses concerned with secondary attack rates, but not to those concerned with index cases.

TABLE 8

Ratios showing the relative frequency with which five classes of individuals introduced common respiratory diseases into the home

Class of Individual	Ratio
Fathers (F)	1.0
Mothers (M)	1.3
School children 6 years of age and over (S6+)	2.2
Preschool children (P)	2.7
School children under 6 years of age (S<6)	3.3

children and school children 6 years of age and older brought home over twice as many infections as did the fathers. The young kindergarten and nursery school children, when present in the family, were the most frequent source of respiratory infections. This order indicates the relative status of each class of individual with respect to his hazard to the home.

Total incidence rates are the combined effects of being infected within and without the home. Therefore, the different rates of introduction of respiratory disease by various classes of individuals should be reflected in the total number of infections suffered by

TABLE 9

Incidence of the common respiratory diseases in members of families containing two children, by class of child

Class of child	Illnesses per person-year				
	F	M	P	S<6	S6+
Both under 6					
P, P	3.27	4.85	6.64	......	......
P, S<6	4.20	5.75	9.81	9.61	......
S<6, S<6	3.67	5.96	......	10.09	......
One under 6					
P, S6+	3.23	5.67	7.96	......	6.47
S<6, S6+	2.69	3.49	......	6.50	6.55
Both 6+					
S6+, S6+	2.02	2.86	......	......	4.52

TABLE 10

Incidence of the common respiratory diseases in members of
families containing three children, by class of child

Class of child	Illnesses per person-year				
	F	M	P	S<6	S6+
Three under 6					
P, P, P	3.16	3.96	6.28	......	......
P, P, S<6	4.92	6.34	8.63	8.59	......
P, S<6, S<6	3.15	6.12	6.12	8.26	......
S<6, S<6, S<6	No families		......	......	......
Two under 6					
P, P, S6+	3.31	5.48	7.88	......	6.48
P, S<6, S6+	3.87	5.23	7.32	6.96	6.56
S<6, S<, S6+	2.44	2.44	......	6.86	4.57
One under 6					
P, S6+, S6+	3.49	4.74	7.24	......	5.11
S<6, S6+, S6+	4.29	4.83	......	5.96	5.10
None under 6					
S6+, S6+, S6+	3.01	4.50	......	......	4.79

their family associates. Tables 9 and 10 were prepared to illustrate this point. In general, the rates for families with either two or three children were higher for those families that had a school child less than 6 years of age, the family member who introduced the relatively greatest number of infections. The results, however, were not consistent. It was expected, for example, that in families with three children under six, the more children there were in school the higher the total attack rates in the various family members would be. It was found that if one child went to school, the incidence rates were higher for each class of person than if none of the three went to school. However, if two of the children were in school, the rates were consistently lower than if one child was in school, and if none of the children attended school, only the mothers' rates were lower.

SPREAD OF THE COMMON RESPIRATORY DISEASES WITHIN THE FAMILY

As stated above, cases which occurred on the first calendar day of episodes were considered as index cases, while cases occurring during

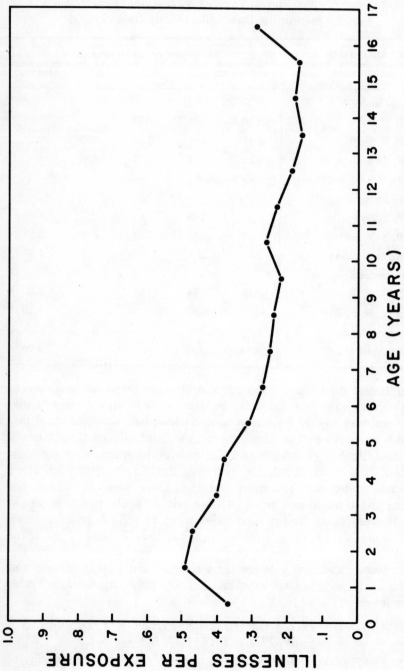

Fig. 14 Secondary attack rates from the common respiratory diseases by age

the 9 succeeding days were taken to be secondary cases. Secondary attack rates were computed by dividing the number of secondary cases by the number of individuals in the families who were exposed to the index cases, that is, the individuals other than the index cases. Figure 14 and Appendix 11, table 1 show the secondary attack rates for various age groups. The ratio was highest at ages 1 and 2 years, at which ages about one-half of the exposures resulted in illness, and gradually decreased thereafter. Fathers not only had the lowest rates of acquiring infection outside of the home but also had the lowest secondary attack rates: only about one exposure in seven resulted in illness. On the average, 25% of all exposures within the home were followed by illness.

Age-specific secondary attack rates for the three classes of children

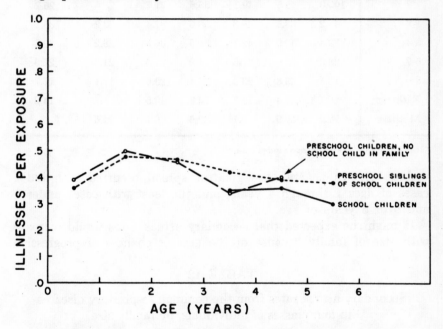

Fig. 15 Secondary attack rates from the common respiratory diseases among children under 6 years of age, by age and class of child

considered above were quite similar (figure 15). Although these three classes of children did not differ in respect to secondary attack rates, they suffered quite different total incidence rates. These facts together imply that excessive contact with the infecting agents, as manifested by a high total incidence, does not reduce susceptibility as measured by secondary attack rates. The general downward trend in secondary attack rates with age implies a reduced susceptibility as age increases beyond the first year of life — a reduction not due to contact with the agents involved but to something else, possibly a nonspecific effect of aging.

However, age-specific secondary attack rates did vary according to the age of the index case to whom the contacts were exposed

TABLE 11

Age-specific secondary attack rates from the common respiratory diseases, by age of index case*

Age of contact (years)	Age of index case (years)						
	<1	1-2	3-4	5-7	8+	Fathers	Mothers
<1	100.0	45.5	49.1	36.6	21.7	23.5	26.2
1-2	43.2	63.5	66.8	58.6	37.4	33.2	30.1
3-4	39.4	40.9	49.3	50.3	36.5	28.2	30.5
5-7	28.9	33.6	27.6	34.9	27.3	21.8	22.0
8+	13.5	23.8	23.2	24.4	23.6	17.1	17.7
Fathers	15.1	17.4	15.7	12.8	10.5	......	14.2
Mothers	22.2	29.9	25.1	22.6	16.1	24.6	......

*Based on episodes with only one index case.

(table 11). In general, the greatest spread occurred with index cases of ages 1 through 4 years, and the least with cases under 1 and over 8 years of age.

It might be expected that secondary attack rates would increase with size of family because of the greater chances of progressive

TABLE 12

Secondary attack rates from the common respiratory diseases in four classes of individuals, by family size

Size of family	Fathers	Mothers	Children <6	Children 6+
3	.18	.31	.39	.16
4	.14	.25	.45	.25
5	.14	.23	.39	.21
6	.13	.20	.40	.25
7	.17	.25	.34	.19
8	.14	.16	.33	.26

spread from one person to another. This was found not to be the case (table 12) possibly because the length of the episode, as defined arbitrarily to be 10 days, may not have been great enough to include a second generation of secondary cases. Secondary attack rates for the family as a whole, without regard to age or relationship, were amazingly constant for families of different sizes (Appendix 11, table 2).

TABLE 13

Number and percentage of cases of the common respiratory diseases occurring on each day of episodes

Day of episode	Number of onsets	Percentage of secondary cases
0	5510	—
1	769	16.2
2	741	15.6
3	716	15.1
4	586	12.4
5	502	10.6
6	440	9.3
7	418	8.8
8	302	6.4
9	264	5.6
Totals	10248	100.0

Intervals between index cases and secondary cases. — Table 13 shows the day of occurrence of the cases in the episodes. Day 0 is the day of onset of the episode, and on that day there were 5510 index cases which occurred in 4951 episodes. The final column shows the percentage distribution of the secondary cases. Approximately one-half of them occurred during the first 3 days after the episode started. The median time of onset was 3.2 days after the midnight following the onset of the index case. Only one-fifth of the secondary cases appeared during the last 3 days of the episodes. There can be no doubt that there was an excessive occurrence of illnesses during the early part of episodes which suggests that the index case was a common source of infection to other members of the family and that the incubation periods were short.

TABLE 14

Median time of onset of secondary cases and the secondary attack
rates from the common respiratory diseases, by age

Age (years)	Median interval* (days)	Secondary attack rates (%)
Fathers	4.0	14
Over 5	3.6	23
Mothers	3.4	23
5	3.1	31
4	2.9	38
Less than 1	2.7	37
3	2.7	40
1	2.6	49
2	2.5	47

*Since all records were kept on a calendar day basis, it was not possible to compute directly the median interval between index and secondary cases. For example, the interval between onset of the index case and a secondary case developing on the next day (day 1 of table 13) might be anywhere between a few minutes and 48 hours. The data of this table show the medians of a series of distributions such as that of table 13. Probably a better estimate of the true medians of index-to-secondary-case intervals would be obtained by adding one-half day to each of these values.

The median time of onset was determined for several classes of individuals. These data are presented in table 14 along with the secondary attack rates for the same classes. It was found that the intervals and the secondary attack rates were inversely correlated, but one cannot put a precise interpretation on either the secondary attack rates or the intervals described. As pointed out above, in no instance was it possible to identify with certainty the source from which a respiratory infection was acquired. Secondary cases as defined here include not only infections acquired from an index case, but also may include second or third passages within the episode and an indefinable number acquired outside the home. Nevertheless, by studying selected family episodes of illness where the situations seemed to be least complicated, it is thought that approximate levels of true secondary attack rates were derived for the several classes of individuals.

The intervals presented in tables 13 and 14 are likewise somewhat poorly defined, for the same reasons which cast some doubt on the absolute levels of the secondary attack rates. In spite of these limitations, the data provide a basis for speculation. Both the rates of secondary attacks and the timing of secondary illnesses are undoubtedly dependent upon many circumstances. Data presented here show that both vary according to the age of the individual. That they also vary according to the age of the index case indicates that every family member is not effectively exposed each time a new infection is introduced into the home. Intensity of contact between the index case and his familial associates is apparently also a pertinent factor in determining secondary attack rates. The inverse correlation between the secondary attack rates and the median time of onset of secondary cases may be due completely to different degrees and frequency of contact between various classes of family members.

In a previous publication (4) an additional hypothesis was presented: that both the secondary attack rates and the incubation periods in various classes of persons reflect relative degrees of immunity. It seems quite likely that if various classes of individuals are adequately exposed to an infectious organism, the attack rates are a reflection of the relative immunity of the individuals in the classes. It is not unreasonable to think that the incubation period may reflect relative immunity. It is known, for example, that with measles which has been modified by increasing the immune status of an individual, a prolonged incubation period may occur (57). It is possible that persons who are relatively immune to respiratory disease may also have longer incubation periods than those who are more susceptible. No direct confirmation of this possibility has been found. Evidence in respect to this hypothesis was sought in reports of experiments in which humans were inoculated with infectious material. Jackson et al. (80) presented data which showed no significant difference between the infection rates of men and women, although the difference they found was in favor of higher infection rates among women. They did not present sex-specific data regarding incubation periods. The Common Cold Research Unit at Salisbury (133) similarly found no significant difference between the infection rates of and incubation periods in men and women volunteers. These observations neither support nor contradict the hypothesis that incubation period is related to immune status in respect to respiratory infection. It is also possible that the results may be due to nonspecific resistance developing with age.

Introductions and secondary attack rates as indices of exposure to common respiratory diseases in the community.—When classes of individuals are arranged in order of their relative risk of introducing infections into the home (table 8), the explanation of several features of this order is not self-evident. Mothers, for example, probably have less contact outside the home than do fathers, yet they introduced more infections than did the fathers;

school children 6 years of age and over have much more contact with the community than do preschool children, yet they introduced relatively fewer infections.

An acceptable explanation of the order of classes of individuals according to their risk of acquiring infection outside of the home is arrived at by taking secondary attack rates as an index of the relative immune status of an individual. Mothers, for example, mothers bring home more infections than do fathers, in spite of family by the fathers (table 8). Judged by secondary attack rates (Appendix 11, table 1) the mothers were .23/.14 or 1.6 times as susceptible as the fathers. It seems reasonable to conclude that mothers bring home more infections than do fathers, in spite of the fact that they are exposed less frequently, because they are more susceptible. It is because of this reasonableness and that of conclusions arising from other comparisons made in this way (table 15) that more confidence can be placed in these assumptions than is warranted *a priori.*

TABLE 15

Comparison of introduction ratios and secondary attack rates for the common respiratory diseases among various family members

Groups compared	Ratio of secondary attack rates	Relative number of introductions
Mothers / Fathers	$\dfrac{.23}{.14} = 1.6$	$\dfrac{1.34}{1} = 1.3$
School <6 / School 6+	$\dfrac{.32}{.23} = 1.4$	$\dfrac{3.26}{2.20} = 1.5$
School <6 / Preschool	$\dfrac{.32}{.43} = 0.7$	$\dfrac{3.26}{2.68} = 1.2$
Preschool / Mothers	$\dfrac{.43}{.23} = 1.9$	$\dfrac{2.68}{1.34} = 2.0$

Table 15 shows a series of comparisons made in this way. The second row compares school children under 6 years of age with older school children. The younger group is 1.4 times as susceptible as the older group. They brought home 1.5 times as many infections. The similarity of these ratios implies equal contact with the community outside the home. This, too, seems reasonable; with equal contact and greater susceptibility the younger school children bring home a greater number of infections.

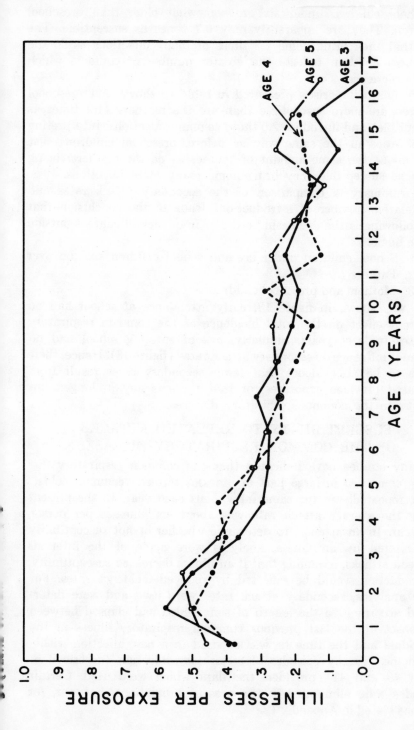

Fig. 16 Secondary attack rates from the common respiratory diseases by age, according to age at time of entry into school

School children under six are somewhat older than preschool children. They are apparently only 0.7 times as susceptible. The fact that they bring home 1.2 times as many infections as do the preschool children reflects the greater number of contacts which they experience.

The final comparison presented in table 15 shows that preschool children are more susceptible than are the mothers (1.9 times as susceptible) and introduce 2.0 times as many infections. Interpreting these ratios in the same way as before, preschool children must have about the same amount of contact as do the mothers; being twice as susceptible they bring home many more infections.

In summary, a comparison of the secondary attack rates and the relative number of introductions leads to the conclusion that the following is the decreasing order of frequency of contact outside of the home:

1. School children under six and school children six and over
2. Fathers
3. Mothers and preschool children

As was shown in figure 13, early attendance at school had no apparent effect on the total incidence of the common respiratory diseases in later years. Similarly, age of entering school had no apparent influence on secondary attack rates (figure 16). Hence, there seems to be no evidence that fewer secondary cases result from increased previous exposures, or that there is any prolonged immunity to the common respiratory diseases.

SUSCEPTIBILITY TO REPEATED ATTACKS OF THE COMMON RESPIRATORY DISEASES

Many studies have indicated that the common respiratory diseases, composed in large part of illnesses termed "common colds," occur repeatedly in the same individuals each year. In the present study the average attack rate was about six illnesses per person per year. In an attempt to determine whether or not susceptibility was altered by an illness, analyses were made of the intervals between attacks, assuming that if an illness decreased susceptibility, the reduction would be reflected by reduced incidence rates. For these analyses, secondary attack rates were used and were determined according to the length of time which had elapsed between the onset of the last previous common respiratory illness in the individual and the time he was exposed to a new infection within the home. Family episodes of respiratory infection (described on pages 40 and 41) provided the data which were used. Certain episodes were eliminated in the present tabulations, however, for reasons stated in Appendix 12.

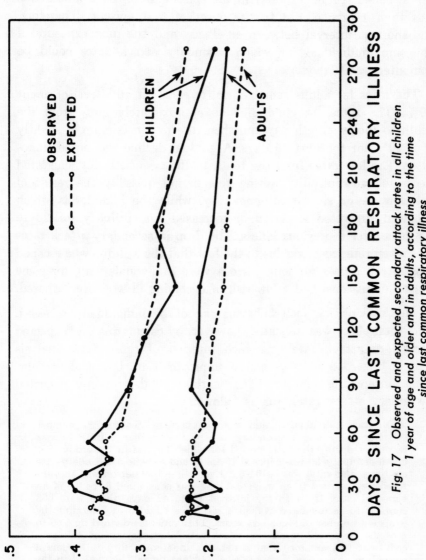

Fig. 17 Observed and expected secondary attack rates in all children 1 year of age and older and in adults, according to the time since last common respiratory illness

Secondary attack rates were determined separately for adults and children over 1 year of age (figure 17; Appendix 11, tables 3 and 4). Because of the definition of an episode, it was not possible for a person to be exposed in an episode if his last illness was less than 10 days prior to the onset of that episode. Therefore, the shortest interval between an illness and the next exposure of the same individual for which secondary attack rates could be computed was 10 days.

The rates for adults remained fairly constant at a level of about 20%. The rates for children were approximately 30% from the tenth to the twentieth day and then rose to a maximum of slightly over 40% for the next 15 days. A gradual decline was noted thereafter. The low rates from the tenth to the twentieth day suggested decreased susceptibility during this period, possibly the result of interference or short-term immunity, while the high levels which followed suggested a period of increased susceptibility for 20 to 35 days after a previous illness. The drop in secondary attack rates was interpreted as being due to the fact that the children who escaped respiratory illness for long periods were individuals who, for some reason or reasons, had a low risk of becoming ill whenever exposed.

The reasons for such behavior cannot be individually assessed. The total effect was indicated, however, by calculating an "expected secondary attack rate" for each interval of time. Such analysis can be regarded only as a first approximation, but it does show some interesting features. The method of determining expected secondary attack rates was as follows:

> For each individual a ratio was computed by dividing the number of times he became a secondary case by the number of times he was a contact during the total period for which he was in the study. For one individual who was exposed 10 times and became a secondary case six times, this ratio was $6/10=0.6$. Every time this person was encountered as a contact to an index case, he was considered to be 0.6 of an expected case. If, as in the interval 40 to 49 days, there were 668 contacts to be tabulated, 668 such ratios were added to determine the expected number of secondary cases. This sum was divided by 6.68 to give the "expected secondary attack rate." In carrying out this procedure it was assumed that a person's inherent ability to become a secondary case upon exposure was constant during his period in the study. (Because this assumption seems least warranted during the first year of life, children under 1 year of age were omitted from the tabulations.) It is recognized that average secondary attack rates do vary with age throughout childhood, and therefore, that this assumption is somewhat contradicted by the data available (see Appendix 11, table 1); no attempt has been made, however, to adjust individual expectancies according to age.

The observed secondary attack rates are contrasted with the expected rates in figure 17. Children had slightly reduced secondary attack rates through the twenty-second day, and slightly excessive rates for the next few weeks. The rates for adults were slightly reduced for the period 10 to 69 days and slightly in excess thereafter. In view of the limitations of the methods of analysis, these differences should not be stressed. Rather, the persistent susceptibility following a recent infection is the impressive feature. Further analyses along these lines seemed unwarranted.

The initial reason for the present tabulations was to determine whether or not in studying the epidemiology of the common respiratory diseases the length of time since the last illness had to be considered as a pertinent variable. In terms of secondary attack rates, at least, it was of minor importance. These observations are consistent with two hypotheses: a) that a majority of the common respiratory diseases are due to agents which produce little or no immunity; and b) that there exist a large number of viruses which produce symptoms of common respiratory disease and which may or may not produce immunity.

A number of observations have suggested that little if any permanent immunity follows any particular common respiratory illness. This may be inferred from the fact that most individuals suffer several times a year with these infections. The observation that both the total incidence and secondary attack rate decrease with advancing age can be interpreted as having no relationship to immunity, but rather to a decrease in the relative susceptibility of a given individual over a period of years associated with some factor or factors in the aging process. The epidemiological studies of Lidwell and Sommerville (93), and of Downes (53) also are compatible with the interpretation that little or no immunity occurs following these respiratory illnesses. On the other hand, the diminution and disappearance of colds or mild respiratory infections among isolated populations as reported by Heinbecker and Irvine-Jones (70) and by Paul and Freese (105) could be interpreted that immunity in such populations does develop and that the infection disappears because of lack of introduction of new strains of virus.

The results of experimental studies in which common colds have been transmitted to volunteers by inoculation of nasal secretions from a patient with an illness have been conflicting. The studies of the Commission on Acute Respiratory Diseases (44) showed no evidence of resistance to infection in volunteers challenged 3 weeks after their initial experimental infection. This result could indicate a lack of immunity or the fact that the challenge dose was sufficiently large to overwhelm any immunity which might have been present. In contrast to this observation are the results of Jackson, Dowling and Anderson (78) and Andrews (28) who demonstrated neutralization of infective secretions by gamma globulin and convalescent sera from patients with common colds. In addition, Jackson and Dowling (79) have demonstrated the existence of five infective nasal secretions isolated in different years which produce homologous immunity but no heterologous immunity. The dominance of one single strain in any particular year or season has not yet been determined but these results suggest that there may be a considerable number of immunologically unrelated viruses that occur singly or together and produce the clinical syndrome of the common cold.

The most reasonable interpretation of these conflicting results would seem to be that there are a number of strains of viruses capable of producing the clinical syndrome of the common respiratory diseases which circulate in open populations with varying frequency throughout the year. It should be pointed out, however, that even though each of these strains produces immunity to itself, the continual high level of occurrence of these minor respiratory illnesses in a population is such that immunity has no apparent effect on the control of this annoying problem.

INDIVIDUAL AND FAMILY VARIATION IN INCIDENCE OF THE COMMON RESPIRATORY DISEASES

Up to now we have been concerned with the *average* incidence of the common respiratory diseases and the manner in which such incidence figures have been influenced by season, age, sex, attendance at school and family composition. We shall now consider not the average figures but the variation in incidence which was observed among individuals and families and also whether or not certain individuals and families were consistent in their behavior from year to year.

In most of the analyses of average incidence it was possible to use all of the data collected. For example, the experience of 2-year-old children consisted not only of those who were observed for the entire period between their second and third birthdays, but also the experience of children who were in the study for only a portion of their third year of life, that is, those who either entered or left the study between their second and third birthdays.

No way was apparent by which the latter children could be included in studies of variation among individuals, and only those portions of the data which represented a complete year of experience in a specified status were included. For example, descriptions of the variation in incidence experienced by 2-year-old children were based on the experience of children who were in the study for that complete year of life. Similarly, when concerned with the variation in the amount of illness recorded for 2-year-old children in families of size four, not only must each child have been in the study for the whole of his third year of life, but in addition, his family size must have remained at four individuals throughout that period. The more specific the class of individual, the more selective was the experience included in the tabulation. The selection, however, did not appear to introduce bias since the average rates for the selected individuals were almost identical with the average rates for the total population.

Table 16 shows the number of common respiratory diseases recorded for individuals at each year of age. The amount of variation among individuals is very striking at each age and overshadows the averages described previously. Similar variation was seen when the data were analyzed separately for each sex.

Figure 18 shows the incidence in the most highly selected groups which were examined in terms of frequency distributions of individual experiences according to age, family size and school status. To be included in this tabulation an individual must have been in the study for the complete period between indicated birthdays, and his school status and family size must have remained unchanged during that period. The height of each bar represents the number of individuals; the tallest bar, for example, represents 11 school children in families of size five, each of whom had five respiratory illnesses between the seventh and eighth birthdays. The most common frequency, depicted by what appears to be a dash (−), represents one child. Again, the impressive feature about these data is the great variation in incidence rates in fairly homogeneous groups of individuals.

The data presented above indicate the fallacy of being concerned solely with *average* annual incidence rates. The latter have clearly shown consistent trends when determined for homogeneous groups selected on the basis of age, sex, family composition and school status. For example, children 8 years of age experienced fewer respiratory illnesses than did 1-year-old children. The variation in frequency of illness in individuals, however, was so great that about one-fifth of the 8-year-old children had more illnesses than the average number of illnesses experienced by children aged 1 year. Similarly, about one-fifth of children aged 1 year had fewer illnesses than the average number for 8-year-old children. Thus, considera-

TABLE 16

Number of individuals having specified number of common respiratory illnesses for each year of age

Age in years	Number of Illnesses																				Total no. of inds.
	0	1	2	3	4	5	6	7	8	9	10	11	12	13	14	15	16	17	18	19	
<1	1	2	4	6	8	6	5	13	9	10	4	1	1	2	1	1					74
1		3		2	7	6	8	12	13	10	9	5	5	6	1	1		1			89
2	1		1	5	3	17	13	13	20	16	10	4	8	4	3	2					120
3		1		2	6	11	17	15	14	11	9	9	7	4	2	1					112
4			6	3	15	6	14	24	16	9	8	13	3	6	2	1					126
5	1	3	2	8	12	17	14	16	14	12	8	4	6	4	5		1				129
6	3	5	7	11	13	11	17	18	13	7	7	5	3	4			1				124
7	1	3	11	10	12	17	20	10	8	11	6	3	2	1	2		1	1			119
8	2	5	8	11	8	12	14	9	14	7	2	4	1	3			1				101
9	3	4	10	9	14	8	11	7	9	6	1	3		3		2					88
10	2	3	5	7	9	12	12	6	8	4	1	1	1	1	1						73
11	2	4	6	12	6	7	10	7	2	2	2	1	1								63
12	1	1	5	6	7	4	9	7	2	1	1	1	1								46
13		4	3	9	1	2	4	3	3	1	1										32
14	1	1	2	3	3	3	3	3	1	1		1									22
15			2	2	1	1	1		1			1									11
16	1		1		1																6
17	1	1																			4
23			2	2																	2
24		1		1	1				1												4

	6	9	15	26	33	45	53	70	80	82	80	76	74	59	50	37	30	24	20	14	12	10	9	6	5	2
				1																						
										1									1						
		1					1			1	1	1													
						1	1																		
					1	1			1																
					1	1													1	1					
			2		1	2	1			1															
			1	1		1		5	2	3	1	1			1					1					
1		1	1	4	2	2	1	6	3	1	1	3	1	1			1			1		1			
		1	2	4	4	3	6	5	1	2	5	6	1	2	3	1	1			1	1				
		1	3	5	3	3	4	4	2	4	5	1	1	1	5	1	3	1			1		1		
		1	1	2	1	4	5	4	8	8	8	6	4	3	1	1	2	1	1			1			
		2	2	3	6	5	6	13	9	11	10	7	9	1	9	1	5	2		1	1		1		1
	1		2	6	9	4	7	12	12	11	7	12	12	5	11	5	3	4	5	3	1	2	2	1	1
1	2	1	3	2	11	10	13	13	9	15	10	10	13	7	8	5	4	3	4	2	2	4	1	1	1
	1	3	3	4	5	6	8	15	14	15	9	17	11	10	6	6	4	5	3		2		2		1
2	1	1	1	1	3	7	6	8	6	9	11	5	9	4	5	3	2	3	1	4	1	1	1	2	
1	2	1			1	1	2	2	7	5	7	6	5	3	2	3	2								
25	26	27	28	29	30	31	32	33	34	35	36	37	38	39	40	41	42	43	44	45	46	47	48	49	50

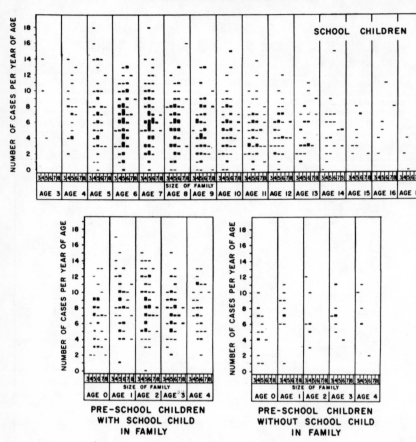

Fig. 18   Number of common respiratory diseases per individual, by year of
age, by relationship and family size

tion of both the average rates and the variation among individuals
is necessary for a presentation of the true picture.

The question of whether or not certain individuals tended to be
consistent from year to year with respect to the number of respiratory illnesses they experienced was examined in a number of
ways. Actually, no completely satisfactory way was determined
for describing the occurrence of illnesses on a time axis. The
analyses to be presented next are concerned with the consistency
with which individuals remained above or below the median incidence
of illness after taking age into account.

Using the data of table 16, the median number of illnesses was
determined for each year of age for children, for the entire group
of fathers, and for the entire group of mothers, ignoring age in
the adults. It was then possible to consider each year of experience

TABLE 17

Distribution of 128 individuals who were observed for 8 years,
according to the number of years the individual had more than
the median incidence of the common respiratory diseases

Number of years in which individual had more than median number of respiratory illnesses	Number of individuals	Expected number of individuals
0	10	0.3
1	8	2.4
2	18	9.9
3	18	23.2
4	12	34.1
5	15	32.0
6	12	18.8
7	15	6.3
8	20	0.9
Total	128	128.0

for each individual and state whether or not it was greater or less
than the median for his group.

Table 17 shows data for individuals who were observed for 8
complete years — each year in this instance extending from one
birthday to the next. There were 128 such individuals having a
total of 1024 person-years of experience. Twenty of them had an
incidence of illness every year which was above median incidence,
fifteen of them had greater than the median incidence in 7 of the
8 years, etc. Altogether 466 (46%) of the 1024 person-years were
classified as being below the median and 558 (54%) as being above
the median. If there were no relationship between the various years
of experience of specific individuals, that is, if the illnesses experienced in this study were distributed at random among these 128
individuals, one would expect 1 individual (corresponding to the
expected number of 0.9) to have all 8 years above the median,
while 20 were observed; only 6 (expected number 6.3) to have
7 years above the median, while 15 were observed, etc.* The excess
of observed over expected numbers at the ends of the distribution
(that is, zero, one, two, seven, and eight years above the median)

---

*These expected numbers were obtained from the terms of $128(.54 + .46)^8$

TABLE 18

Distribution of individuals according to number of complete years in study and the number of years in which more than the median incidence of common respiratory diseases was experienced

Number of years in which individual had more than median number of respiratory illnesses	Number of years observed											
	4		5		6		7		8		9	
	Obs.	Exp.	Obs.	Exp.	Obs.	Exp.	Obs.	Exp.	Obs.	Exp.	Obs.	Exp.
0	11	3.5	6	1.1	2	0.1	6	0.2	10	0.3	2	1.1
1	10	13.3	6	6.5	3	0.9	3	1.3	8	2.4	4	3.8
2	11	19.1	17	16.0	1	2.7	5	4.5	18	9.9	7	6.0
3	8	12.2	7	19.5	2	4.3	0	8.9	18	23.2	3	5.4
4	11	2.9	12	11.9	0	3.8	6	10.4	12	34.1	2	3.2
5			10	2.9	2	1.8	3	7.4	15	32.0	2	1.2
6					4	0.4	6	2.9	12	18.8	0	0.3
7							7	0.5	15	6.3	0	0.1
8									20	0.9	1	0.0
9											0	0.0
Totals	51	51.0	58	58.0	14	14.0	36	36.0	128	128.0	21	21.0

indicate that some individuals do tend to have either a low or a high number of illnesses recorded year after year.

Separate computations were made for individuals observed for other periods of time and are presented in table 18. All of the groups showed the same tendency as described in the preceding paragraph; that is, certain individuals tended to be more consistent in respect to their illness experience than would be expected on the basis of chance.

Two obvious questions were whether or not the various members of a given family tended to have a similar level of incidence of common respiratory disease and whether or not families as a whole maintained a relatively constant level of incidence over a period of years. Several approaches were used to derive quantitative statements in answer to these questions. The one which seems most simple in concept and descriptive of the data has been described by Miller (21).

The analysis was based on the experience of the 47 families which entered the study between 1948 and 1950 and remained in it for at least 5 years. There were 196 persons in the families at the time of their enrollment, and the number of common respiratory illnesses was determined for each of these for each of the first 5 years under observation. In order that both age and length of time in the study might be taken into account in the analysis, each person-year of experience for children was specified according to year in the study (i.e., first, second, third, fourth, or fifth year after enrollment) and according to age at the beginning of the year. (Actually, age at the time of the first respiratory illness was taken as the age during the first year, and this was increased by 1 year at each anniversary of the enrollment date. This method of stating age was used because it was mechanically easiest to accomplish and introduced only a slight error.) Adults were placed into one of two groups: mothers or fathers. There was a total of 21 groups.

The distributions of respiratory illnesses were transformed in the following way: for each group, the mean number of common respiratory illnesses and the standard deviation were computed, the mean was subtracted from each observation, and each such difference was divided by the standard deviation. In this way, the number of common respiratory diseases for each person was expressed as the number of standard deviations above or below the mean for the group. When tested by the chi square test it was concluded that the 21 distributions of indices were similiar, so that a relative position in one group corresponded closely to the same relative position in another group. A person's relative position within his group, then, was indicated by the annual index for that

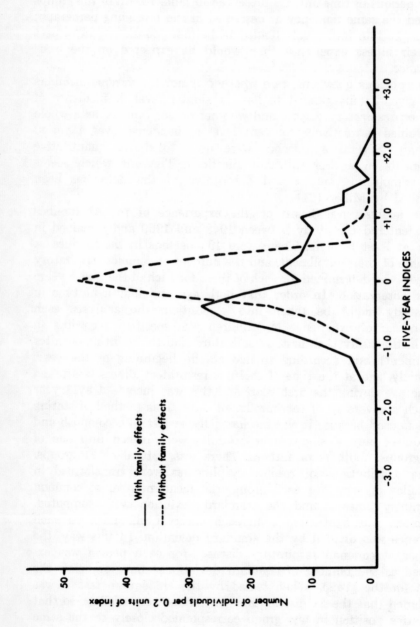

Fig. 19 Frequency distributions of 196 individuals according to their 5-year indices (common respiratory diseases), with and without family effects

person. An index of his standing during the entire 5-year period was obtained by averaging his five annual indices. Annual family indices were obtained by averaging the indices of the members of the respective families, and a 5-year family index was obtained by averaging the five annual family indices.

The analysis was presented in considerable detail by Miller (21). Briefly, after standardizing for the variables listed above, there was a tendency for members of the same family to have similar levels of incidence of common respiratory disease, and a given family tended to remain at the same relative incidence level over the five-year period. Thus some families tended to have consistently high levels, while others had consistently low levels of incidence.

Figure 19 demonstrates the tendency for members of the same family to have similar levels of incidence. This figure shows (1) the distribution of the 196 individual 5-year indices, and (2) a distribution of numbers obtained by subtracting the 5-year family index from each individual 5-year index. The second distribution is that of individual indices with the family effects removed.

TABLE 19

Distribution of families by the number of positive and negative signs of their annual indices

Number of signs		Number of families	Expected number of families
+	−		
5	0	9	0.66
4	1	4	4.43
3	2	6	11.95
2	3	7	16.14
1	4	7	10.89
0	5	14	2.94
Totals		47	47.00

Evidence on the year-to-year consistency of the annual family indices is presented in table 19, which classifies the families according to the number of positive and negative signs of their annual indices. For example, there were nine families with five positive annual indices, four families with four positive indices and one negative index, and so forth. The last column of table 19 shows the expected number of families for each combination of signs if the signs had been distributed at random. There was a considerable excess of families having five positive or five negative annual indices and a corresponding deficiency of families having both positive and negative indices. Another analysis showed that there was no concentration of positive signs among the larger families and that the year-to-year consistency was not due to size of family.

In summary, there was a striking amount of variation from individual to individual in the incidence of the common respiratory diseases at each year of age which was superimposed upon a downward trend in average rates with increasing age. Some persons tended to have either a high or low number of illnesses year after year. To some extent this tendency reflected the fact that certain families had either a consistently high or low level of incidence. The explanation of these findings is not known. Differences among families in the manner of recording illnesses may have contributed to the findings; such recording differences were judged by the staff to have been minor. If one or more family members consistently had a large number of infections from sources outside the home, this fact, coupled with the high secondary attack rates, could contribute to the year-to-year consistency of incidence rates both for families and for individual family members.. Prior experience, innate susceptibility or resistance, and other common hereditary or environmental influences may have played major roles. The influence of such factors cannot yet be sharply defined.

CLINICAL ASPECTS

In the early days of the study it was thought that the group of illnesses designated as the common respiratory diseases could be subclassified on a combined clinical and epidemiological basis and that such subdivision might have etiological significance. Accordingly, attempts were made to define such "entities" as the common cold, acute respiratory disease (ARD), and influenza-like illnesses, and to classify the illnesses in such terms. Even though it was possible to select certain illnesses and label them, for example common colds, as the study progressed it became increasingly obvious that such a clinical classification for all the illnesses in this group was arbitrary and artificial and had little or no apparent relationship to etiology. Attempts were therefore made to derive a meaningful classification based on symptoms. One such attempt is presented here.

Four symptoms were selected for analysis: coryza, sore throat, hoarseness, and cough. Coryza was considered to be present in any illness characterized by sneezing, nasal discharge and obstructed nose, occurring singly or in combination. Sore throat included complaints of sore or irritated throat. Hoarseness and cough are self-explanatory. The illnesses included in this analysis are those which occurred in the years 1948 through 1954 and which were diagnosed as common respiratory diseases. The occurrence of one or more of the above four symptoms was determined for each illness.

TABLE 20

Percentage of common respiratory illnesses in which specific symptoms were present, by age

Symptoms	Age					
	<1	1 - 5	6 - 18	Fathers	Mothers	Total
Coryza	95.5	91.7	86.5	81.5	81.9	87.4
Sore throat	4.9	15.0	37.6	61.3	69.7	36.3
Hoarseness	9.4	18.5	18.0	21.9	30.8	20.6
Cough	51.2	56.4	46.3	42.7	48.3	50.3

Table 20 (also Appendix 13, table 1) shows the frequency with which the four symptoms occurred and table 21 (also Appendix 13, table 2) presents the frequency with which various combinations of symptoms were encountered in 10,563 cases observed during the period; 571 cases were excluded either because the record was inadequate or because one or more symptoms from a preceding illness were still present and it was therefore impossible to state the characteristics of the illness induced by the new infection. An additional 63 cases were excluded for miscellaneous reasons.

The relative frequency with which these symptoms and combinations of them were encountered varied with age. Coryza was the most frequent symptom in each age group studied, but its occurrence varied from being present in 95% of illnesses in children under 1 year of age to 82% of illnesses in adults. This may be a true difference or it may reflect the difficulty of recognizing respiratory infection in an infant if coryza is absent. For example, those illnesses in adults which were characterized by only sore throat had practically no counterpart in infants. Cough was the second most commonly encountered symptom and showed the least variation with age of all the localizing symptoms. Fathers recorded the lowest proportion of common respiratory diseases with cough (43%) while children 1 to 5 years of age showed the highest proportion (56%). Cough was, apparently, a symptom which was easily recognized in

TABLE 21

Percentage of common respiratory illnesses in which specific combinations of symptoms were present, by age

| Symptoms* | | | | Age | | | | | |
Coryza	Sore throat	Hoarseness	Cough	<1	1-5	6-18	Fathers	Mothers	Total
x	x	x	x	0.8	3.7	5.6	11.7	18.2	7.8
x	x	x	o	0.2	0.6	2.4	3.2	4.6	2.1
x	x	o	x	1.4	4.8	10.3	14.2	14.0	8.9
x	x	o	o	1.6	3.0	10.7	17.3	18.2	9.5
x	o	x	x	6.8	9.6	5.2	2.9	3.2	6.3
x	o	x	o	1.2	2.4	2.4	1.3	1.4	2.0
x	o	o	x	39.3	32.9	19.2	8.4	7.4	21.9
x	o	o	o	44.3	34.6	30.7	22.5	14.9	28.9
o	x	x	x	0.0	0.4	0.7	1.6	1.4	0.8
o	x	x	o	0.0	0.3	0.8	0.7	1.0	0.6
o	x	o	x	0.4	0.4	1.2	2.0	2.0	1.1
o	x	o	o	0.6	1.8	5.9	10.6	10.2	5.5
o	o	x	x	0.2	0.7	0.5	0.2	0.5	0.5
o	o	x	o	0.2	0.6	0.4	0.3	0.4	0.4
o	o	o	x	2.3	3.8	3.7	1.7	1.7	3.0
o	o	o	o	0.8	0.3	0.4	1.4	0.8	0.6
Total				100.0	100.0	100.0	100.0	100.0	100.0

*x = Present; o = Absent

infancy as a sign of respiratory disease (51%). Sore throat and hoarseness varied considerably among age groups; both increased in frequency with age, so that 70% of illnesses in mothers were characterized by sore throat and 31% by hoarseness.

With these differences in the relative frequency of individual symptoms, it is to be expected that the frequency with which the various combinations of symptoms were encountered would also vary. In infancy the most common illness was that in which coryza was the only localizing symptom (table 21); the next most common was the combination of coryza and cough. Together these two types constituted 84% of all illnesses in infancy. In older children the same two types of illness were also most frequently encountered, but they constituted only 50% of the illnesses in children 6 years of age and older. In general, the older the individuals, the more complex were the symptom groupings; infants had 1.6 symptoms per illness and this increased to 1.9 for children six and over. Fathers had an average of 2.1 and mothers an average of 2.3 symptoms per illness. The degree to which this reflects the fact that the mother did most of the recording remains unanswered.

Various tabulations were made (Appendix 13, table 3) based on table 21 showing the association between symptoms. As might be expected, the relationships are very complex. Some of the more simple relationships are enumerated here:

1. Persons with coryza had a lower incidence of sore throat than did individuals without coryza. This was true in each age group.

2. The correlations between coryza and hoarseness and between coryza and cough were not constant when the several age groups were considered.

3. There was a consistently positive correlation between the presence of sore throat and hoarseness.

4. There was no consistent pattern of relationship between sore throat and cough.

5. Hoarseness and cough were highly correlated: if hoarseness was present, the incidence of cough was much higher than if hoarseness was absent; this was true in every age group.

The correlation of more than two localizing symptoms was not carried out extensively. Table 22 is presented to show the relationship between hoarseness and sore throat and cough. Hoarseness and cough were highly related, but sore throat seemed to have little effect on this relationship; that is, sore throat was independent of cough while hoarseness and cough tended to go together.

Fever was taken as the objective measurement of a general constitutional reaction to infection. An attempt was made to have the mothers determine and record the temperature at 4:00 P.M. on days

TABLE 22

Number of common respiratory illnesses by age groups, according to presence or absence of combinations of hoarseness, sore throat, and cough

Age	Hoarseness*	Sore throat*	Cough* x	Cough* o	Total	% with cough
<1	x	x	4	1	5	80.0
	x	o	36	7	43	83.7
	o	x	9	11	20	45.0
	o	o	213	231	444	48.0
1-5	x	x	169	39	208	81.3
	x	o	424	123	547	77.5
	o	x	210	197	407	51.6
	o	o	1501	1425	2926	51.3
6-18	x	x	164	83	247	66.4
	x	o	149	73	222	67.1
	o	x	299	434	733	40.8
	o	o	597	811	1408	42.4
Fathers	x	x	194	57	251	77.3
	x	o	45	23	68	66.2
	o	x	235	406	641	36.7
	o	o	147	348	495	29.7
Mothers	x	x	372	108	480	77.5
	x	o	70	35	105	66.7
	o	x	303	540	843	35.9
	o	o	172	298	470	36.6

*x = Present; o = Absent

when individuals were ill and at other times of the day as indicated. In general the temperature was not taken unless the mother felt that fever was present and thus in many illnesses the actual temperature was not recorded. Based on a firm belief that the mothers were a very conscientious group, we were quite satisfied to consider the absence of an entry as indicating that the temperature did not

TABLE 23

Percentage of common respiratory illnesses with fever, for each combination of localizing symptoms

Symptoms*				Total no. cases	Fever present	
Coryza	Sore throat	Hoarseness	Cough		Number	%
x	x	x	x	820	182	22.2
x	x	x	o	225	32	14.2
x	x	o	x	941	182	19.3
x	x	o	o	1008	117	11.6
x	o	x	x	667	162	24.3
x	o	x	o	213	11	5.2
x	o	o	x	2310	403	17.4
x	o	o	o	3052	191	6.3
o	x	x	x	83	16	19.3
o	x	x	o	63	9	14.3
o	x	o	x	115	24	20.9
o	x	o	o	580	98	16.9
o	o	x	x	57	13	22.8
o	o	x	o	48	2	4.2
o	o	o	x	320	36	11.3
o	o	o	o	61	23	37.7
Total				10,563	1501	14.2

*x = Present; o = Absent

TABLE 24

Percentage of common respiratory illnesses with fever, according to the presence or absence of sore throat and cough

Symptoms*		Total no. cases	Fever present	
Sore throat	Cough		Number	%
x	x	1959	404	20.6
x	0	1876	256	13.6
0	x	3354	614	18.3

*x = Present; o = Absent

exceed 100°F. Therefore a recorded temperature of 100° or higher was interpreted as fever, and a recorded temperature of less than 100° or no record of a temperature was interpreted to indicate the absence of fever.

Of the total 10,563 illnesses, 14.2% had fever (table 23). Of those illnesses characterized by coryza as the only localizing symptom, by hoarseness alone, or by coryza and hoarseness, relatively few had an associated fever (4-6%). If the remaining cases are classified according to the presence or absence of sore throat and cough

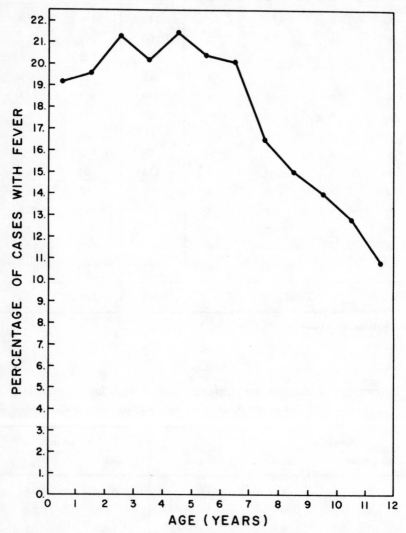

Fig. 20   Percentage of cases of the common respiratory diseases in which fever was present, by year of age

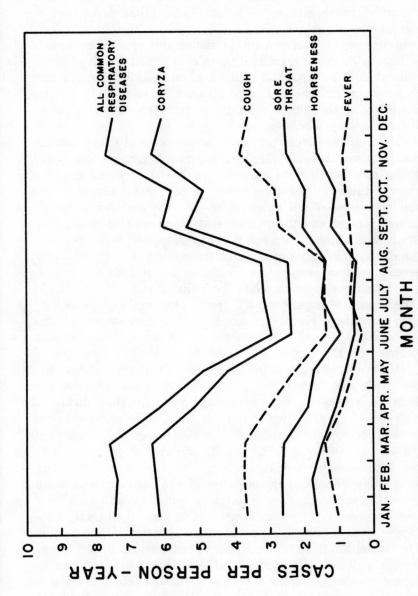

Fig. 21 Incidence of the common respiratory diseases in which various
symptoms were present, by month (1948-1954)

(table 24), it is apparent that fever was associated with cough, whether or not sore throat was present.

In summary, cough appeared to be the localizing symptom most frequently associated with fever. In the absence of cough, a larger percentage of those with sore throat (13.6%) had fever than if sore throat was absent (4-6%).

The occurrence of fever was quite constant during the first 6 years of life (figure 20 and Appendix 13, table 4); during each of these years about 20% of respiratory illnesses were febrile. Beyond this age there was a gradual decline to about 11% at age 11. Among parents 5.1% of the illnesses of the mothers and 6.6% of those of the fathers were febrile.

The relationship between season of occurrence and the symptoms present is shown in figure 21. The uppermost curve of this figure shows the month-by-month variation in incidence of all common respiratory diseases over the 7-year period. Also shown is the seasonal incidence of all common respiratory diseases in which coryza was present and the incidence of those common respiratory diseases in which cough, sore throat, hoarseness, and fever occurred. The groups of illnesses represented in these curves are not mutually exclusive; a common respiratory illness in which both coryza and cough occurred, for example, would be included in both curves.

In the combined experience of 7 years the incidence of each of the four respiratory symptoms was highest in the winter months (November-March) and showed a trough of low incidence during the summer months (June, July, and August). The incidence of cases with fever was greatest in late winter (February and March). Illnesses with sore throat and fever differed somewhat from the others in their behavior during the summer since their incidence was higher in July and August than in June. The upswing in the incidence of the common respiratory diseases in September included a sharp increase in the incidence of all four respiratory symptoms, but not in the incidence of fever.

The monthly variations in incidence of the common respiratory diseases with each of the four respiratory symptoms and with fever were not completely consistent from year to year when each year's experience was examined separately. In general, however, the patterns resembled those of the combined experience of all 7 years.

That the patterns of occurrence of sore throat and of fever resemble one another and differ from the patterns of the other symptom groups is suggested in figure 21. The differences stand out more clearly in figure 22 which shows the seasonal variation in the percentage of common respiratory diseases in which each of the four respiratory symptoms and fever occurred. Illnesses with

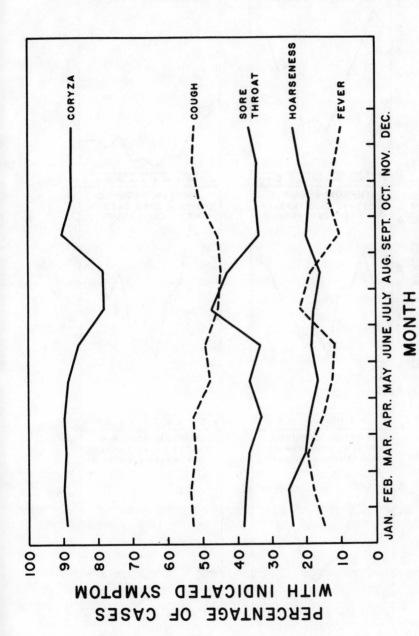

Fig. 22 Percentage of cases of the common respiratory diseases in which specific symptoms were present, by month (1948-1954)

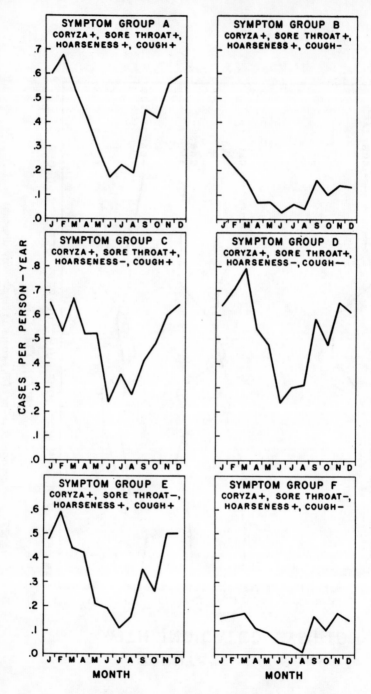

Fig. 23   Incidence of the common respiratory diseases by month,
according to symptom group (1948-1954)

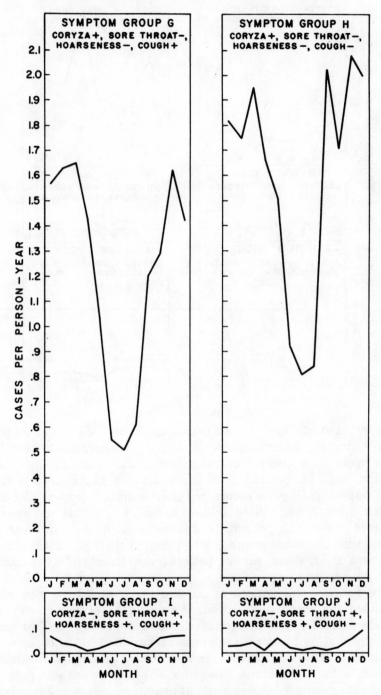

Fig. 23(B) (Continued)

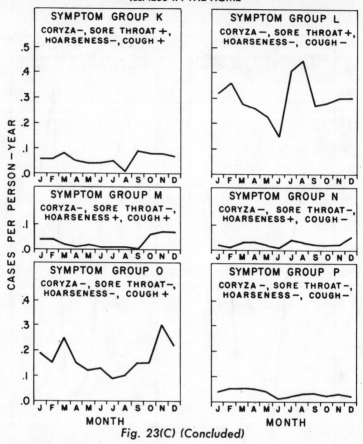

Fig. 23(C) (Concluded)

sore throat made up a larger percentage during July and August than during any other months. Similarly, illnesses accompanied by fever made up a larger percentage during July than during other months, while the percentage of febrile illnesses in August was also high, approximating the occurrence of fever in late winter. Coryza, on the other hand, and to a lesser extent, hoarseness and cough, occurred in a smaller percentage of illnesses during July and August than during the other months. When each of the 7 years was examined separately, these seasonal patterns were found to be consistent from year to year.

The various combinations of the four major symptoms were also examined for seasonal variation. As would be expected with 12 months and 16 illness categories, the data are complex. Two relationships, having to do with the seasonal variation in the occurrence of coryza and of sore throat, are noteworthy. First, the incidence of each of the eight illness categories in which coryza was present (figure 23, groups A-H) was, without exception, lowest in June, July and August. In contrast, the non-coryzal categories had quite variable summer incidence rates, and for none of them were all three summer months the three lowest in incidence. Second, most of the illness categories in which sore throat occurred (figure 23, groups A-D and I-L) showed, to a greater or lesser extent, a midsummer increase in incidence; this increase was most marked for those cases of common respiratory disease with sore throat only (category L).

TABLE 25

Percentage of common respiratory illnesses with specified symptoms in which fever was present, by season, 1948-1954

Symptoms	February — March			July — August			Rest of year		
	Total no.	Fever present		Total no.	Fever present		Total no.	Fever present	
		No.	%		No.	%		No.	%
Cough	1088	288	26.47	453	92	20.31	3772	638	16.91
Sore throat	767	154	20.08	454	132	29.07	2614	374	14.31
Hoarseness	466	115	24.68	167	40	23.95	1543	272	17.63
Coryza	1859	353	18.99	789	127	16.10	6588	800	12.14

The seasonal variation in the association of fever with each of the four respiratory symptoms is summarized in table 25. In both the February-March and July-August periods all respiratory symptoms were acompanied by fever more frequently than at other times of the year. During February and March there was about the same relative increase in the frequency of fever accompanying each of the four respiratory symptoms. In July and August, on the other hand, the increased frequency of fever with sore throat was much greater than with other respiratory symptoms. Etiological data regarding febrile summer cases are meager but suggest that they were caused by a variety of agents including adenoviruses, Coxsackie viruses, polioviruses and ECHO viruses.

Complications of the common respiratory diseases were tabulated when they were known to exist (Appendix 13, table 5). Otitis media was the most frequently encountered complication, and was recorded in 1.9% of the illnesses, a figure which is probably too low since this diagnosis was made only on the basis of a direct examination of the ear drum. In general, the data regarding complications left much to be desired. Mothers were not specifically requested to record complications except as "other" symptoms. Usually an individual was not examined by a physician more than once during an illness. In addition, whether a condition was to be considered as a complication, as part of the illness, or as an unrelated associated process was entirely a matter of clinical judgment.

COMMON RESPIRATORY DISEASES DURING THE FIRST YEAR OF LIFE

The common respiratory diseases occurring during the first year of life were studied with particular care since it was thought that these illnesses might show the least complicated clinical and etiological patterns and that their epidemiological behavior might reflect transmission in the home to the greatest extent. Their clinical characteristics and epidemiological aspects are described in this section.

CLINICAL CHARACTERISTICS

Symptoms of the first respiratory infection.—There were 80 newborn babies who had their first respiratory illness while in the study and in most instances these illnesses were mild. The first respiratory infection in every baby was classified as a common respiratory disease rather than a specific infection such as pneumonia, influenza, streptococcal infection or nonbacterial tonsillitis or pharyngitis.

From the standpoint of symptoms alone (figure 24), nasal discharge was most frequent, occurring in 85% of the 80 illnesses. Furthermore, in all but three instances, this first infection was accompanied by one, two, or all three of the following coryzal symptoms: sneezing, nasal discharge and obstructed nose. Cough was recorded in 30 of the cases (38%). Other symptoms such as hoarseness, fever, conjunctival discharge, excess mucus in the throat (or "sputum"), and wheezing were rarely noted. Thus, the principal response of the respiratory tract to the first infection appeared to be rhinitis. It was difficult to judge whether or not cough was due to mucus or to tracheitis or bronchitis.

There were 15 illnesses characterized by a single symptom. These illnesses were considered to be respiratory infections because there were either "fresh colds" in the family or the symptom was so pronounced that there did not seem to be any other reasonable explanation. The most frequent syndrome consisted of sneezing, nasal discharge and obstructed nose. There were four babies with conjunctival discharge. In one instance only, an older sibling experienced conjunctivitis along with other respiratory symptoms and fever at the same time as the baby. While the other three babies had conjunctivitis in association with respiratory symptoms, members of their families were experiencing common colds without conjunctival involvement.

It is questionable whether the six infants with febrile illnesses were experiencing a simple common cold. Throat cultures in all in-

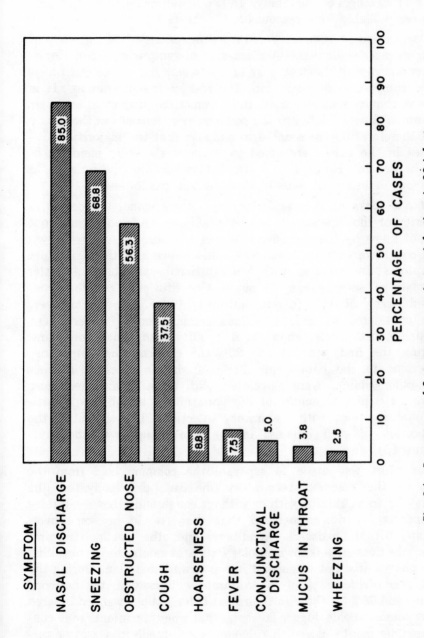

SYMPTOM

NASAL DISCHARGE — 85.0

SNEEZING — 68.8

OBSTRUCTED NOSE — 56.3

COUGH — 37.5

HOARSENESS — 8.8

FEVER — 7.5

CONJUNCTIVAL DISCHARGE — 5.0

MUCUS IN THROAT — 3.8

WHEEZING — 2.5

PERCENTAGE OF CASES

Fig. 24   Percentage of first common respiratory infections in 80 infants in which specified symptoms were present

stances failed to grow any of the usual pathogenic bacteria. In three instances febrile respiratory illnesses occurred simultaneously in other members of the family. In two instances immunization procedures probably were responsible for the fever.

Comparison of common respiratory infections of 73 infants and their next-older siblings.—A discussion of symptoms of respiratory infections during the first year of life seems out of context unless some comparison is made with the rest of the population. It is known that the incidence of the common respiratory diseases in infants is closely related to the occurrence of illnesses in the family and therefore it is reasonable to suppose that the majority of illnesses in the babies are allied to those of the older members of the household. Hence it was decided to compare the illnesses in newborn infants with those of their next-older silblings.

If one looks at the respiratory symptoms alone, the degree of severity of the illnesses cannot be readily appreciated because one cannot know by the exclusive study of a syndrome such as coryza and cough whether an illness was mild or severe. If the respiratory symptoms are coupled with constitutional symptoms, a better estimate of severity can be made. Constitutional reactions consisted largely of fever (a temperature of 100°F. or over) but were also considered to include various combinations of feverishness, chilliness, listlessness, anorexia, irritability, and aches and pains. During the first year of life 20% of the common respiratory infections in the babies and 21% of similar illnesses in their next-older siblings were associated with constitutional reactions. During the first 2 months of life none of the infants had constitutional reactions with respiratory infections, but thereafter the proportion of such illnesses in the two groups was the same (figure 25).

An effort was made to separate the common cold from the rest of the common respiratory diseases, principally on the basis of a frank rhinitis with or without cough and other respiratory symptoms. It was recognized that there would be some overlapping with influenza-like syndromes and other common respiratory infections of unknown etiology such as nonbacterial tonsillitis and pharyngitis, but in general it was a workable plan. During the first year of life, 83% of the respiratory illnesses in the newborn babies and 76% of those in their next-older siblings were considered to be common colds. Figure 26 shows that when the infants were considered by month of age this diagnosis was made in a greater percentage of illnesses in the newborn infants than in those of their next-older siblings, but the difference was not very great.

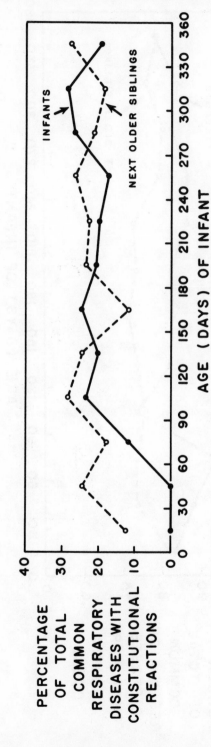

Fig. 25 *Percentage of total common respiratory diseases with constitutional reactions among 73 infants and their next older siblings, by age of infant in 30-day periods*

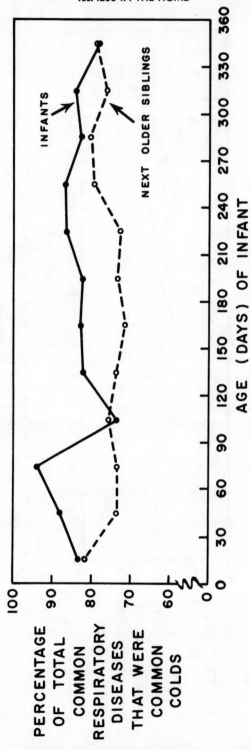

Fig. 26   Percentage of total common respiratory diseases that were
"common colds" among 73 infants and their next older siblings,
by age of infant in 30-day periods

Also, 15% of the common colds in both groups were associated with constitutional reactions. It is interesting to note that approximately 44% of the remainder of the common respiratory diseases in both groups were accompanied by constitutional reactions. A number of these illnesses could have been influenza or adenovirus infections. In broad terms, one can say that babies with common respiratory infections did not appear to be more or less ill in a general way than their next-older siblings, and what differences in symptoms there may have been could be attributed to the ability of older children to be articulate about the way they felt.

The involvement of the respiratory tract in these illnesses appeared to be limited to the nasal mucosa and the pharynx in many instances, and cough, when present, seemed to arise from excess secretions from these areas. A small group of newborn infants and next-older siblings, however, developed a complication, such as conjunctivitis, otitis media, sinusitis, or bronchitis, which in some cases appeared to be a continuum of the original disease. In others, a secondary bacterial infection could not be easily excluded. Needless to say, it was difficult to decide on the basis of clinical examination alone whether or not a true bacterial invasion had occurred, but the index of suspicion was always high when a purulent drainage or a temperature of 101° F. or over was present.

There were 10 infants who had conjunctivitis in association with a common respiratory infection during the first year of life and only one of them had fever. This was a boy who had practically recovered from primary atypical pneumonia when he became ill again with coryza, conjunctivitis, and exacerbation of cough. By the twelfth day, his temperature had risen to 104° F. so he was admitted to the hospital. Physical and roentgenographic examination revealed a recurrence of pneumonia and the presence of otitis media. The total leucocyte count was 8000. *Staphylococcus aureus* was cultured from the throat. Penicillin and sulfadiazine were administered. He recovered uneventfully.

Throat cultures were taken at the time of illness from seven of the other nine babies and only one yielded pathogenic bacteria: a group A, nontypable streptococcus that had been carried previously. No cultures were taken from the conjunctivae of any of these infants. Two other babies were given antibiotic therapy.

Among the next-older siblings, there were six cases of conjunctivitis in association with respiratory illness and two of these were febrile. One of them had coryza and cough followed by a temperature of 100.6° F. on the third day of illness and conjunctivitis on the fifth day; the other developed coryza and cough followed by conjunctivitis on the third day of illness and bronchitis with a temperature of 102° F. on the fourth day. Throat cultures in all instances were free from known pathogenic bacteria. No cultures were taken from the conjunctivae. None of these children received antibiotic therapy.

Eight infants had otitis media and seven of them had an associated constitutional reaction: six had temperatures ranging from 102° to 104° F. and one a record of feverishness, listlessness and irritability. Two of the infants with fever developed suppuration. Seven of the eight babies were given antibiotic therapy. Throat cultures were not rewarding except for *Staphylococcus aureus* in the boy with pneumonia described above. Cultures were not made of the purulent drainage from the ears.

There were 18 cases of otitis media among the next-older siblings. One child had three attacks, two children had two attacks, and the rest of the cases were single episodes. Seven children had fever ranging from 100.6° to 103° F. and two children developed suppuration. Antibacterial therapy was administered in nine cases. Pathogenic bacteria were grown from the throat cultures in seven instances: pneumococci in three; *Staphylococcus aureus* in one; a group A, nontypable streptococcus in one; group A, type 6 streptococcus in one; and groups B and F streptococci in one. Cultures were not made of the discharge from the ears. These data seem to provide justification for the administration of antibiotics to chidren with otitis media and fever. The fever tends to be high, and it seems reasonable to suppose that a bacterial complication has supervened.

Finally, there were four next-older siblings who had the following findings in association with respiratory infections: sinusitis in one, external otitis in one, and cervical adenitis in two. The child with sinusitis (a diagnosis made principally on the basis of a prolonged thick nasal discharge) proved to have a type 19 pneumococcus in the throat culture; the case of external otitis had group A, type 4 streptococcus in the throat culture, an organism which the child had been carrying; and the children with cervical adenitis were also each carrying a group A streptococcus, one being type 12, and the other nontypable.

In summary, the first illness in newborn infants was mainly a rhinitis. Cough occurred in about one-third of the cases and fever was uncommon. During their first year of life, common respiratory infections in newborn infants and their next-older siblings did not differ in the degree of severity as judged by the percentage with constitutional reactions. For the same period of time, common colds were slightly more frequent in the babies than in their next-older siblings. Both groups had a few cases with complications such as otitis media and conjunctivitis.

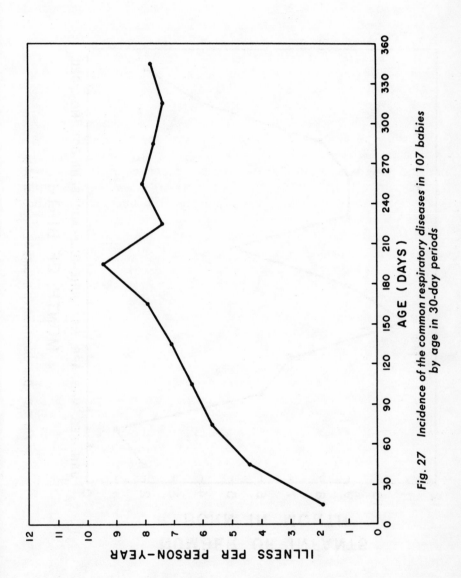

Fig. 27 Incidence of the common respiratory diseases in 107 babies by age in 30-day periods

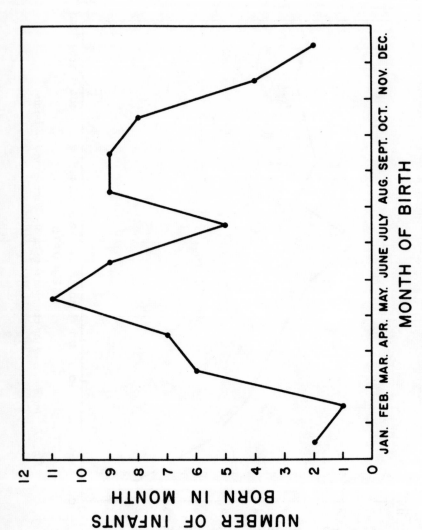

Fig 28   Distribution of 73 infants by month of birth

EPIDEMIOLOGICAL ASPECTS

Number of infants in study.—The analyses presented here are based on two groups: (1) The 107 children who were in the study for at least a part of their first year of life. Of these, 83 were born after their parents were in the study and 24 were infants less than one year of age when their families joined the study. Actually, there were 84 babies born into the study, but one baby, because of severe eczema, spent most of his first year of life away from home and was excluded from all of the analyses. (2) The 73 babies who remained in the study throughout their first full year of life.

Incidence of the common respiratory diseases by month of age.— The incidence of the common respiratory diseases in 107 infants (figure 27 and Appendix 7, table 1) according to periods of 30 days of age rose from a minimum of 1.9 cases per person-year while under 30 days of age to a maximum of 9.4 cases per person-year during the sixth month of age. Thereafter the rates ranged from 7.3 to 8.1

TABLE 26

Incidence of the common respiratory diseases during the first year of life of 73 infants, by periods of 30 days of age:
September-April and May-August

Period number	September - April			May - August		
	Number of illnesses	Number of person-days	Cases per person-year	Number of illnesses	Number of person-days	Cases per person-year
1	9	1170	2.81	3	1020	1.07
2	21	1214	6.31	4	976	1.50
3	29	1296	8.17	5	894	2.04
4	33	1560	7.72	5	630	2.90
5	35	1745	7.32	4	445	3.28
6	47	1922	8.93	5	268	6.81
7	54	1836	10.74	8	354	8.25
8	36	1626	8.08	9	564	5.82
9	36	1459	9.01	10	731	4.99
10	27	1226	8.04	14	964	5.30
11	34	1215	10.21	11	975	4.12
12	35	1204	10.61	11	986	4.07
13*	4	192	7.60	2	185	3.95
Total	400	17,665	8.26	91	8992	3.69

*Days 361-365 of age

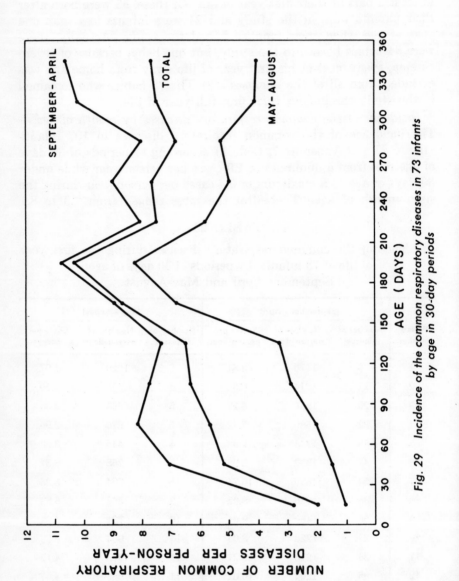

Fig. 29   Incidence of the common respiratory diseases in 73 infants by age in 30-day periods

cases per person-year. For the entire first year of life there were 6.8 common respiratory illnesses per person-year. On the average, then, infants developed new illnesses every 2 months.

Of particular interest is the increasing incidence from birth to 6 months of age. That this was largely due to seasonal effects rather than a function of age, is apparent from the following analyses based upon the 73 children followed throughout their complete first year of life.

Over the years of study it had been established that the occurrence of common respiratory infections in the population was cyclical in nature, with the time of high incidence being September through April, the "high season," and the time of low incidence being May through August, the "low season." The dates of birth (figure 28) of the 73 infants in the study during their first full year of life were not uniformly distributed throughout the year and indeed were so unevenly distributed as to have a marked effect on the month-of-age-specific incidence rates. Table 26 and figure 29 show that infants during the first year of life had more common respiratory infections during each month of age in the "high season" than in the "low season." The graphs of incidence during each "season" both show a peak of occurrence during the seventh month of life. This appeared to be the time of greatest susceptibility. While the rates of infection during the "low season" slumped sharply after the seventh month of life, the incidence of the common respiratory diseases during the "high season" continued at a level of eight or more illnesses per person-year. Furthermore, except for the first 30 days of life, illnesses in each month of age during the "high season" exceeded seven cases per person-year, and only a slight upward trend in rates was noticeable after the second month of life. Thus the impression of gradual build-up of susceptibility during the first six months is dispelled when the season of the year is also taken into account.

Even the low rates during the first few weeks of life do not necessarily imply a relative immunity during that period. In these families it was customary to set aside a nursery for the newborn baby and during the early weeks of life most of the infant's time was spent in this area. During the first month at least, the mother (or practical nurse) was usually the only person in constant attendance. Furthermore, she would keep away children with colds and other infections. In fact, some mothers wore face masks if they, too, became ill. After several weeks the baby would spend more time "in the bosom of the family"—in a crib or playpen "downstairs" and in the arms of other members of the household. It appears,

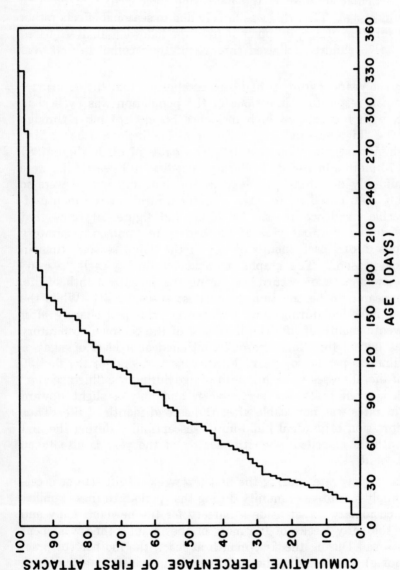

Fig. 30   Cumulative percentage of 73 children who have experienced
an attack of the common respiratory diseases by day of age.

therefore, that the newborn child was isolated from contagious diseases as far as is practical during the first few weeks of life.

Figure 30 shows the cumulative incidence of first attacks of the common respiratory diseases among the 73 infants. Within the first 30 days of life, 18% of newborn babies had their first infection; by 60 days, 41%; by 90 days, 58%; by 120 days, 75%; by 180 days, 93%; and by 329 days, all of them had been ill. The source of infection during the first 3 months of life at least was usually some other member of the household.

Secondary attack rates by month of age.—The secondary attack rate, that is, the percentage of times infants acquired a common respiratory infection following its introduction into the household by some other member of the family, was determined for each 30-day period of age (see Chapter VI, p. 45). During the first month the rate was 9% (table 27). In the second month the rate increased sharply to 31%. During the remainder of the year, on the average, 39% of the times that another member of the family "brought home"

TABLE 27

Secondary attack rates from the common respiratory diseases in 73 infants by periods of 30 days of age: all episodes

30 day period	Number of secondary cases	Number of exposures	Illnesses per exposure
1	4	47	.09
2	14	45	.31
3	13	53	.25
4	17	49	.35
5	17	46	.37
6	24	49	.49
7	25	50	.50
8	27	54	.50
9	16	41	.39
10	22	49	.45
11	12	32	.38
12	14	44	.32
13*	1	6	.17
Total	206	566	.36

*Days 361-365 of age.

a respiratory infection, the baby, too, would develop a cold. The highest secondary attack rates were during the sixth to eighth months. These rates are thought to measure susceptibility better than the total incidence rates. Their level certainly implies no great immunity after the first month of life, and the low rate in that month may reflect the greater precautions described above.

Once an infection has been introduced into the household, the path of spread becomes obscure. A measure of the risk to the infant was obtained, however, according to which member of the family introduced the infection (the index case). Table 28 shows the pro-

TABLE 28

Secondary attack rates from the common respiratory diseases among 73 infants according to age of index case: single index case episodes

Age of index case	Number of exposures	Number of secondary cases	Illnesses per exposure
Less than 7 years	277	120	.43
7 years and over	96	25	.26
Fathers	56	12	.21
Mothers	82	23	.28
Total	511	180	.35

portion of times an infant became infected when a child less than seven, seven or over, a father or a mother introduced the infection into the home. The baby became ill most often when a child less than seven introduced the infection. For the entire first year of life, 43% of the times that a child less than seven was the index case, the baby was infected.

Relationship of last common respiratory infection in mother before delivery to onset of first illness in infant.—An analysis of the common respiratory diseases during the first year of life would not be complete without some reflection upon the inherent resistance of the host. From the above description, it seems quite clear that during the first 30 days of life babies do not acquire respiratory infections with the frequency that they do after this time. The possibility of protection by maternal antibodies stimulated by recent infection in the mother was examined by comparing the number of

days before delivery that the mother had her last common respiratory infection with the number of days after birth that her baby

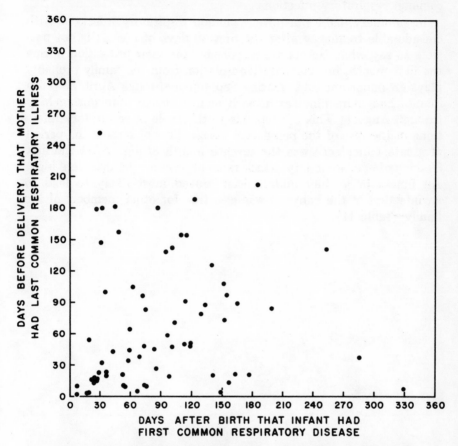

Fig. 31   Correlation between the number of days before delivery that
mother's last common respiratory illness occurred and age of infant at time
of its first common respiratory illness—69 mothers and infants

was first ill with respiratory disease (figure 31). This information
was available for 69 of 73 mothers of the newborn infants in the
study. In each of the remaining four mothers no common respiratory
infection occurred from the time of her entry into the study to the
birth of the child. There appeared to be no correlation between
the two intervals, certainly no negative correlation as might be
expected. There were 11 instances in which mothers were ill within
30 days before delivery and the babies were ill within 30 days after
delivery. It is impossible to say that these were examples of failure
of transmission of protective antibodies. The infections observed in
the parent before delivery and in the infant after delivery may have

been caused by different viruses. The question of passive immunity will have to await precise knowledge of the causes of this group of common respiratory infections.

In summary, babies acquired common respiratory infections with considerable frequency after the first 30 days of life. It is not possible to say what factors are responsible for their protection during the first month, but comparative isolation from the family probably plays an important role. During September through April, newborn infants had more illnesses in each month of age than during May through August. This corresponds to the cycle of respiratory infections in the rest of the population. Regardless of season, the period of greatest incidence was the seventh month of life. After the first 30 days of age, secondary attack rates in newborn infants were high. An illness in a child under seven proved most likely to lead to an infection in the baby, as was also true for other members of the family (table 11).

Chapter VII
STREPTOCOCCAL INFECTIONS

The diagnosis of streptococcal tonsillitis and pharyngitis was made on the basis of a combination of clinical and bacteriological evidence. In general it required both the presence of those clinical findings commonly considered to be characteristic of these infections and the identification of a recently acquired group A streptococcus. Serological tests were not done in most instances and therefore were not considered as part of the evidence required to make the diagnosis. No attempt was made to differentiate between tonsillitis and pharyngitis.

INCIDENCE

INCIDENCE BY AGE

During the entire period of the study 437 illnesses were diagnosed as streptococcal tonsillitis and pharyngitis (table 3); 369 of these occurred among the children. Figure 32 and Appendix 14, table 1 show that the attack rates increased from birth to a peak during the ages 5 to 7 years, then decreased with advancing age. No case of streptococcal respiratory disease was diagnosed during the first year of life. The peak rate of 1.1 cases per 1000 person-days, maintained during the 3-year span including ages 5, 6, and 7 years, indicates that during this period of life 40% of the population were ill each year with these infections. For adults the incidence rate was relatively low— 0.17 cases per 1000 person-days.

Figure 33 shows the cumulative incidence expressed as cumulative average number of cases per person. By about 5.8 years of age children had experienced an average of one case per child, by 8.5 years, two cases, and by the thirteenth birthday, three cases per child. These are, of course, average values. A study of individual experiences was not made except to the limited extent shown in Appendix 5, table 1. As indicated there, the greatest number of streptococcal illnesses experienced by any one individual was eight, although many escaped completely.

SEASONAL OCCURRENCE

Figure 34 shows the seasonal pattern of occurrence of these illnesses. Because of small numbers, data are not presented for each month of the study, but the totals for all Januaries, all Februaries,

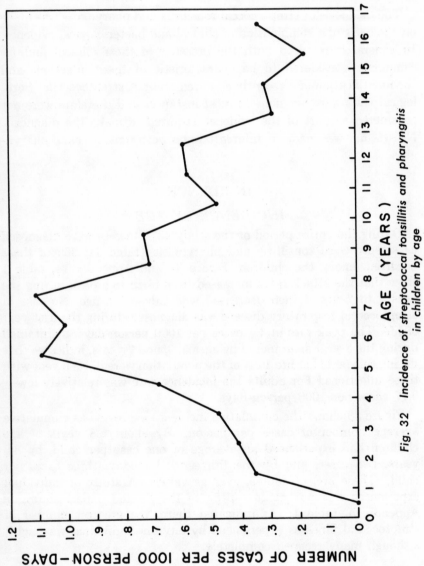

Fig. 32 Incidence of streptococcal tonsillitis and pharyngitis
in children by age

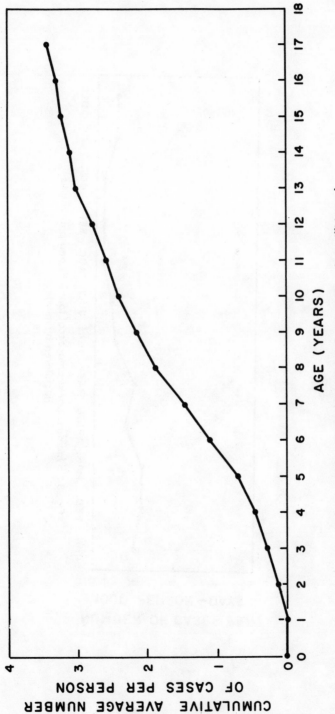

Fig. 33 Cumulative incidence of streptococcal tonsillitis and pharyngitis in children by age

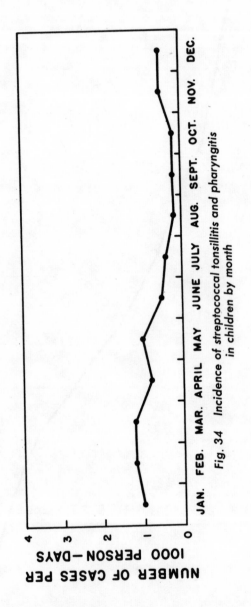

Fig. 34 Incidence of streptococcal tonsillitis and pharyngitis in children by month

etc., are shown. The pattern of high rates in January through May and low rates during the summer was found for each age individually, the magnitude of the swings varying with the total attack rate for the respective age groups. Thus in those months of generally high incidence, children aged five, six, and seven had rates that were higher than those for children of all other ages, while children in all age groups had an equally low level of incidence during the summer.

DETAILED STUDY, 1948-1952

A more detailed epidemiological study was made for the period January 1, 1948, through July 1, 1952 (19). The study was concerned with the frequency of acquisition of group A streptococci, the illnesses that occurred coincidentally with acquisition, and the factors influencing spread within families. Since specific therapy could have had an influence on spread, special attention was given to the recording of details of the treatment, if any, which was given under the direction of the family physician. In some instances antibiotics were administered, generally in amounts now known to be inadequate for eradication of streptococci. When drugs were administered, the therapeutic regimens were so variable, both in type of drug and in dosage, that comparisons were impossible. Moreover, no effect on duration of the carrier state could be found. Accordingly, therapy was ignored for the purpose of the analyses presented here, and the details of therapy have been omitted.

ACQUISITION OF GROUP A STREPTOCOCCI

Acquisition of a group A streptococcus was defined as the detection of a type (or of a nontypable strain) which had not been found in throat cultures from that individual during the preceding 10 weeks. While this definition was somewhat arbitrary, it was based on the distribution of intervals between successive positive cultures. If one of the cultures taken during the 2 weeks immediately preceding an apparent acquisition was overgrown, or if one of the routine weekly cultures in this period had been missed, the acquisition was eliminated from consideration. In cases in which two or more types were acquired simultaneously, each was counted as an acquisition.

Types of streptococci. In 189 of 490 acquisitions of group A streptococci, the streptococci could not be typed, either because they had no type-specific M substance or because they were types other than the 33 for which antisera were available. Types 12, 4, 5, 1 and 6 predominated in that order, and types 2, 11, 13, 19, 28, 31, 33, 41, and 44 were also identified. Acquisitions were most numerous during January through June, and there was considerable variation from month to month (figure 35). There was some correlation between the acquisition rates for typable and nontypable streptococci during the

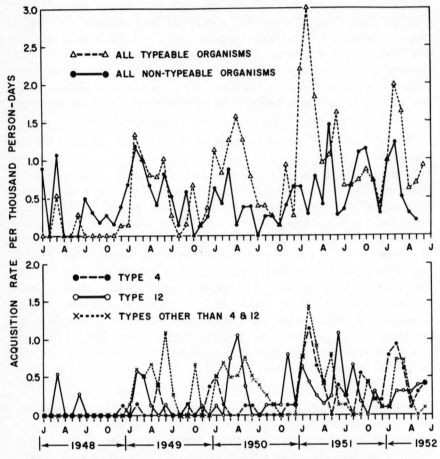

Fig. 35   Acquisition rates for group A streptococci by month and year

year. The occurrence of different types varied considerably from time to time, suggesting that short epidemics occurred briefly in the population and that these were caused by the introduction of a specific type. This is illustrated by the acquisition rates of types 4 and 12, also shown in figure 35.

Relationship of age and sex to acquisition of streptococci.—The rate of acquisition varied according to age and school status (table 29), being highest among young school children and lowest among the preschool children who had no school siblings. Adults had approximately the same risk of acquiring streptococci as the latter group. There were also differences among the groups in the relative frequency of typable as contrasted with nontypable organisms (table 30). Less than half of those acquired by the fathers were typable; among the remaining groups more than half were typable. Similar

TABLE 29

Acquisitions of group A streptococci by age and school status

Age	School status	No. of acquisitions	No. of person-days eligible to acquire*	No. of acquisitions per 1000 person-days
<6 years	Preschool**	14	34,080	0.4
<6 years	Preschool‡	113	69,115	1.6
<6 years	School	94	30,851	3.0
6 years or older	School	173	80,896	2.1
Mothers		54	83,326	0.6
Fathers		42	82,534	0.5
Total		490	380,802	1.3

*Person not considered eligible to acquire streptococcus until 70 days of observation had occurred.
**Not siblings of school children.
‡Siblings of school children.

tabulations showing the relative occurrence of the various types of typable streptococci (types 4 and 12 and all others) were examined; no special selection of a type for a segment of the population was noted. There was no difference in the acquisition rates of males or females, either in children or adults.

ILLNESSES AT TIME OF ACQUISITION OF STREPTOCOCCI

The study of the relation of illness to acquisition of streptococci was limited to the 379 acquisitions occurring more than 30 days from another acquisition. Illnesses that occurred within the 13-day period starting with the sixth day before and ending with the sixth day after the day the acquisition was detected (except illnesses that obviously could not be related to the organism, such as bursitis, bee sting, herpes and lacerations) were studied in relation to these acquisitions.

The illnesses which occurred concurrently with the acquisitions of streptococci were classified according to a rigid set of criteria. Furthermore, to evaluate these criteria it was felt desirable to examine the occurrence of illness in a group of individuals who did not acquire streptococci. This group, designated as the control group, was selected by a matching process. For each acquisition a

TABLE 30

Acquisitions of typable and nontypable group A streptococci
by age and school status

Age	School status	Typable acquisitions		Nontypable acquisitions		Total
		No.	%	No.	%	
< 6 years	Preschool*	10	71	4	29	14
< 6 years	Preschool**	67	59	46	41	113
< 6 years	School	57	61	37	39	94
6 years or older	School	108	62	65	38	173
Mothers		40	74	14	26	54
Fathers		19	45	23	55	42
Total		301	61	189	39	490

*Not siblings of school children.
**Siblings of school children.

list was prepared of all individuals of corresponding age on the date
of acquisition. With the use of a table of random numbers, one of
these was selected. If such a subject had acquired a group A streptococcus within the 6 days before or in the 30 days after this date,
he was eliminated and another individual was selected by the same
process.

Thus, each person who had acquired a group A streptococcus was
matched with a corresponding person of the same age (in years)
who had not acquired a group A streptococcus, and the illnesses
among those who had acquired streptococci were compared with the
illnesses occuring in the control group on the corresponding dates.
Illnesses in both groups were classified as follows:

Streptococcal tonsillitis and pharyngitis. An illness that included
one or more of the following symptoms and signs: sore or injected
throat, exudate, enlarged and tender anterior cervical lymph nodes, or
nodes showing a definite enlargement since a recent observation.

Other illness. Illnesses in which none of the above symptoms and
signs were present.

No illness. Cases in which no symptoms or signs were recognized
by the mother, nurse or physician.

TABLE 31

Illness rates in individuals who acquired group A streptococci and in a control group

Classification	Streptococcal illness		Other illness		Acquisitions without illness	
	No. of cases	No./100 acquisitions*	No. of cases	No./100 acquisitions*	No. of cases	No./100 acquisitions*
Persons acquiring streptococci	164	43	109	29	148	39
Control group	21	6	102	27	266	70

*Percentages here and in succeeding tables do not necessarily add up to 100, for some patients had more than one illness during the 13-day period.

The data of table 31 show that the rate of streptococcal illness in the acquisition group was 43 per 100 acquisitions.* The incidence of other illness in the acquisition group was 29%. No illnesses were associated with 39% of the acquisitions. The occurrence of illness was much greater in the group acquiring streptococci than in the control group. There were only 21 cases in the control group which met the clinical criteria for streptococcal pharyngitis. This gives some measure of the validity of the definition used, since these 21 cases probably were not of streptococcal origin. The agreement between the number of other illnesses (109) in the acquisition group and the total illnesses (123) in the control group implies that the diagnostic criteria were reliable, and that the excess of illness in the acquisition group was true streptococcal illness.

In 114 of the 164 streptococcal illnesses in the acquisition group, cultures of the throat on blood agar plates at the time of illness showed group A streptococci in a quantity of not less than 10 colonies. Streptococci were estimated to contribute from more than 10 colonies to 25% of the growth on the plates in 49 of the 114 illnesses and more than 25% of the growth in 65 of them. In 50 cases, cultures at the time of illness were lacking or showed either no streptococci or fewer than 10 colonies.

To determine whether or not the ability to cause illness was related to the type of streptococcus acquired, all illnesses occurring among adults and children were compared according to type of organism. Among children there was little difference between the relative frequency and types of illness that followed acquisitions of types 4 and 12 (table 32). However, a greater incidence of streptococcal illness occurred after types 4 and 12 than after other typable organisms. Sixty-six percent of type 12 and 58% of type 4 acquisitions were followed by streptococcal illnesses. In contrast, only 35% of the acquisitions of all other typable organisms were followed by streptococcal illnesses; this was comparable to the 36% of the acquisitions of nontypable organisms followed by such illnesses. The data regarding types 4 and 12 in adults were too few to be presented separately and they are combined in table 33. Again, a greater proportion of acquisitions of types 4 and 12 was followed by streptococcal illness than was true for the acquisition of nontypable strains. The miscellaneous other types, however, acted more like types 4 and 12 than like the nontypable streptococci.

---

*This figure does not express exactly the proportion of acquisitions followed by a streptococcal illness since in eight cases acquisition was related to two illnesses judged clinically to be separate streptococcal infections occurring within the 13-day period. The true proportion of streptococcal illnesses per 100 acquistions is thus 156:379, or 41%. Since this difference is so small, the ratio of illnesses per 100 acquisitions has for convenience been considered equivalent to the illness rate.

TABLE 32

Illness rates among children according to type of group A streptococcus acquired

Type of streptococcus	No. of acquisitions	Streptococcal illness		Other illness		Acquisitions without illness	
		No. of cases	No./100 acquisitions	No. of cases	No./100 acquisitions	No. of persons	No./100 acquisitions
4	52	30	58	24	46	12	23
12	61	40	66	19	31	15	25
Other	65	23	35	13	20	30	46
Nontypable	119	43	36	43	36	45	38
Totals	297	136	46	99	33	102	34

TABLE 33

Illness rates among adults according to type of group A
streptococcus acquired

Type of streptococcus	No. of acquisitions	Streptococcal illness		Other illness		Acquisitions without illness	
		No. of cases	No./100 acquisitions	No. of cases	No./100 acquisitions	No. of persons	No./100 acquisitions
4 and 12	23	9	39	2	9	12	52
Other	24	11	46	5	21	10	42
Nontypable	35	8	23	3	9	24	69
Totals	82	28	34	10	12	46	56

These data indicate, therefore, that if acquisition of a pathogenic organism occurs in either adult or child, it produces clinical illness, on the average, approximately 40% of the time. Types 4 and 12 were most likely to produce such illness among children. Moreover, recognized illness developed approximately one and a third times as frequently in children as in their parents.

INTRODUCTION AND SPREAD OF STREPTOCOCCI IN THE FAMILY

To study the introduction and spread of streptococci in families, it was necessary to define, somewhat arbitrarily, the criteria to be used as indicating a new acquisition for the family. An introduction into the family was defined as occurring when some member of the family acquired a group A streptococcus after the whole family had been free of that organism for 10 consecutive weeks. The person involved was designated as the index carrier whether or not there was an associated illness. Analyses were restricted to acquisitions involving typable streptococci. In five instances, the index person had simultaneously acquired two strains of streptococci. These simultaneous acquisitions were tabulated separately. Family contacts of index carriers were defined as the other members of the families of the index carriers from whom throat cultures had been regularly obtained both before and after the acquisition of the streptococcus by the index carrier. Family contacts who acquired the type of streptococcus introduced into the family by the index person were considered to be secondary carriers. If the same organism was subsequently reintroduced into the family, the introduction was eliminated from the present analyses. Nontypable organisms were excluded from consideration since secondary carriers could conceivably have acquired different types that could not be identified. There were 125 index carriers who acquired a typable organism. In five additional instances, typable organisms were introduced simultaneously by two or more members of the family unit.

The relative risk of becoming index carriers for each class of individual — which may be interpreted as the relative risk of acquiring infections outside the home — was computed according to the method described for common respiratory diseases (Appendix 10). The frequency with which fathers were index carriers was assigned a value of one, and then the risk for each class of subject was computed taking into account the composition of the various families. Table 34 shows that mothers introduced 1.1 as many infections, preschool children introduced an average of 3.8 as many infections, and school children 6 years of age or

TABLE 34

Ratios showing the relative frequency with which five classes of individuals introduced typable group A streptococci into the home

Class of individual	Relative no. of index carriers
Father	1.0
Mother	1.1
Preschool child	3.8
School child, 6+ years of age	4.8
School child, < 6 years of age	6.0

older, 4.8 as many infections as the fathers. School children less than 6 years old had the greatest relative number of introductions per person (6.0).

A secondary carrier was defined as a member of the family who acquired the same type within 10 weeks of introduction. Since the numbers were relatively small, the illnesses occurring among secondary carriers were not analyzed. If the index case had a streptococcal illness (Appendix 14, table 2) approximately 25% of the other members of the family acquired the same organism. Children acquired the organism more readily than did their parents. Among children 3 and 4 years old, 50% acquired the organism. Fathers became carriers least frequently. If the index carrier escaped having streptococcal illness, the secondary carrier rates were much lower (Appendix 14, table 3). The over-all rate was only 9%. Again, children 3 and 4 years of age were infected most frequently. There were no appreciable differences among rates for the other age groups in the family units. So far as may be learned from relatively small numbers, the class of the index case did not make any difference in the resultant rate of parasitization (Appendix 14, table 4).

Exact data on the intervals between acquisition by an idex carrier and later acquisitions within the family cannot be determined. Cultures were obtained at weekly intervals unless illness occurred, when a culture was obtained as soon as possible. The average number of days elapsing between the index acquisition and the first secondary positive culture was 15. Figure 36 shows the spread within families. This figure concerns episodes occurring among families who acquired type 4 streptococci. Apparently spread of the organism in family units may be slow. In family 40, for example, once introduction of the organism occurred, the strain persisted for 126 weeks; individual 3 of the family did not become parasitized until 100 weeks after the organism was introduced into the family.

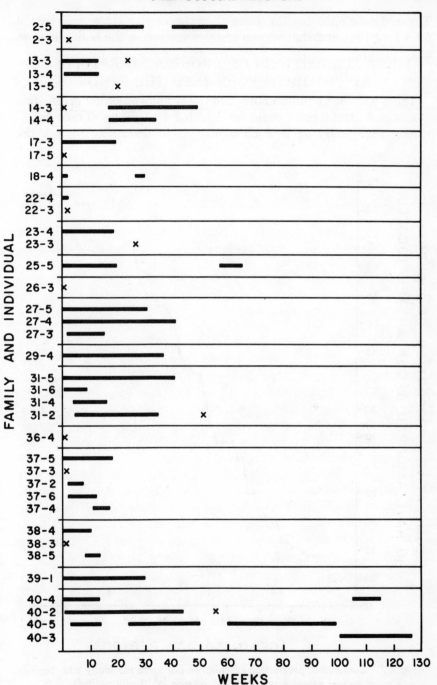

X = ACQUIRED THE ORGANISM AND THEN NO LONGER OBSERVED

Fig. 36   Family episodes of infection with type 4, group A streptococci

These data emphasize the facts that the carrier state may persist for a long time and that spread of the organism in the family is slow.

FIRST ACQUISITIONS OF GROUP A STREPTOCOCCI BY CHILDREN BORN INTO THE STUDY

There were 82* children born into the study whose first acquisition of group A streptococci could be detected by culture. These acquisitions were analyzed in such a way as to determine by age the

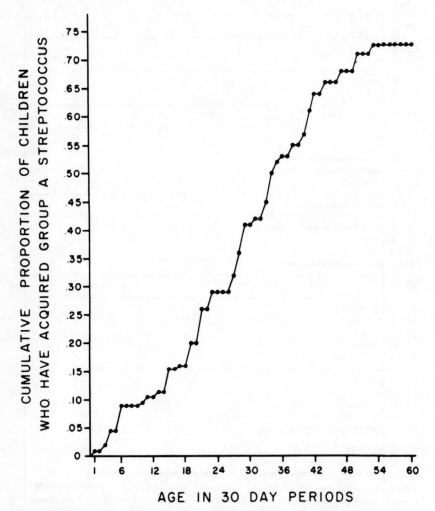

Fig. 37   *Cumulative proportion of children born into the study who have acquired group A streptococci, by age in 30-day periods*

*Two additional children were excluded from this analysis because one died in the post-natal period and one was away from home during the first year of life.

cumulative proportion of children who had had an experience with these organisms. The results are presented in figure 37. At the end of the first year, approximately 12% had acquired a group A streptococcus; at the end of the fourth year, 68%; and at the end of 5 years, 75%. The principal source of the organisms was an older sibling.

Respiratory illness was present in 48 of the children at the time acquisition was detected. Because symptoms could not be easily evaluated in these young children, fever was considered to be the most reliable evidence of a generalized reaction: 20 children were afebrile and 28 had fever ranging from 100.4° F. to 104° F. Of the febrile group, 14 had enlarged and inflamed tonsils but only 5 had exudate on the tonsils and pharyngeal walls. In five children, relapse occurred from 2 to 7 days after apparent recovery. All of these five children had been febrile in the first episode and they had fever again during relapse (from 101° F. to 104.8° F.). Group A streptococci similar to those originally acquired were recovered from all of them at the time of recurrence—three had type 4 and two had nontypable strains. Because of the small number of illnesses, clinical characterization was considered not to be of appreciable value. Acquisition of group A streptococci occurred in nine children less than 1 year of age. No illnesses occurred in these children although in each of the three families streptococcal illnesses due to the same type occurred at the same time in two older siblings. Thus there is a suggestion that the acquisition of group A streptococci during the first year of life may be an innocuous event.

POST-STREPTOCOCCAL ILLNESS

A diagnosis of post-streptococcal illness was made 67 times during the study (Appendix 5, table 1). This category, admittedly ill-defined, was used to include several types of illness:

1. One case of questionable rheumatic fever which was not preceded by a recognized streptococcal infection.

This 6-year-old girl had an illness during the first week of June, 1949, characterized by feverishness, sneezing, hoarseness, cough, wheezing and low grade fever (99.5°-100°F.). The illness was considered to be a mild attack of asthma, to which she was subject, and lasted for 6 days. There was no clinical evidence of tonsillitis and pharyngitis, and group A streptococci were not found in any of the repeated throat cultures. Twenty-one days later she complained of fatigue and pain in the left groin and hip. These symptoms persisted and intensified so that 3 days later she awakened at 5 A.M., complaining that because of the pain she could not turn over in bed or walk. There was soreness and questionable swelling of the left buttock without redness or heat. She had no fever, rash or involvement of other joints. She was admitted to the hospital later that day. The pertinent findings were pain and limitation of motion of the hip in all directions and an area of tenderness to deep palpation over the middle of Poupart's ligament. There were no other abnormal findings. The urine, hemoglobin, and erythrocyte count were normal, the total leucocyte count 10,500 with 77% neutrophiles, 19% lymphocytes, 3% monocytes, and 1% eosinophiles. The sedimentation rate was slightly elevated (20 mm./hr.). Radiographic examination of the hip showed no abnormalities. The pain and limitation of motion subsided with bed rest and she was asymptomatic at discharge home on the fourth hospital day. Physical examination the following day showed no abnormalities. She developed a daily low grade fever (99°-100°F.), however, which persisted for 3 weeks, during which time she was confined to bed by her pediatrician. Recovery was complete and there was no evidence of cardiac involvement.

This illness does not meet the criteria for the certain diagnosis of rheumatic fever, although the possibility was entertained. The diagnosis in the hospital was acute non-suppurative arthritis of unknown cause.

2. **Two cases of acute glomerulonephritis which followed the onset of acute streptococcal tonsillitis and pharyngitis by 13 and 20 days, respectively.**

a. This patient was a 4-year-old girl (Case no. 7 in table IV, ref. 107) who became ill on November 1, 1950, with sore throat, anorexia, vomiting, cough, and temperature of 102°F. On physical examination she did not appear to be acutely ill. The pharynx and tonsils were red and injected and spotty exudate was present on the left tonsil. There was slightly tender, bilateral, anterior cervical adenopathy. No other abnormalities were noted. The following day she was afebrile and she appeared to be fully recovered 2 days later. No specific therapy was given.

Cultures of the throat on November 2 revealed group A streptococci, type 12. She had had no known previous streptococcal infections nor had she harbored a group A streptococcus while in the study. The first detection of group A, type 12, streptococci in this family was in a throat culture obtained on October 25, 1950, from an older sibling. These organisms were also found in cultures from a younger sibling on October 30, from the mother on November 20, and from the father on November 23. The two siblings continued to carry the organisms until mid-February, 1951, the mother until May, 1951, and the father until December, 1951. The patient's cultures were positive until November 20, when she was treated with penicillin. She did not re-acquire the organism thereafter.

The patient remained well until November 12, when she developed an acute illness of 5 days' duration, characterized by headache, listlessness, anorexia, cough, vomiting and fever up to 103°F. On physical examination she appeared to be moderately ill, the pharynx and tonsils were slightly injected without exudate, the anterior cervical nodes were enlarged and tender, and a few scattered sonorous rhonchi were heard in the chest. She recovered without treatment and was symptom-free for 2 days.

On November 19, she voluntarily remained in bed, although she had no specific complaints, and her mother noted that her face was "puffy." She had no fever and the only abnormal findings were periorbital and facial edema, a blood pressure of 132/56, slight albuminuria, and hematuria (80 RBC/HPF). She was kept in bed for 3 weeks. The hematuria gradually subsided during the next 2 months and she was well without residual findings by mid-February, 1951.

Each of the other four members of the family had respiratory illnesses in association with the acquisition of the type 12 streptococcus. The illness in the youngest sibling was clinically a common cold. The illnesses of the oldest sibling, the mother and the father were mild but clinically characteristic of streptococcal tonsillitis and pharyngitis. Each of them subsequently developed microscopic hematuria but no other manifestations of acute glomerulonephritis.

b. This patient, a 3½-year-old boy, developed an acute febrile illness on March 12, 1953, while away from home on a trip with his family. He was seen by a local physician who diagnosed the illness as tonsillitis and administered an injection of 400,000 units of penicillin and 0.5 gm. of streptomycin which was followed by clinical improvement. On his return to Cleveland 4 days later he appeared to be well and examination revealed only minimal spotty exudate on the tonsils, lymphoid hyperplasia of the pharyngeal wall and enlarged submental glands. Cultures of the throat revealed no group A streptococci. Eight days later, however, he developed facial edema and microscopic hematuria. His blood pressure was normal. Cultures of the throat at this time revealed group A, type 12, streptococci. The edema persisted for 6 days and the hematuria for 5 weeks. There were no other indications of nephritis and his activity was not restricted. He continued to carry type 12 streptococci until June, 1953. His previous experience with streptococci was as follows: in January, 1950, he acquired a group A, type 4, organism which he carried intermittently until November, 1951; in October, 1950, he acquired another group A streptococcus, which could not be typed with the sera available, and carried this organism intermittently until May, 1952; on May 7, 1952, he had a febrile illness diagnosed as a streptococcal tonsillitis and pharyngitis lasting 4 days. Cultures revealed a group A streptococcus which was not typable.

Two illnesses considered as streptococcal infections occurred in the five other members of the family. On March 24, 1953, the mother had an illness characterized by headache, feverishness, chilliness, anorexia, generalized aching, sneezing and cough, sore throat, and fever (102° F.). The pharynx and tonsils were injected and exudate was found on the tonsils. Anterior cervical lymphadenopathy was present. Throat cultures revealed group A, type 12, streptococci. The illness lasted 7 days. Three doses of penicillin (300,000 units) were given on March 25, 26, and 27. Microscopic hematuria followed the illness. Cultures thereafter showed no streptococci. The father had a febrile illness with sore throat on April 5 and 6, 1953, for which he was given penicillin on both days. Cultures revealed no streptococci. Urinalysis showed microscopic hematuria.

No streptococcal illnesses developed in the remaining three children although the two older children harbored group A streptococci: type 6 in one child and type 12 in the other. Both developed microscopic hematuria. The youngest child did not harbor group A streptococci during this time.

3. Three cases in which aching or sore knees, tendons, or muscles followed the onsets of streptococcal infection by 9 days, 17 days, and 39 days, respectively.

a. This patient was a 6½-year-old girl who developed a characteristic febrile streptococcal pharyngitis and tonsillitis on February 28, 1948, which lasted 12 days. Cultures at the onset of illness showed that she had acquired a group A streptococcus which could not be typed with the sera available. Sore throat and fever resumed on March 24 and lasted 8 days. On March 6, she developed fever (102°F.), pinpoint exudate on the tonsils and aches in the joints, particularly of the feet. These symptoms lasted only 24 hours. She continued to harbor nontypable group A streptococci intermittently until January, 1949. Antistreptolysin determinations showed a rise in titer from 50 units before to 159 units after the illness. Neither streptococci nor streptococcal illness occurred in other members of the family.

b. This 4-year-old girl developed an illness on May 16, 1950, coincidental with the acquisition for the first time of a group A streptococcus, type 1. The illness, which lasted 5 days, was characterized by feverishness, fever, irritability, listnessness, anorexia, sore throat, enlarged and injected tonsils, acutely red pharynx and bilateral tender anterior cervical adenopathy. On the thirteenth day she had recurrence of fever, muscular aches and pains and persistent adenopathy. These lasted for 7 days, followed by complete recovery. Tonsillectomy and adenoidectomy were performed on June 8. She continued to harbor the type 1, group A streptococcus until July, 1950.

Her younger sibling acquired a group A, type 5 streptococcus on April 11, 1950, which she carried for a year without apparent streptococcal illness. Neither parent harbored streptococci.

c. This patient was a 7-year-old girl whose first recognized streptococcal infection occurred on March 27, 1949, and was due to a group A, type 6, streptococcus. She continued to harbor this organism, as did most of her younger siblings, until January 7, 1950, when she had the sudden onset of an illness characterized by headache, feverishness, chilliness, listlessness, anorexia, obstructed nose, sore throat, vomiting, and temperature of 103°F. On examination she showed large and injected tonsils with spotty exudate, injected pharynx with lymphoid hyperplasia and tender cervical adenopathy. Cultures of her throat showed a group A streptococcus which could not be typed with the sera available. She made an apparently complete recovery and was well until January 23, when she complained of aches and pains in her legs without other manifestations of illness. On June 1, 1950, she acquired a group A, type 1, streptococcus without illness. Her antistreptolysin titer rose from 50 to 250 units following her illness in 1949 and increased to 317 units following the illness in 1950. No other members of the family had clinical streptococcal illness.

4. One case of thrombophlebitis which occurred 10 days after the onset of acute streptococcal tonsillitis and pharyngitis.

This 8½-year-old girl became ill on November 29, 1948, with headache, feverishness, nasal discharge, anorexia, sore throat, cough, and a temperature of 100.6°F. which rose the following day to 104°F. Physical examination showed a moderately ill patient who was flushed, had slight injection of nasal mucous membranes, tonsils and pharynx, spotty exudate on the tonsils and anterior cervical adenopathy which was initially not tender and later became tender. Examination of the blood and urine was normal. Cultures of the throat revealed a group A hemolytic streptococcus which could not be typed. The illness lasted 7 days. Three days later there was a recurrence of headache, feverishness, sore throat, tender cervical adenopathy, and temperature of 100°F. She complained of generalized aching and pain in the upper right arm and shoulder. Physical examination again revealed spotty exudate over the tonsils and tenderness to palpation over the area of venous drainage from two inches below the elbow to the axilla. There was no redness or swelling. She was admitted to the hospital for a period of 4 days. She was afebrile and the symptoms gradually subsided. No definite evidence of thrombosis could be determined. Examination of the blood and urine was normal. Sedimentation rate was normal. Cultures of the throat showed a group A streptococcus which could not be typed. She complained of the same symptoms for one day after discharge and then was well. In February of 1949 a group A, type 1, streptococcus was recovered from her throat.

The mother had an illness diagnosed as streptococcal tonsillitis and pharyngitis on December 12, 1948, associated with a group A streptococcus which was not typable. She received treatment with penicillin and was well 4 days after the onset. Three other members of the family harbored a group A nontypable streptococcus until February and March of 1949 when they acquired a group A, type 1, streptococcus without evidence of clinical streptococcal illness.

5. Sixty cases characterized by the subsequent occurrence of a combination of one or more of the following symptoms: fever, sore throat, cervical adenitis, otitis media, and miscellaneous respiratory symptoms. These occurred up to approximately a month after the onset of the initial streptococcal illnesses.

The exact frequency with which acute symptoms suggestive of streptococcal tonsillitis and pharyngitis reappeared should not be inferred from these 60 cases. For example, there were five additional instances which were classified as acute streptococcal infections, but which in reality followed by less than a month an illness of the same diagnosis. In these cases there was no laboratory evidence of a newly acquired streptococcus and they, therefore, were indistinguishable from the 60 cases in class 5 above. Furthermore, as shown in Appendix 14, table 5, the relative frequency with which this diagnosis was made varied by calendar year. On the other hand, recurrence of the acute symptoms of fever, sore throat, cervical adenitis, etc., is not unusual in the month following an initial streptococcal illness.

Despite the low occurrence of serious post-streptococcal complications, the observations of these families aided in establishing the etiological role of nephritogenic group A streptococci, especially types 12 and 4, in acute glomerulonephritis and in establishing the degree of hematuria that should be considered as significant (107, 124). In addition, observations on the entire family made possible a diagnosis of hereditary familial nephritis which could not otherwise have been made on the basis of the clinical findings (137).

SPECIAL STUDY OF POST-STREPTOCOCCAL COMPLICATIONS

A small group of persons who acquired group A streptococci were followed intensively, along with a control group. In addition to the routine examinations, special procedures were carried out. Details of this study are included in Appendix 15. No definite evidence of post-streptococcal activity indicative of rheumatic fever was observed in this small series of cases.

Chapter VIII

RELATION OF TONSILLECTOMY TO INCIDENCE OF CERTAIN ILLNESSES IN CHILDREN

The question of whether or not an excessively large number of common respiratory infections in a child constitutes an indication for tonsillectomy continues to receive a variety of answers. Similarly, evidence on the relationship between the occurrence of streptococcal respiratory disease and the presence or absence of tonsils is conflicting (42). The data of the present study were examined to see whether or not the presence of tonsils was related to illness. Some of these data have been presented elsewhere (8). The illnesses which were studied in this respect were: 1) the common respiratory diseases; 2) streptococcal tonsillitis and pharyngitis*; 3) nonbacterial tonsillitis and pharyngitis; 4) fevers of unknown origin; and 5) infectious gastroenteritis.

The term tonsillectomy is used loosely, because in most instances it was not known whether both tonsils and adenoids, or only one of these had been removed surgically. The fact that an operation

---

*No attempt was made here to differentiate between tonsillitis and pharyngitis.

TABLE 35

Age-specific incidence rates of several diagnostic groups of illnesses in children according to status with respect to tonsillectomy

Diagnostic group	Tonsillec-tomy	Age group (years)			
		3-5	6-7	8-9	10+
Common respiratory diseases	Yes	23.2	19.4	17.3	13.9
	No	20.6	15.7	14.3	14.2
Nonbacterial tonsillitis and pharyngitis	Yes	0.44	0.47	0.09	0.15
	No	0.55	0.33	0.42	0.25
Streptococcal tonsillitis and pharyngitis	Yes	0.39	0.37	0.40	0.28
	No	0.81	1.36	0.98	0.73
Fevers of unknown origin	Yes	0.44	0.23	0.23	0.16
	No	0.49	0.53	0.29	0.21
Infectious gastroenteritis	Yes	5.74	6.22	5.35	3.46
	No	5.35	5.52	5.06	4.10

*Illnesses per 1000 person-days.

118

had been performed for this general purpose, however, was accurately recorded.

Table 35 and Appendix 16, table 1 show the age-specific incidence rates for the several groups of illnesses separately for children who had had tonsillectomies and for those who had not had the operation. These data are restricted to children 3 years of age or older, because only one child under 3 years of age had had a tonsillectomy. The age-specific incidence rates for the common respiratory diseases were approximately the same for both groups of children, although there were slightly higher rates among those who had had the operation than among those who had not. The same was true of infectious gastroenteritis. There was no consistency in the relationship between tonsillectomy and the rates for nonbacterial tonsillitis and pharyngitis: in three of the four age groups those who had not had the operation had the higher rates; for the 8-9 year old group this difference was quite marked. Illnesses where only constitutional symptoms were noted showed, in each of the four age groups, an excess among those who had not had the operation, although the excess

TABLE 36

Age-adjusted incidence rates of common respiratory illnesses in which specific symptoms were present, children 3 years of age and older, according to status with respect to tonsillectomy, 1948-1954

Symptom	Present	Absent	Illnesses per 1,000 person-days	
			Children who had had tonsillectomy	Children who had not had tonsillectomy
Coryza	x		16.2	14.6
		x	2.1	2.1
Sore throat	x		5.6	4.7
		x	12.7	12.0
Hoarseness	x		3.6	3.0
		x	14.7	13.7
Cough	x		9.9	8.2
		x	8.4	8.5
Fever*	x		3.7	3.1
		x	15.8	14.5

*The data used in computing the age-adjusted rates regarding fever include the cases which had inadequate information with respect to localizing symptoms and were therefore omitted in computing the other age-adjusted rates of this section. The total age-adjusted rates, including all cases, were 19.5 cases per 1,000 person-days for children who had had tonsillectomy and 17.6 for those who had not.

was not very great. The greater incidence of streptococcal tonsillitis and pharyngitis among those not having had a tonsillectomy was marked and consistent.

The apparent decrease in nonbacterial tonsillitis and pharyngitis in the group who had had tonsillectomy was not great; it was not thought worthwhile to investigate this further on a purely statistical basis. Similarly the difference noted for fevers of unknown origin was relatively small and not significant. The two other groups of illnesses, the common respiratory diseases and streptococcal tonsillitis and pharyngitis, were subjected to further analyses.

THE COMMON RESPIRATORY DISEASES
SYMPTOMS

The relation between status with respect to tonsillectomy and symptoms of the common respiratory diseases was studied using the classification presented on pp. 66-67. Age-adjusted incidence rates were computed for several symptom groups, separately for those who had had tonsillectomy and for those who had not. As pointed out on page 67, some of the cases (5.4%) could not be classified because of inadequate information; this led to some inaccuracy in the age-adjusted rates, but probably had little influence on the com-

TABLE 37

Age-adjusted incidence rates for the common respiratory illnesses among children 3 years of age and older, for each combination of localizing symptoms, according to status with respect to tonsillectomy, 1948-1954

Symptom groups*				Illnesses per 1,000 person-days	
Coryza	Sore throat	Hoarseness	Cough	Children who had had tonsillectomy	Children who had not had tonsillectomy
x or o	x	x	x	1.1	0.9
x or o	x	x	o	0.4	0.3
x or o	x	o	x	2.0	1.4
x or o	x	o	o	2.0	2.1
x or o	o	x	x	1.4	1.3
x or o	o	x	o	0.6	0.5
x or o	o	o	x	5.4	4.7
x	o	o	o	5.3	5.5

*o = Absent; x = Present

parisons which are of interest in the present section. The age-adjusted rates were for children 3 years of age or over.

The total age-adjusted rate for children who had had tonsillectomy was 18.3 cases per 1,000 person-days; the corresponding rate for those whose tonsils were intact was 16.7 cases per 1,000 person-days. Table 36 shows similar rates for the various localizing symptoms associated with these illnesses, and for fever. There was no symptom which showed an excessive occurrence in the group who had not had tonsillectomy. Table 37 shows the rates for some of the combinations of symptoms. In general, no major differences in the age-adjusted rate of occurrence of symptoms in the two groups of children were found, and the differences which did occur reflected only the higher total incidence rates among children who had undergone tonsillectomy. The clinical symptoms of the common respiratory diseases were essentially the same in children who had undergone tonsillectomy and those who had not.

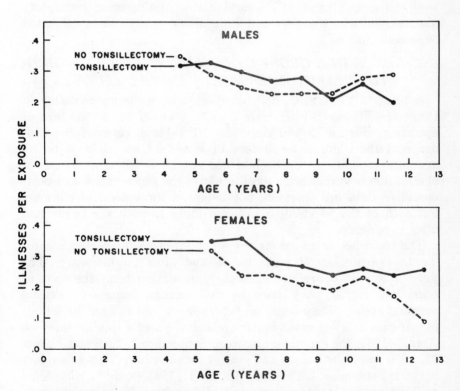

Fig. 38   Secondary attack rates for the common respiratory diseases in children by age and sex, according to status with respect to tonsillectomy

SECONDARY ATTACK RATES

The total average incidence rates given above reflect the total occurrence of illness, while secondary attack rates may be indicative of relative susceptibility. The secondary attack rates supposedly are based on reaction to known exposure to an index case, while total incidence rates are determined by the frequency of exposure to any source of infection.

Age-specific and sex-specific secondary attack rates in family episodes (as defined on page 41) of the common respiratory diseases are presented in figure 38 and Appendix 16, tables 2 and 3, separately for those who had had previous tonsillectomy and those who had not. With minor exceptions, the secondary attack rates were consistently higher for those who had had the operation. This implies that children who had had the operation were more susceptible to the common respiratory diseases than were those who had not had the operation. This finding is consistent with age-specific incidence rates given in table 35. In view of the analysis presented in the following section, this difference seems to mean that children who had a high inherent susceptibility to the common respiratory diseases and who therefore had more illnesses, were those subjected to tonsillectomy.

INCIDENCE IN A GROUP OF CHILDREN WHO HAD THEIR TONSILLECTOMIES WHILE IN THE STUDY

A total of 59 children had tonsillectomies while participating in the study. These children were 2 to 11 years of age at the time of operation. Figure 39 and Appendix 16, table 4, consider the incidence of the common respiratory diseases in these children before and after operation. Each child did not have the same length of observation before as after tonsillectomy; the preoperative and postoperative data are therefore not balanced for individual children, but each of the 59 children did contribute to both the before and after experience.

The incidence rates among the 59 children are presented according to the number of years before and after tonsillectomy. The years referred to are not elapsed years dating from the time of operation; rather, they refer to the common respiratory disease seasonal cycles. They begin on September 1 and end on the following August 31. For example, for a child who had a tonsillectomy on April 1, 1950, the experience between September 1, 1949 and August 31, 1950 would be classed as "year of tonsillectomy"; his experience between September 1, 1948 and August 31, 1949 would be considered as "first year before tonsillectomy", and so forth. The year of tonsillectomy is further divided into the time before and the time after

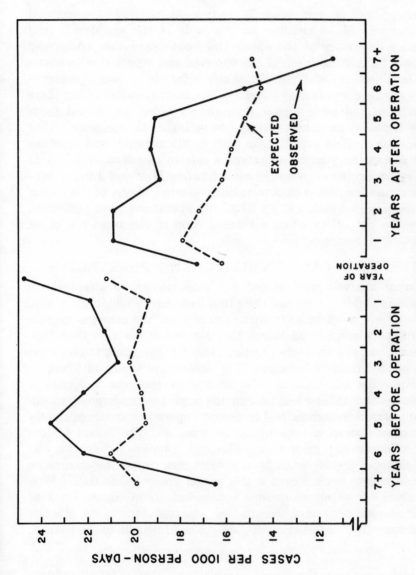

Fig. 39   Observed and expected incidence of the common respiratory diseases before and after tonsillectomy in 59 children

the operation so that, for the hypothetical person whose tonsillectomy was performed on April 1, 1950, the period from September 1, 1949 through March 31, 1950 is included as "year of tonsillectomy before operation" and the period from April 1, 1950 through August 31, 1950 as "year of tonsillectomy after operation."

The expected rates in figure 39 are those that would have occurred in this group of 59 children on the basis of the age-specific and season-specific rates of the entire childhood population (Appendix 16, table 4). A comparison of the observed and expected rates shows that tonsillectomy did not materially alter the average incidence of the common respiratory diseases. The average rates among these 59 children had been higher than the expected for several years before tonsillectomy and continued to be higher than expected after the operation. The abrupt drop both in the expected and observed rates during the year of operation is due to two factors: 1) 17 of the 59 tonsillectomies were performed during May and June so that the preoperative period of observation consisted chiefly of the winter months of high incidence; 2) 32 of the operations were performed before the age of six when a marked drop in the incidence of all respiratory illnesses occurs.

STREPTOCOCCAL TONSILLITIS AND PHARYNGITIS

Further analysis was carried out with respect to streptococcal illnesses in children who had their tonsillectomies while in the study. This analysis was similar to that presented for the common respiratory diseases in figure 39 except that November 1, rather than September 1, was chosen as the starting point for describing the seasonal cycle of streptococcal infection. The results are shown in figure 40 and Appendix 16, table 5. The data show that the incidence of streptococcal tonsillitis and pharyngitis in persons undergoing tonsillectomy was consistently higher prior to operation and consistently lower after operation than would be expected. The reason for the high incidence just prior to tonsillectomy (approximately two and one-half times the expected figure) is not clear unless the occurrence of acute streptococcal illness in this period finally led to the decision to operate. It seems reasonable to conclude from these data that tonsillectomy, performed because of repeated attacks of streptococcal tonsillitis and pharyngitis, should be of benefit to the patient.

COMMENTS

Attack rates from the common respiratory diseases for all children in the present study were no lower among those who had had their tonsils removed than among those who had not had this operation (table 35). This finding is consistent with the studies reported by

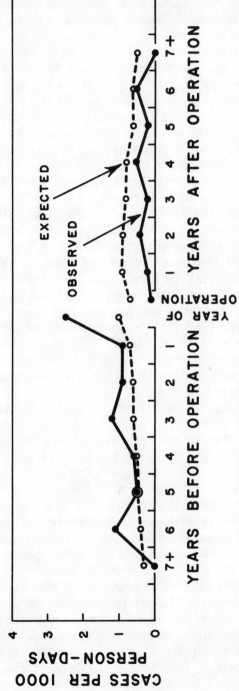

Fig. 40 Observed and expected incidence of streptococcal tonsillitis and pharyngitis before and after tonsillectomy in 59 children

the Medical Research Council (96) and by Patton (104), both of which were conducted among older children in boarding schools and were based on records of illnesses resulting in absence from classes. These two studies, as well as the present one, are free from the inaccuracies inherent in those that rely on memory.

The subgroups employed here (tables 36 and 37) provide an index of the severity of illness based on the presence or absence of certain symptoms. The attack rates of each of these various types of upper respiratory disease were almost identical for the two groups of children. This is in agreement with the findings of the Medical Research Council. Patton found that colds and bronchitis occurred somewhat more frequently in those whose tonsils had been removed, whereas tonsillitis occurred less frequently and pharyngitis with about the same frequency as in those who had not had tonsillectomy. Mertz (99), using another index of severity, found the incidence of disabling respiratory illnesses (those causing interruption in daily activities) and the duration of disability to be very similar among children who had had tonsillectomy and those who had not.

The observation that the attack rates for the common respiratory diseases were no lower among children who had had tonsillectomy than among children who had not had this operation (table 35), is not, in itself, evidence that the operation was of no value in reducing the incidence of these infections. Without knowledge of the attack rates before operation and without considering age-specific incidence, it is impossible to determine whether or not illness rates were changed after tonsillectomy.

The data for the 59 children who underwent tonsillectomy while in this study do, however, provide direct evidence that the operation did not influence the incidence of the common respiratory diseases. These children, on the average, had an excessively high rate before and continued to have an excessively high rate after operation. This is at variance with the results reported by the Medical Research Council. The 364 boys who underwent tonsillectomy while under observation in that study had, on the average, more than the expected number of nasopharyngeal infections before tonsillectomy but fewer than expected after operation. There are certain notable differences, however, between the Medical Research Council study and the present one: the age distribution of the boys observed both before and after tonsillectomy in the former study is not given, but it is unlikely that any were under 7 years of age at the time of operation; in contrast, 39 of the 59 children reported upon here were under seven at the time of operation. The nasopharyngeal infections reported in the Medical Research Council study included only illnesses requiring absence from classes for a day or more, whereas in the present study any symptom abnormal for the child concerned was considered sufficient to designate the presence of an illness. The former study did not exclude streptococcal and nonbacterial tonsillitis and pharyngitis, whereas these were excluded from the common respiratory diseases considered here. Although the seasonal distribution of the period of observation before and after tonsillectomy in the Medical Research Council study was not stated, it is possible that seasons characterized by a high incidence of the common respiratory diseases were not equally divided between preoperative and postoperative periods. This factor was found to be important in the present study in evaluating the rate of illness immediately after tonsillectomy and has been taken into account here by the use of rates adjusted for age and season. The relative importance of these factors in explaining the lack of agreement between the findings of these two studies is not known.

In a somewhat different type of investigation, Kaiser (86, 87) conducted parallel follow-up examinations on two groups of children of comparable ages. Both were reported to have had the same indications for tonsillectomy, but for various reasons the operation was performed only on the children in one group. These children were examined and questioned about illnesses 1, 3, and 10 years after tonsillectomy had been performed. At the same time the group of children who had not had this operation were examined and questioned. The data presented are difficult to interpret. Kaiser (87), referring to common colds, otitis media, sinusitis and laryngitis, concluded, "It cannot be demonstrated that the tonsils are often a causative factor in these infections; consequently tonsillectomy does not offer a solution for their eradication save in exceptional cases." The findings of the present study are consistent with this conclusion.

With respect to streptococcal tonsillitis and pharyngitis, however, the situation appeared to be quite different. The data for all the children in the study (table 35) show that in each age group from 3 to 10 years or older, the incidence of streptococcal illness was lower in those children who had had tonsillectomies than in those who had not. In most instances the information regarding the operation was based on history and is possibly open to some degree of error for this reason. The analysis of streptococcal illnesses in children who had their tonsillectomies while in the study, however, gave strong support to the difference in incidence rates in the total group of children. The incidence of streptococcal tonsillitis and pharyngitis in persons undergoing tonsillectomy was consistently higher prior to the operation and consistently lower after the operation than would be expected (figure 40). This finding does not agree with that of Chamovitz *et al.* (42), who reported no difference in the occurrence of streptococcal infections in young adult males who did or did not have a history of tonsillectomy. We have no clear explanation for the differences reported in these two studies. It would be difficult to explain the differences on the basis of prior exposure to various types of group A streptococci and the subsequent development of immunity. It may be, however, that age plays a significant role; for example, the lymphoid tissue of the tonsils and adenoids gradually decreases with increasing age and in many instances this decrease amounts to what might be called a "physiological tonsillectomy and adenoidectomy." Thus if these structures truly play a role in susceptibility to streptococcal infections, adults who have not had tonsillectomies may resemble, physiologically, children who have had tonsillectomy more than they do children who have had not the operation.

Chapter IX
ETIOLOGY OF THE COMMON RESPIRATORY DISEASES

As pointed out in Chapter VI, attempts to classify the common respiratory diseases on a clinical basis were unsatisfactory and gave little indication of possible etiological groupings. Many attempts were made to isolate viruses in animals and fertile eggs. Apart from the influenza viruses, these attempts were unsuccessful during the first part of the study. The development of a practical method of tissue culture by Enders, Weller, Robbins and others (60, 121, 123), however, made possible a new approach and resulted not only in the isolation of many new viruses but also in convenient procedures for identifying and typing viruses and for the preparation of suitable antigens for serological and other uses. Accordingly, it was possible to study the relation of certain of the new viruses to the common respiratory illnesses both by isolation attempts and serological studies in current cases and by retrospective serological studies using the stored serum specimens.

This chapter deals with viruses encountered or utilized during the study, namely, adenoviruses, polioviruses, Coxsackie viruses, and parainfluenza viruses. The data concerning influenza and the epidemic of poliomyelitis in 1952 are presented in Chapters X and XII.

ADENOVIRUSES

The isolation and identification of the adenoviruses were reported in late 1953 and early 1954 by Rowe et al. (113), and by Hilleman et al. (72, 73). The relationship of type 4 adenovirus to acute respiratory disease (ARD) of military recruits was promptly confirmed (23, 50, 65) and it was further found that this type appeared to behave quite differently in civilian than in military populations. Extension of work with adenoviruses in this study confirmed the observations of Bell and co-workers (30) relating type 3 adenoviruses as well as certain other types to acute nonbacterial tonsillitis and pharyngitis and provided considerable information regarding the role of this group of viruses in the common respiratory disease problem. The data are presented under two headings: a) the occurrence and distribution of antibodies, and b) the occurrence of illness.*

OCCURRENCE AND DISTRIBUTION OF ANTIBODIES

Surveys for neutralizing antibodies to the adenoviruses were carried out in order to gain an impression of the extent of infection

---
*Laboratory methods are described in Appendix 3.

with these viruses. The assumption was made that the presence of
neutralizing antibody to a specific type indicated prior clinical or
inapparent infection with that type even though the data could not
be related to any particular illness.

Type 4 adenovirus.—As already indicated (Chapter VI), we had
been unsuccessful in detecting the occurrence of illnesses resembling "acute respiratory disease of recruits" (ARD) in the families
by clinical or epidemiological means. When type 4 adenovirus was
shown to be a cause of the recruit disease, therefore, we turned to
serological surveys to determine whether the antibody status of the
population would give a clue as to whether or not type 4 infections
were occurring, and if so, to what extent. Accordingly, 157 sera
obtained routinely in the spring of 1954 were screened for the
presence of type 4 neutralizing antibody in a titer of 8 or more
(table 38). None of the 73 children (aged 1 to 18 years) had this

TABLE 38

Percentage of individuals tested who had neutralizing antibody for
type 4 adenovirus, Spring, 1954

| | No. tested | Antibody present* | |
		No.	%
Children	73	0	0
Mothers	43	6	14.0
Fathers	41	20	49.0

*Present at final serum dilution of 1:8, which indicates a titer of 8 or more.

antibody. Thus, the serological data for these children indicated
that an agent which produces epidemic disease in military recruits
probably had not infected the child members of this civilian population during their lifetime—a maximum of 18 years. Fourteen percent of the mothers and 49% of the fathers had this antibody.
The sex difference noted could not be attributed to exposure
to ARD during military service (10). Further study showed that
type 4 antibody had been present in serum specimens obtained
4 to 6 years previously from 22 of the 26 adults with antibody.
Although sporadic type 4 infections subsequently have been described in civilians, this curious and puzzling difference between
civilian and military populations has persisted without explanation.

Types 1-7 adenoviruses.—During the following year the observations regarding type 4 were confirmed and data regarding the prev-

alence of neutralizing antibodies were extended to the first seven types (table 39). Antibodies for types 1, 2 and 3 were present in

TABLE 39

Percentage of individuals tested who had neutralizing antibodies for adenoviruses types 1 through 7, Spring, 1955

Virus type	Adults			Children		
	No. tested	Antibody*		No. tested	Antibody*	
		No.	%		No.	%
1	120	39	32	138	51	37
2	120	59	49	138	70	51
3	120	53	44	140	57	41
4	55	16	29	70	0	0
5	120	36	30	138	14	10
6	120	18	15	138	20	14
7	65	15	23	68	8	12

*Present at final serum dilution of 1:8, which indicates a titer of 8 or more.

from one-third to one-half of both the adults and children. Antibodies for types 5 and 7 were somewhat more common in adults. In general, the proportion of persons showing specific antibodies for these types increased with age (figure 41). Type 2 antibody was most common, being closely followed by antibodies for types 1 and 3. Antibody to type 7, another type responsible for epidemic acute respiratory disease in military recruits, was absent in children under 5 years and then increased in frequency with age. The cumulative occurrence of antibodies against one or more types was illustrated by dividing the children into three age groups and grouping those over 15 with the adults (figure 42), following the design used by Huebner et al. (75). More than 80% of children 1 to 5 years of age showed antibodies against one or more types. A gradual increase in number of persons having multiple type-specific antibodies occurred with increasing age, but there was little additional increase between the 11 to 15-year-old group and the adults.

The availability of serial serum specimens collected at intervals in previous years provided a unique opportunity for the measurement of the time and frequency of acquisition of type-specific adenovirus antibodies in the first 5 years of life (15). At the time this study was

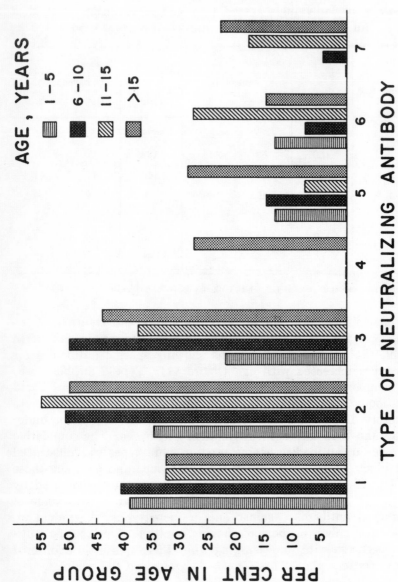

Fig. 41   Percentage of individuals with type-specific neutralizing antibodies for adenoviruses by age

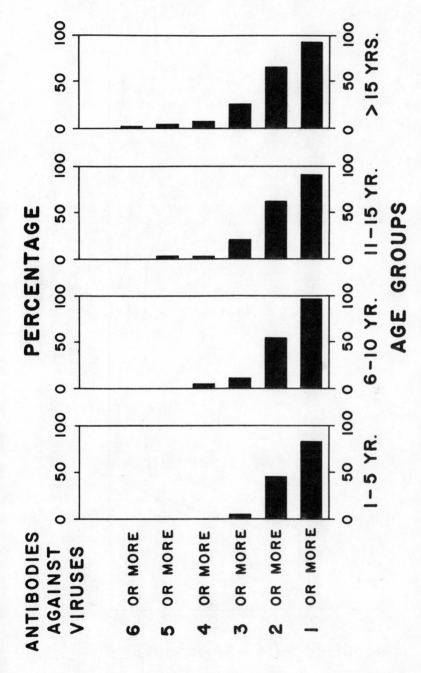

Fig. 42 Cumulative percentage distribution of individuals according to the number of adenoviruses to which they had neutralizing antibodies, by age

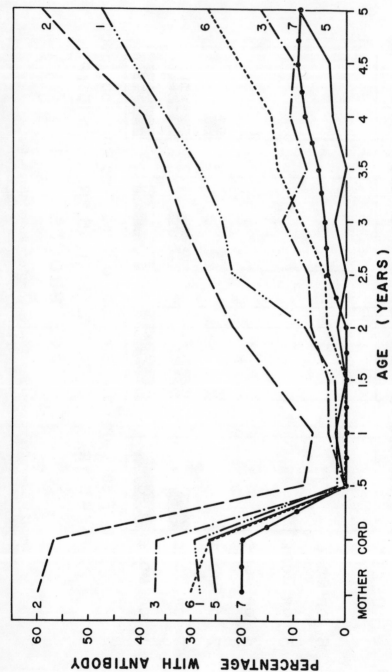

Fig. 43 Disappearance of maternally transmitted and acquisition of type-specific adenovirus antibodies in first 5 years of life

made, 81 children had been born into the population of families. Serum specimens had been collected from the mother during the third trimester of pregnancy or at term, from the umbilical cord at birth, and from the child at intervals of approximately 6 months thereafter (Figure 43 and Appendix 17). Sera from these children and their mothers were tested for neutralizing antibodies against six of the first seven types. Type 4 was excluded because the serum tests had shown that children had no antibody to it. The antibody pattern of the newborn infants' cord blood mirrored the mothers' pattern, indicating placental transmission of adenovirus antibodies. By 6 months of age these maternal antibodies had disappeared. After the first year of life there was a steady increase in the percentage of children with type 2 antibody, and by the age of 5 years the percentage with antibody was the same as that in the maternal group. Antibodies for types 1 and 6 were also acquired at rather constant rates, producing curves with slopes similar to that for type 2. The antibody prevalence for the 5-year-old children exceeded the mothers' level for type 1 antibody. Acquisition of antibody to type 6 was much less common but, again, almost as many 5-year-old

TABLE 40

Percentage of individuals tested who had neutralizing antibodies for adenoviruses types 8-18, Fall, 1957

Virus type	Adults			Children		
	No. tested	Antibody*		No. tested	Antibody*	
		No.	%		No.	%
8	120	7	6	0	....	....
9	120	1	1	0	....	....
10	120	4	3	0	...	....
11	120	14	12	188	7	4
12	120	16	13	188	17	9
13	120	0	0	0	....	....
14	120	19	16	188	14	7
15	120	12	10	188	2	1
16	120	3	2	0	....	....
17	120	0	0	0	....	....
18	120	44	37	188	6	3

*Present at final serum dilution of 1:8, which indicates a titer of 8 or more.

children as their mothers had type 6 antibody. Type 3 antibody was slowly acquired; 17% of the children, slightly less than half the mothers' level, possessed type 3 antibody at age five. By this age only 10% of the children had acquired antibodies to types 5 or 7. Assuming that type-specific antibody reflects prior infection, these data, plus those presented in table 39, indicate that infections with types 1, 2, and 3 were fairly common in childhood, type 1 and 2 infections occurring early but about half the type 3 infections occurring after age five. Infections due to type 4 were absent and those due to types 5 and 7 were relatively infrequent in the first 5 years of life; only 20 to 30% of adults had been infected with these types.

Types 8 to 18 adenoviruses.—Sera collected in the fall of 1957 were screened at a final dilution of 1:8 for neutralizing antibodies to adenoviruses types 8 to 18 (table 40). The sera from children were not tested against types 8, 9, 10, 13, 16 and 17 because the percentages of adults demonstrating antibodies to these types were so small. Approximately one-third of the adults had antibody to type 18 and from 10 to 15% of them had antibodies to types 11, 12, 14 and 15. From 1 to 10% of the children showed antibodies to these five types. The data indicate that these higher types of adenoviruses, with the possible exception of type 18, were not common causes of infection in this population.

OCCURRENCE OF ILLNESS

Study of specific illnesses, combining virus isolations with serological procedures, provided information regarding the clinical syndromes induced by adenoviruses and contributed additional data relative to the frequency of such infections.

TABLE 41

Isolation of adenoviruses and serological findings in cases of nonbacterial tonsillitis and pharyngitis, Summer, 1954

Virus type	Isolations from the 16 cases tested	Serologic response as measured in specimens drawn in spring and fall		
		No. tested	Increases in titer*	
			No.	%
2	1	269	8	3
3	6	289	38	13
5	0	271	9	3

*From less than 8 to 8 or greater.

Epidemic occurrence.—It has long been recognized that certain forms of pharyngitis, with or without exudate, probably were of viral etiology and epidemics of nonbacterial exudative pharyngitis have been described (45). An illness characterized by fever, headache, and sore throat occurred in epidemic form in the family study population during July and August of 1954. Clinically recognized infections occurred mainly in children and only rarely in adults. The illness was manifested by erythema, edema, lymphoid hyperplasia and, usually, patches of exudate on the tonsils or pharyngeal wall. Conjunctivitis was noted in only an occasional case. Group A streptococci were not present. Pharyngeal swabs from 16 cases were tested for the presence of virus and serum specimens collected from the population before and after the epidemic were tested for increases in titer of neutralizing antibodies to types 2, 3, and 5 adenoviruses (table 41). An adenovirus was isolated from seven of the cases tested; six of the seven strains belonged to type 3. When the serum specimens which spanned the summer were tested, a few type 2 and type 5 infections were detected, and 38, or 13%, of 289 individuals were shown to have increases in titer of type 3 antibody.

The correlation between illness and antibody rise to type 3 adeno-

TABLE 42

The development of neutralizing antibody to type 3 adenovirus in individuals with and without nonbacterial tonsillitis and pharyngitis, Summer, 1954

	Number of persons	Antibody response			
		Increase in titer*		No increase in titer	
		No.	%	No.	%
Pharyngitis	63	32	51	31	49
No pharyngitis	226	6	3	220	97
Total	289	38	13	251	87

*From less than 8 to 8 or greater.

virus is shown in table 42. Of the 289 persons whose sera were tested, 63 had illnesses compatible with a diagnosis of nonbacterial tonsillitis and pharyngitis and 226 remained well. Thirty-two, or 51% of those ill, showed a significant rise in antibody titer; 31, or 49%, did not. In contrast, only 3% of those who were not ill showed antibody rises. Looking at the table in the other direction it may be seen that 32, or 84%, of the 38 individuals having antibody rises had illnesses while only 12% of those who showed no antibody rises were ill. Thirty-three of the 38 individuals with antibody rises were children, of whom 31 were ill; 4 of the 5 adults with antibody rises remained well.

It is thus apparent that a large proportion of persons showing antibody rises to type 3 adenovirus had clinical illnesses, that the inapparent infection rate was low (2%), and that no children had inapparent infections. Two of the 31 illnesses among those not showing antibody responses to type 3 showed antibody rises to type 2; the remaining illnesses were presumably due to other adenovirus types or to other agents.

The data were then examined to determine whether or not any relation could be found between the presence of antibody prior to the epidemic and the occurrence of overt clinical illness. A "susceptible" individual was defined as one who had no detectable antibody in his serum at a dilution of 1:8. Total attack rates were determined for the susceptibles and for those whose initial titers were 8 or greater. In addition, secondary attack rates were determined in 15 families in which an index case could be clearly distinguished on the basis of a characteristic clinical illness followed by an antibody rise.

The results (table 43) show that both the total and secondary attack rates were approximately three times as great among "susceptible" children as among those whose initial antibody titers were

TABLE 43

Incidence of adenovirus type 3 tonsillitis and pharyngitis in the total population and secondary attack rates in 15 families in relation to neutralizing antibody status

	Antibody titer prior to epidemic	Total attack rate			Secondary attack rate*		
		No. persons at risk	Pharyngitis		No. persons at risk	Pharyngitis	
			No.	%		No.	%
Children	Less than 8	129	44	34	30	19	63
	8 or greater	31	3	10	4	1	25
Adults	Less than 8	71	9	13	15	4	27
	8 or greater	58	7	12	15	3	20

*One index case in each family episode has been excluded.

8 or more. In contrast, the presence or absence of antibody in adults had no apparent effect on attack rates. Additional data on these points were subsequently collected by studying the intrafamilial spread of sporadic adenovirus infections.

Sporadic infections.—Sporadic infections were detected during a study designed to determine the importance of adenoviruses as etiologic agents in respiratory disease (10). Pharyngeal swabs were collected from September, 1954 through June, 1955 and serum specimens that spanned approximately the same period were tested for increases in titer of neutralizing antibodies for types 1 through 7

TABLE 44

Virus isolations in HeLa cell cultures from pharyngeal swabs,
September 1954-June 1955

Time interval	How collected	Number tested	Virus isolations	
			Kind	No.
9/27 - 10/2	All persons	45 (35 from illness)	Poliovirus	3
10/4 - 10/19	Selected illnesses	4	Poliovirus	2
11/1 - 11/30	All respiratory illnesses	147	Poliovirus Coxsackie Adenovirus	1 4 5
12/6 - 1/5	Selected illnesses	16	....	0
1/17 - 1/29	All respiratory illnesses	106	Adenovirus	3
1/31 - 6/31	Selected illnesses	223	Adenovirus	2
Total		531	Poliovirus Coxsackie Adenovirus	6 4 10

(tables 44 and 45). As a beginning, swabs were collected from all members of the population during the period of high prevalence 3 weeks after the opening of school. The sudden increase in respiratory disease rates at this time is somewhat reminiscent of the behavior of acute respiratory disease (ARD) in military recruits. Since 45 of the 318 swabs collected did not yield adenoviruses, however, the others were not tested. During two subsequent periods, the month of November and 2 weeks in January, specimens were collected from all individuals with respiratory symptoms. At other times selected illnesses were cultured.

TABLE 45

Increases in titer of neutralizing antibodies for adenoviruses between Fall, 1954 and Spring, 1955

Virus type	Adults			Children			Total		
	No. tested	Increase* No.	%	No. tested	Increase* No.	%	No. tested	Increase* No.	%
1	120	2	1.7	132	9	6.8	252	11	4.4
2	119	2	1.7	134	1	0.7	253	3	1.2
3	120	2	1.7	137	5	3.6	257	7	2.7
4	55	0	0	70	0	0	125	0	0
5	120	2	1.7	138	3	2.2	258	5	1.9
6	120	2	1.7	136	6	4.4	256	8	3.1
7	65	0	0	66	0	0	131	0	0

*From less than 8 to 8 or greater, or from 8 to 32 or greater.

Only 10 adenoviruses were isolated from 531 specimens, a yield of about 2% (table 44). That the low virus isolation rate reflected a true measure of the importance of adenoviruses as causes of respiratory disease in this civilian population was confirmed by the serological studies (table 45). The percentage of persons showing increases in titer to any one of the seven types ranged from 0 to 5%, with children showing a few more increases than adults. In all, there were 35 different rises detected. If each antibody increase is accepted as indicative of symptomatic infection, a very crude measure of the frequency with which adenoviruses caused respiratory illness can be obtained. The number of nonbacterial respiratory diseases that occurred during the interval between the date of the fall serum specimen and 2 weeks before the date of the spring specimen was tabulated for each individual tested. During these intervals, 267 individuals had 862 respiratory illnesses. At most, 35, or 4%, of these illnesses could be attributed to infection with adenoviruses. Since certain of the antibody rises may have represented heterotypic responses, this is a maximum estimate. Subsequent studies of civilian populations by other investigators provided remarkably similar estimates (25).

An additional 190 pharyngeal swabs were collected between July, 1955 and May, 1957 as follows: 1955—91; 1956—62; 1957—37. These specimens were collected from selected cases and, in general, those thought clinically to be possible adenovirus infections. The

TABLE 46

Viruses isolated from swabs collected at time of respiratory symptoms

	Time period		Total
	July & August 1954	September 1954 – May 1957	
Specimens tested	18*	721	739
Viruses‡	7	29	36
Poliovirus (all type 1)	0	5**	5**
Coxsackie (Group B, 3)	0	7	7
Adenoviruses			
Type 1	0	2	2
Type 2	1	1	2
Type 3	6	10	16
Type 5	0	2	2
Type 6	0	1	1
Type 15	0	1	1

*From 16 individuals.

**One additional strain was isolated from a 3-year-old child in family 29 who had no symptoms at time swab was obtained.

‡If multiple isolations were made during a single illness, the isolation was counted only once. Thus the 36 viruses isolated came from 36 separate illnesses.

processing of these swabs added seven adenoviruses and three Coxsackie viruses to those previously detected. Table 46 summarizes the total experience with specimens inoculated into cultures of continuous cell lines in an attempt to isolate adenoviruses. Two-thirds of the adenovirus isolates were type 3, and more detailed information is presented to illustrate the behavior of infection with this type. The findings in three families from whom type 3 viruses were isolated are detailed in tables 47, 48 and 49.

In family 29 (table 47), the 4-year-old daughter developed coryza associated with a mild cough. Three days later, her 14-year-old sister developed conjunctivitis and pharyngitis; type 3 virus was recovered from both eye and throat. The parents and 11-year-old boy re-

TABLE 47

Type 3 adenovirus infections in Family 29

Subject (age)	Date of onset	Symptoms	Specimens for virus		Serum	
			Date	Result	Date	Titer
4 years	10/2/55	Nasal discharge and obstruction, throat cough	None		10/29/54 10/16/55	<8 128
14 years	10/5/55	Conjunctivitis, nasal discharge and obstruction, sore throat, pharyngeal injection, cervical adenopathy	10/8/55 Pharynx Eye	++	3/26/55 10/16/55	<8 512
Father		None	None		3/26/55 10/30/55	<8 <8
Mother		None	None		3/28/55 10/16/55	<8 512
11 years		None	None		3/26/55 10/16/55	<8 32

TABLE 48

Type 3 adenovirus infections in Family 40

Subject (age)	Date of onset	Symptoms	Specimens for virus		Serum	
			Date	Result	Date	Titer
4 years	7/10/56	Sneezing, nasal discharge, hoarseness, cough, anorexia, feverishness, abdominal pain (on vacation)	7/26/56	0	None available	
Mother	7/10/56	Sore throat, headache, nasal discharge, cough, hoarseness, cervical adenopathy, aches in joints of hands (on vacation)	7/26/56	0	3/19/56 7/26/56 10/28/56	32 32 32
7 years	7/15/56	Sore throat, anorexia, vomiting, abdominal pain, feverishness (on vacation)	7/25/56	0	4/11/56 7/26/56 10/28/56	<8 >32 64
9 years	7/21/56	Anorexia, headache, abdominal pain, conjunctivitis, cervical adenopathy, exudative pharyngitis, sore throat, T. 101°F	7/25/56	+	7/26/56 10/28/56	<8 64
11 years	7/29/56	Sore throat, hoarseness, anorexia, headache, malaise, conjunctival injection, cervical adenopathy, spotty exudate, T. 101.5°F	7/26/56	+	7/26/56 10/28/56	<8 32
Father		No illness	None		3/10/56 8/4/56 10/28/56	<8 16 64

TABLE 49

Type 3 adenovirus infections in Family 77

Subject (age)	Date of onset	Symptoms	Specimens for virus		Serum	
			Date	Result	Date	Titer
Mother	9/10/55	Irritated throat, hoarseness, throat cough	None		9/10/55 4/22/56	<8 32
Father	9/15/55	Throat cough	None		9/10/55 4/22/56	32 32
3 years	9/15/55	Nasal obstruction, pharyngeal injection, cervical adenopathy, T. 102.5°F	None		8/27/54 4/22/56	<8 128
4 years	9/22/55	Headache, irritated throat, slight pharyngeal injection, T. 103.5°F	None		9/10/55 4/22/56	<8 512
6 years	9/22/55	Headache, palpebral and pharyngeal injection, T. 104°F	9/26/55	+	9/10/55 4/22/56	<8 128
11 years		None			9/12/55 4/22/56	32 32
12 years		None			9/10/55 4/22/56	>32 128

mained well. Because of the spacing of the serum specimens it was not possible definitely to relate antibody increases to illness and virus isolation. A review of the family's charts suggested that it was reasonable to assume such a relationship. Of the two clinical illnesses, one resembled the common cold and the other typical pharyngoconjunctival fever. The mother and the 11-year-old child had inapparent infections; the father escaped.

As shown in table 48, the episode in family 40 began while the family was on vacation. The symptoms recorded for the first three cases are similar to those confirmed in the next two as adenovirus infections, but pharyngeal swabs were not collected until long after the onset. This is particularly unfortunate in the case of the mother, for she had type 3 antibody prior to these symptoms and may have represented an example of the occurrence of infection in the presence of antibody. The father had an inapparent infection.

The episode in family 77 (table 49) began with mild illness in the mother and was followed by a milder illness in the father; one already had antibody and the other developed antibody in the serum drawn 7 months later. Here again, the limitations of data derived from sera so spaced are shown. Three younger children had acute febrile illnesses characterized by pharyngitis; one of these developed palpebral injection. The two older children, both of whom already had type 3 antibody, remained well.

In all there were six such episodes. Sera were available from 30 of the 34 members of the six families with sporadic type 3 infections. Six individuals already had antibody; one of these reported respiratory symptoms. Seventeen of the 24 susceptibles (71%) developed increases of antibody titer; fourteen (58%) had symptoms. Seven persons, 29%, escaped infection; six of the seven were adults. Three of the susceptibles (12.5%) had inapparent infections. Among susceptibles, as determined by the absence of neutralizing antibody at a level of 8, the secondary attack rate for illness was 8 of 18 or 44%; for antibody increase, 11 of 18 or 61%. These attack rates among exposed susceptibles are similar to those noted during the 1954 summer epidemic. It is obvious that in these individual family outbreaks the family unit experienced an "epidemic" although none was evident in the general population.

The above data indicated quite clearly that immunity or resistance to infection was correlated with the presence of type-specific antibody in the sera of exposed persons and that susceptibility was correlated with the absence of detectable antibody. On the other hand, the question might be raised as to why so many persons who were apparently susceptible and were in intimate contact with infected persons in the home did not themselves become infected as indicated by the occurrence of illness or the development of anti-body. In a previous publication (51) the question was raised as to whether the manner and ability of the virus to spread and produce disease could be related to certain characteristics of adenoviruses in the laboratory. The type 3 adenovirus is adsorbed to cells at a relatively slow rate and in tissue culture relatively few cells combine with the virus. Furthermore, only a small percentage of the virus is liberated from the cells in which it propagates. In order to obtain a maximum yield of virus it is necessary to disrupt the cells, which contain approximately 30 times more virus than is found in the supernatant fluid. Despite the appearance of cytopathic change, the infected cells remain alive and continue to metabolize at a normal or slightly increased rate. The fact that these viruses adsorb ineffi-ciently and dissociate poorly from the cells in which they multiply may be an important factor in the epidemiology of the disease and may explain the failure of illnesses to occur in persons without detectable antibody who are repeatedly exposed to infected indi-viduals. The ability of adenoviruses to spread and produce disease, despite these characteristics, may be a reflection of their remarkable stability over a wide range of pH and temperature.

Viruses which do not kill cells which they infect but do initiate pathologic changes, should produce self-limited and mild disease. This appears to be the case with adenovirus type 3. In addition, viruses which are stable, do not kill cells which they infect, and cannot readily dissociate from such cells, should be ideal agents to initiate latent infections in the hosts in which they multiply. It is clear from the available evidence that most of the adenoviruses do effect a symbiotic relationship with man whereby they persist in a "masked" state for long periods in cells of the respiratory tract. This may be a normal consequence of infection, perhaps conferring long-lasting immunity, or conversely, perhaps permitting recurrent illnesses and infections from an endogenous source. Thus, although clinically recognized disease is caused by certain of the adenoviruses, latent infections may be the rule for most of the agents of this group. It is realized that certain types of adenoviruses—such as types 4 and 7—have the laboratory properties described above for other types, yet they cause epidemic disease, especially in military recruits. The property of these viruses for epidemic spread cannot yet be described in terms of their definable characteristics under laboratory conditions.

During these studies neither rectal swabs nor stool specimens were processed for adenoviruses. Thus, no conclusions can be reached regarding the distribution of the higher types (31, 112, 114) in this population. However, an interesting family outbreak of conjuncti-

TABLE 50

Type 15 adenovirus infections in Family 76

Subject (age)	Date of onset	Symptoms	Specimen for virus Date	Specimen for virus Result	Serum Date	Serum Titer
4 years	8/26/55	Conjunctivitis which persisted until 9/15, T. 103.4°F on day of onset	None		5/8/55 11/18/55	<8 128
5 years	8/29/55	Conjunctivitis for 3 days, nausea and abdominal pain for few hours on 8/31, afebrile	8/29 (eye) 8/31 (pharynx)	+ +	5/8/55 9/8/55 4/22/56	<8 8 >64
3 years	8/30/55	Conjunctivitis which persisted until 9/12, nasal obstruction	8/31	0	8/18/55 11/21/55	<8 32
Mother	8/30/55	Conjunctivitis, left eye, on 9/5 to 9/7, coryza, irritated throat, non-productive cough	None		8/18/55 11/18/55	<8 8
1 year	9/3/55	Conjunctivitis, 9/7 to 9/24, nasal discharge, cough	None		8/18/55 11/18/55	<8 32

vitis in 1955 was related to type 15 adenovirus, the prototype for this virus having been first isolated by Murray and associates (101) from patients with acute conjunctivitis in Saudi Arabia in that same year. Data relative to the illnesses occurring in this family at the time type 15 adenovirus was isolated from one of the children are summarized in table 50. The mother and four of the children all had conjunctivitis; all developed increases in titer of neutralizing antibody. The parents were divorced several months later and it is not known to what extent the father was exposed to cases in the family. No convalescent-phase serum was available from him. Conjunctivitis persisted for from 3 days to 3 weeks. It was unilateral in one case; bilateral in the others. The 4-year-old child was described as having palpebral and bulbar conjunctival injection and puffy eyelids on the left and palpebral injection only on the right. No members of the family developed chronic ocular changes.

Since the completion of these studies a number of additional human adenovirus types have been identified, and detailed investigations of selected population groups continue to increase knowledge and understanding of the disease relationships and epidemiological behavior of this important group of agents. Two of the major contributions of the Cleveland study in the adenovirus field were 1) the demonstration that the epidemiology of types 4 and 7 adenovirus infections differs in civilian and military populations, and 2) the collection of data on which to base judgments regarding the general use of adenovirus vaccine (15, 25, 61, 126). Although infections with types 4 and 7 are a common cause of morbidity and hospitalization in military populations, epidemics due to these types are rarely seen in civilian populations. As demonstrated by the data presented above and those reported by others (71, 75) adenovirus antibodies are common and increase in frequency with age, an indication that many of these types commonly infect man. How often these infections are inapparent is not known, nor has the duration of natural or vaccine-induced immunity been established. On the basis of our data it was estimated that a polyvalent adenovirus vaccine, even if it were completely effective, would result in only a 6% reduction in the number of respiratory illnesses experienced by the average child during the first 10 years of life. It may be necessary to revise this estimate in the future when comparable data relative to the new types become available, but the basic conclusion remains the same.

POLIOVIRUSES

As indicated in table 46, six strains of poliovirus were isolated from pharyngeal swabs collected at the time of respiratory illnesses

TABLE 51

Type 1 poliovirus in Family 29

Subject (age)	Date of onset	Symptoms	Virus isolation	Titer of antibodies in serum			
				Date	Type 1	Type 2	Type 3
Mother	9/29/54	Irritated throat	10/1/54 +	4/1/53 4/15/54 10/24/54 12/22/54	<5 <5 >5 >320	>5 NT* >5 >5	<5 NT* 5 <5
10 years	10/2/54	Constitutional**, T. 101°F., abdominal pain	10/1/54 +	4/1/53 4/15/54 10/24/54 12/29/54	<5 <5 >5 200	>5 NT* >5 >5	<5 NT* <5 <5
Father		None	10/1/54	5/10/53 4/11/54 10/24/54 1/6/55	<5 <5 >5 128	<5 NT* <5 >5	<5 NT* <5 <5
13 years		None	10/1/54 +	4/1/53 4/15/54 10/24/54 12/29/54	<5 <5 >5 >320	>5 NT* >5 >5	<5 NT* >5 5
4 years		None	10/1/54	4/1/53 4/15/54 10/24/54 12/29/54	<5 <5 >16 >320	>5 NT* >5 >5	<5 <5 NT* <5

*Not tested.
**Fever and malaise.

TABLE 52

Type 1 poliovirus in Family 83

Subject (age)	Date of onset	Symptoms	Virus isolation	Date	Titer of antibodies in serum		
					Type 1	Type 2	Type 3
3 years	10/6/54	Nasal obstruction and cough	No specimen	3/19/52 2/26/55	<5 >320	<5 <5	<5 <5
5 years	10/18/54	Anorexia, nasal obstruction, sore throat, vomiting, T. 104°F.	10/19/54 +	No serum			
7 years	10/19/54	Nasal obstruction, irritated throat, T. 102°F.	10/19/54 +	4/21/53 9/2/54 2/26/55	<5 <5 200	<5 NT* <5	<5 NT* <5
Mother		None	No specimen	4/21/53 9/30/54 2/26/55	<5 <5 16	<5 NT* <5	<5 NT* <5
Father		None	No specimen	4/26/53 9/11/54 3/16/55	<5 <5 <5	>5 NT* >5	<5 NT* <5

*Not tested.

in three families. All were type 1 and all were isolated during the months of October and November 1954 at which time no cases of paralytic poliomyelitis were reported in the community (9). These family epidemics are summarized in tables 51-53.

Pharyngeal swabs were collected from all members of Family 29 (table 51) on October 1, 1954. Those from the mother and the 10-year-old child were processed because they had respiratory symptoms within 3 days of the routine collection of the specimens. When polioviruses were isolated, specimens from the other three members of the family were examined. Virus was isolated from the 13-year-old daughter who had reported no symptoms. Neutralization tests indicated that type 1 antibody had appeared in serum specimens obtained 3 weeks after the collection of the throat swabs. Titration of subsequent sera demonstrated that significant increases in titer of type 1 antibody developed in all five members of the family.

Type 1 polioviruses were isolated from two children in Family 83 (table 52) from specimens collected in mid-October. At this time, only persons with selected respiratory illnesses were being cultured. No sera were available from one of these children; the other child and a younger sibling showed significant increases in titer of type 1 antibody. The mother had a very slight increase in titer; the father gave no serological evidence of infection. The grippelike illnesses in the two older children were consistent with severe common colds or acute respiratory disease. It is of some interest that these two girls were scheduled for tonsillectomy, the operation being cancelled because of the development of the symptoms noted.

In November an effort was made to collect pharyngeal swabs in broth from all persons with respiratory symptoms. It is unfortunate that one was not obtained from the father of Family 80. Type 1 poliovirus was isolated from one of the two children (table 53). Serological evidence of infection with type 1 virus developed in both children; the mother and father escaped infection.

In the absence of the laboratory studies, it is likely that the illnesses observed in families 29, 80, and 83 would have been classified as belonging to the heterogeneous group of common respiratory diseases. Indeed, it is possible that the symptoms recorded were due to unidentified respiratory viruses, and were not produced by the polioviruses shown to be present in the throats. Virus is present in the throat during the acute stage of poliomyelitis (135) but inapparent infections have usually been recognized by stool surveys. Several investigators (33, 34, 138), by examination of stools, respiratory secretions and blood, have documented the importance of the family unit in the spread of poliomyelitis. Of particular interest here is the fact that polioviruses were present in the throats of the

TABLE 53
Type 1 poliovirus in Family 80

Subject (age)	Date of onset	Symptoms	Virus isolation	Date	Titer of antibodies in serum		
					Type 1	Type 2	Type 3
3 years	10/28/54	Anorexia, vomiting (twice), T. 102°F.; patient febrile for 3 days	No specimen	4/15/53	<5	<5	<5
				1/25/55	160	<5	<5
Father	11/5/54	Coryza, mild pharyngeal injection	11/5/54 +	5/10/53	<5	>5	<5
				9/11/54	<5	NT*	NT*
				1/25/55	<5	>5	<5
	11/3/54	Irritated throat	No specimen				
6 years	11/8/54	Coryza	11/8/54	4/15/53	<5	<5	<5
				5/26/55	>320	<5	<5
Mother		None	No specimen	4/15/53	>5	>5	>5
				9/11/54	<5	NT*	NT*
				1/25/55	9	>5	<5

* Not tested.

members of these families in the fall at a time when paralytic disease had disappeared from the community and, further, that none of the concomitant illnesses resembled clinical poliomyelitis. Although the symptoms that did occur cannot necessarily be attributed to the virus, sufficient viral antigen was produced to stimulate antibody production.

Since the polioviruses had not caused either paralysis or recognizable nonparalytic disease, they were submitted to Dr. Albert B. Sabin because of his interest in finding avirulent strains. The virulence of two of these strains was tested in cynomolgus monkeys. The strain from Family 29 caused partial paralysis in some of the monkeys given large amounts of virus by the intracerebral route. The strain from Family 80 produced histologic lesions but no paralysis after intracerebral inoculation in 10 monkeys; on intraspinal inoculation of $10^{5.5}TCD_{50}$ this strain resulted in paralysis in two of four monkeys. Dr. Sabin (115) commented as follows:

"Unpublished studies on a large number of strains of poliomyelitis viruses indicate the existence of a wide spectrum of pathogenicity for primate neurons. At the most severe end of the spectrum are strains that readily multiply in and damage chimpanzee as well as monkey neurons. In the middle of the spectrum are viruses that, though still paralytogenic for monkeys by intracerebral as well as by spinal inoculation, are not paralytogenic for chimpanzees even after direct spinal inoculation of 10^6TCD_{50} or more. At the most attenuated end of the spectrum are strains that not only are avirulent by intracerebral inoculation in monkeys but also require the direct spinal inoculation of more than 10^5TCD_{50} to produce a localized nonprogressive paralysis in an occasional monkey... The small proportion of paralytic infections in human beings suggests that human neurons are either even more resistant than those of chimpanzees or at worst of a similar order of resistance. The quantitative tests... performed in monkeys with the poliomyelitis strains recovered from families 29 and 80 indicate that they belong at the attenuated end of the spectrum that would be expected to be nonparalytogenic for chimpanzees in the maximum dosage."

COXSACKIE VIRUSES

During the course of studies on the etiology of the common respiratory diseases, no strains of Group A Coxsackie viruses were isolated, which is not surprising since suckling mice were not employed routinely. Some illnesses occurred which may well have been herpangina but were considered as nonbacterial tonsillitis and pharyngitis for purposes of classification. Coxsackie virus, Group B, type 3, however, was encountered in three families and serological studies were carried out with Coxsackie virus, Group A, type 21.

PHARYNGITIS

During the testing of pharyngeal swabs, three strains of Coxsackie Group B, type 3 virus, were isolated. Two were obtained

TABLE 54

Occurrence of infection with Group B, type 3, Coxsackie virus in Family 85

Subject (age)	Date of onset	Symptoms	Specimen for virus		Serum	
			Date	Result	Date	Antibody titer
3 years	7/17/55	Fever, abdominal pain, diarrhea	None		7/11/55	<8
					2/17/56	>512
7 years	7/18/55	Fever, conjunctival injection, pharyngeal exudate, abdominal pain	7/19/55	+	7/11/55	<8
					10/6/55	256
5 years	7/21/55	Fever, sore throat, pharyngeal exudate, abdominal pain	7/22/55	+	7/11/55	<8
					10/6/55	>512
Father		None	None		7/3/55	<8
					9/29/55	32
Mother		None	None		7/11/55	<8
					10/6/55	64

from siblings in July, 1955 and one from a child ill in September, 1956. The isolations are perhaps of more than usual interest because in each instance the specimen was obtained from an individual with an illness resembling nonbacterial pharyngitis, the symptoms of which are ordinarily associated with Group A, but not usually with Group B, virus infection.

The course of events in the family with two virus-positive cases is outlined in table 54. Three children had fever and abdominal pains; two showed pharyngeal exudate; one had conjunctival injection. All five members of the family, including the asymptomatic parents, developed increases in titer of antibody to the virus isolated from the 7-year-old child.

The 1956 isolate was from an 11-year-old boy ill with sore throat, anorexia, nausea, vomiting, headache, and a temperature of 100° F. In this family, only the individual from whom virus was isolated developed an increase in titer of antibody, although four other members tested had no antibody in their earlier sera.

PLEURODYNIA

In contrast to the above illnesses resembling pharyngitis, a family episode of infection with Coxsackie virus, Group B, type 3, occurred in which the illnesses resembled pleurodynia. This episode (table 55) afforded an excellent illustration of the spread of Coxsackie virus infections among the members of a household. During a 10-day period, seven of the eight members of the family became ill, only the 3-month-old infant having no recognized illness. The clinical manifestations were strikingly similar as the disease progressed through the family, the illness being characterized by fever, headache and such respiratory symptoms as coryza, sore throat, cough and chest pain. The adults were better able to describe the pain as a generalized aching throughout the muscles of the thorax. Viruses isolated from three of the children were identified as Coxsackie, Group B, type 3. All the six subjects tested showed significant increases in their antibody titers for this virus. Whereas the illnesses were similar in character, the disease was not recognized clinically as pleurodynia until the causative agent was identified. Similar illnesses were not observed in other families.

SEROLOGICAL STUDIES WITH COXSACKIE VIRUS, GROUP A, TYPE 21 (COE VIRUS)

Sera collected in the fall of 1957 were tested for neutralizing antibody to Coxsackie virus, Group A, type 21. Antibody in a titer of 8 or greater was found in the sera of 22% of 59 fathers and 13% of 60 mothers. Only 1 of 167 children had detectable antibody.

TABLE 55

Coxsackie virus, group B, type 3, in Family 37

Subject (age)	Date of onset	Symptoms	Pharyngeal swab		Serum	
			Date	Virus Present	Date	Antibody titer
10 years	10/31/54	Headache, malaise, coryza, cough, chest pain, T. 101°F.	11/2/54 11/5/54	+ +	10/10/54 12/17/54	<4 256
Father	11/3/54	Headache, coryza, irritated throat, cough, aches in back and chest, feverish	11/5/54	−	10/10/54 12/31/54	<4 16
6 years	11/3/54	Headache, malaise, sore throat, chest pain, feverish	11/5/54	−	10/10/54 12/17/54	<4 64
9 years	11/6/54	Headache, malaise, sore throat, chest pain, T. 103°F.	11/9/54	+	10/10/54 12/17/54	<4 256
Mother	11/7/54	Malaise, listlessness, T. 102°F.	11/9/54	+	(No serum)	
1 year	11/9/54	Headache, malaise, sore throat, chest pain, T. 101°F.	11/9/54	−	10/10/54 12/16/54	<4 256
13 years	11/10/54	Headache, malaise, coryza, sore throat, pains in chest, shoulders and trunk, feverish	None		10/10/54 12/16/54	<4 256
3 months		None	None		(No serum)	

These data suggest that the Coxsackie virus A-21 was not a frequent cause of disease in this population.

PARAINFLUENZA VIRUSES

Although no systematic attempts were made to isolate parainfluenza viruses while the study was in progress, serological studies were carried out subsequently to determine the prevalence of parainfluenza neutralizing antibodies and thus to gain some indication of the frequency with which they caused infection.

PARAINFLUENZA VIRUS, TYPE 1

Sera from the fall of 1957 were tested for neutralizing antibody to

TABLE 56

Occurrence of type 1 parainfluenza virus neutralizing antibody in sera collected in the Fall of 1957

Subjects	No. Tested	Percent of individuals with indicated titer of antibody			
		<8	8	16	32 or $>$
Parents	118	24	13	25	38
Children:					
0 - 4 years	19	100	....	....	....
5 - 9 years	72	81	3	8	8
10 - 14 years	68	54	9	28	9
15+	23	61	13	13	13

parainfluenza virus, type 1 (table 56). Antibody titers of 8 or greater were not found in the sera of children 4 years of age or younger, suggesting that the virus had not been prevalent during the period from 1953 to 1957. The percentage of individuals with detectable antibody increased with age, so that by 14 years of age approximately one-half of the children had antibody and among adults the proportion increased to three-fourths. No sex difference in titers was found in adults.

A comparison was made between the antibody titers of sera collected in 1947-48 and 1957 from the same 76 parents (table 57). Forty-nine of the 57 persons (86%) who had had antibody titers of 8 or greater in 1947-48 also had antibody titers of 8 or greater in 1957; this indicates either that antibody persists for relatively long periods or is maintained by repeated infections. Twelve of the 19

TABLE 57

Comparison of type 1 parainfluenza virus neutralizing antibody
titers in sera collected from same parents in 1947-48 and in 1957

Titer in 1947-48	Titer in 1957		Total
	Less than 8	8 or greater	
Less than 8	7	12	19
8 or greater	8	49	57
Total	15	61	76

persons (63%) who had had no detectable antibody in 1947-48 and
were therefore presumably susceptible, had titers of 8 or greater in
1957. This indicates a high infection rate.

These data therefore suggest that parainfluenza virus, type 1,
was highly active in this population at one or more periods during
the study.

PARAINFLUENZA VIRUS, TYPE 2

Limited studies were done with the parainfluenza 2 virus and
sera collected in 1957, neutralization being indicated by hemadsorp-

TABLE 58

Occurrence of type 2 parainfluenza virus neutralizing antibody
in sera collected in 1957

Age group	No. of sera tested	% of individuals with indicated titer of antibody			
		<8	8	16	32 or>
Adults	124	56	4	34	6
Children	104	68	6	18	8

tion-inhibition. The results shown in table 58 demonstrate that
antibody titers of 8 or greater were found in approximately one-third
of the children and one-half of the adults.

PARAINFLUENZA VIRUS, TYPE 3

More extensive studies were done with parafluenza virus, type 3.
The prevalence of antibody in all members of the population was
determined, as was the time of appearance of antibody during the

first 5 years of life, in a manner analogous to the serological studies with adenoviruses (Appendix 17).

Preliminary work showed that the neutralization test was a more sensitive indicator of the presence of antibody than was either the hemagglutination-inhibition test or the complement-fixation test, though there was close correlation between the results of all three tests. The neutralization test was therefore used in all experiments.

TABLE 59

Occurrence of antibody to type 3 parainfluenza virus in sera collected in 1957

Age group (years)	No. tested	Neutralizing antibody titer					
		<8		8 - 32		>32	
		No.	%	No.	%	No.	%
0 - 4	21	5	24	3	14	13	62
5 - 9	75	1	1	16	21	58	77
10 - 14	68	0	....	6	9	62	91
15+	23	0	....	2	9	21	91
Parents	119	0	....	13	11	106	89

Occurrence of antibody.—The sera obtained in the fall of 1957 were tested at final dilutions of 1:8 and 1:32. Table 59 shows the results. It can be seen that a high percentage of all individuals had antibody to the virus. In the 0-4 year age group 76% of individuals had a titer of 8 or greater, and 99-100% of older groups had antibody of this titer. An indication of the amount of antibody possessed by these individuals was obtained by determining the occurrence of antibody titers greater than 32. Titers of this magnitude were found in 62% of the 0-4 year age group, in 77% of the 5-9 year age group, and in 89-91% of all older groups. Thus almost all members of the population had antibody to parainfluenza virus, type 3; this antibody was usually present in significantly high titers and developed early in life.

Acquisition of antibody in the first 5 years of life.—The exact time of appearance of antibody was determined by testing the sera of children born into the study. Cord sera and matching maternal sera were available for 41 children. Sixty-five children had one or more sera collected at 6 months of age or later. For a variety of reasons, few children had complete sets of sera for the first five years of life.

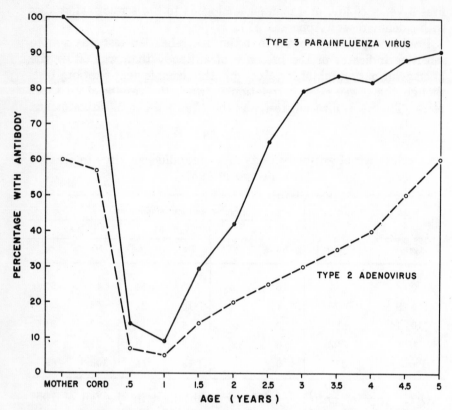

Fig. 44 *Disappearance of maternally transmitted and acquisition of active antibodies to type 3 parainfluenza virus and type 2 adenovirus in the first 5 years of life*

The results of this study are shown graphically in figure 44. Antibody was present in all of the mothers' sera and in 37 of the 41 cord sera. By 6 months of age only 2 of the 14 tested had antibody. It is possible that in one of these infants this represented maternal antibody, because the serum at 1 year of age contained no detectable antibody; the antibody level of the other at 1 year of age was unknown. The percentage of individuals with antibody remained low at 1 year of age (9.5%), but thereafter rose rapidly, reaching 65% by 2½ years of age. By 3½ years approximately 85% of the children had antibody.

Figure 44 compares the acquisition of parainfluenza virus, type 3, antibody with the acquisition of type 2 adenovirus antibody. Type 2 was chosen for this comparison because a higher percentage of individuals possess antibody for this type than for other adenovirus types and because type 2 antibody developed earlier in life.

It is evident that an even higher percentage of individuals have parainfluenza virus type 3 antibody and that this antibody is developed earlier in life. If may be concluded, therefore, that infections with parainfluenza virus, type 3, are commoner and occur at an earlier age than infections with adenovirus, type 2, as well as with the other types of adenovirus.

Chapter X
INFLUENZA

The study was carried out during the decade when the A1 or A-prime set of influenza viruses was generally prevalent. Strains of this set first appeared in 1947, the FM1 strain being their prototype at that time, and persisted until replaced by Asian (A2) strains in 1957. Influenza infections were recognized in the population in 5 of the first 6 years of the study. Influenza A1 viruses were isolated in 1949, 1950, 1951, and 1953; influenza B viruses were isolated in 1950 and 1952. Thus, measurement of the occurrence and recurrence of influenza in the same individuals and families was possible over a period of years (16). Further, it was possible to examine simultaneously the importance of two variables—immunity and antigenic variation—in relation to recurrent infections with members of the A1 set of viruses. In addition to the opportunity provided for intensive study of epidemic illnesses in 1950, 1951, and 1953, there was the opportunity to examine sera collected at 6-month intervals since 1948. These serologic studies spanned a 6-year period, and provided information regarding the pattern of antibody response exhibited by the individuals in the population during and between epidemics.

Moreover, the population was ideally suited for the collection of data regarding the impact of Asian influenza during its initial epidemic appearance in the U.S. in the fall of 1957 (17), and the study, which had been terminated in May, 1957, was reestablished for this purpose. By superimposing intensive clinical and laboratory observations on an existing epidemiologic framework, clinical and serological attack rates could be determined and measurements made of the influence of this new influenza virus on the bacterial flora of the upper respiratory tract. Further, the clinical characteristics of the illnesses produced by the A2 strain and those produced by the previous A1 strains could be compared.

In other analyses, the term "common respiratory diseases" was used to designate those respiratory illnesses from which a specific etiological agent was not isolated or which did not present a distinct clinical picture, such as nonbacterial tonsillitis and pharyngitis. Influenza was diagnosed only when a virus was isolated. The group of common respiratory diseases thus included "influenza-like" illnesses which were not proved by laboratory confirmation. For the purpose of the influenza studies the common respiratory illnesses were reclassified into two groups. The term "influenza-like" was used to designate those illnesses characterized by abrupt onset of fever, headache, myalgia, and other constitutional manifestations, and with symptoms referable to the throat and lower respiratory tract. The remaining undifferentiated respiratory infections characterized by symptoms such as sneezing, nasal discharge, irritated throat, hoarseness and cough were designated as "other common respiratory diseases."

THE INFLUENZA A1 YEARS

VIRUS ISOLATIONS

Periods during which specimens were collected are shown in Appendix 18, table 1, and details are given in Appendix 18. Only two strains of influenza virus B were isolated from individual specimens, one in 1950 and one in 1952; no further analysis was made of data relative to these isolations.

During the three A1 epidemic years influenza viruses were detected in the population for the following periods: in 1950, for 14 weeks from February 25 to May 25; in 1951, for 5 weeks from February 16 to March 23; in 1953, for 7 weeks from January 14 to February 24. In two of these years, 1950 and 1951, specimens were collected routinely at weekly intervals throughout the epidemic (1950) or at the peak of the epidemic (1951), in the search for carriers or inapparent infections. Virus was isolated only once from specimens collected from asymptomatic individuals.

In the three epidemic periods noted, A1 strains were isolated from 71 individuals, 30 adults and 41 children. Viruses were isolated from one person in 2 different years, 1950 and 1953. Thus, 70 individuals, representing 40 families, were infected as demonstrated by virus isolation studies, but recurrent infection in the same individual apparently was rare. A rather constant percentage of families yielded

TABLE 60

The isolation of type A1 influenza virus in three different years

| Year | No. | Families | | No. | Individuals | |
| | | Virus isolated | | | Virus isolated | |
		No.	%		No.	%
1950	57	14	24.6	257	18	7.0
1951	54	15	27.8	245	31	12.7
1953	68	18	26.5	325	22	6.8

virus in each of the 3 years (table 60). Of the 14 families with
virus in 1950, 11 were still in the study in 1951, and virus was
isolated from 1. Ten of the 1950 virus-positive families were still
under observation in 1953, and viruses were isolated from three. Of
the 15 families with virus in 1951, 14 were in the study in 1953,
and viruses were isolated from 4. Of the 18 families with viruses
in 1953, 17 had been observed in both 1950 and 1951, and viruses were
obtained from 7 in one of these years. In each instance the numbers
observed are the numbers expected if the virus isolation rates for
the given years are applied to the various families in the groups,
except in the case of the 1950 positive families where three isolations would have been expected in 1951. Thus, on the basis of
presence of virus in the families, there was a slight suggestion that
those families infected in 1950 were spared in 1951, but not in 1953.
On the basis of presence of virus in families, those families infected
in 1951 showed no evidence of "family immunity" in 1953.

CLINICAL ILLNESSES

Data from the 3 years 1950, 1951, and 1953 were compared to
examine the response of the population to the demonstrated
presence of influenza A1 virus. First, the clinical diagnoses were
tabulated on the basis of the symptoms reported by the individuals

TABLE 61

The clinical diagnoses in 71 individuals from whom type A1
influenza virus was isolated

Clinical diagnosis	Percent with diagnosis		
	1950	1951	1953
Influenza-like	57.9	83.9	68.2
Other common respiratory disease	36.8	9.7	18.2
Pneumococcal pneumonia	0	3.2	0
Streptococcal pharyngitis	0	0	4.5
Nonbacterial tonsillitis and pharyngitis	0	0	4.5
Roseola	0	3.2	0
Gastroenteritis	0	0	4.5
No illness	5.3	0	0

from whom the viruses were isolated (table 61). Then the illnesses
occurring in these persons and the members of their families in

an arbitrary period beginning 7 days before and ending 7 days after the isolation of virus were tabulated (table 62).

TABLE 62

The occurrence of illness in families at time of isolation of type A1 influenza virus

	1950		1951		1953	
	No.	%	No.	%	No.	%
Individuals	64	100.0	73	100.0	107	100.0
Illnesses						
Total	48	75.0	56	76.7	61	57.0
Respiratory disease	45	70.3	53	72.6	58	54.2
Influenza-like illness	18	28.1	42	57.5	35	32.7

Influenza A1 strains produced somewhat more severe illnesses in 1951 than in either 1950 or 1953, both in the individuals from whom viruses were isolated and in the members of their families. Of all the individuals exposed to virus in the families in 3 different years, about the same percentage developed respiratory symptoms. Thus, the occurrence of A1 infections in the community in the 2 preceding years (1949 and 1950) did not reduce the clinical manifestations of the disease in 1951. Indeed, a greater percentage of individuals had "influenza-like" illnesses in 1951 than in 1953 after an interval of 1 year during which influenza A1 infections were not recognized clinically or by isolation.

Although analysis of virus isolation data alone showed little or no evidence of immunity, and the clinical expression of influenza-like infection did not diminish in the total population in successive epidemics, the clinical data suggest that natural infection did confer some degree of immunity. When the occurrence of influenza-like illnesses during the three epidemic periods was tabulated in relation to the previous virus experiences of the individual's family (table 63), it was apparent that the occurrence of influenza-like illnesses in the members of a given family during one epidemic was influenced by whether or not influenza virus had been isolated from that family during the preceding epidemic. Of those individuals in virus-positive families in 1950, 6% had influenza-like illnesses in 1951. In contrast, of those not in demonstrated contact with the virus in 1950, 24% had such illnesses in 1951. Of those individuals living in families from which virus was isolated in 1951, 6% had influenza-like

TABLE 63

The occurrence of influenza-like illnesses according to whether
or not influenza virus had been demonstrated in members of the
same families during the preceding epidemic

Virus present in families		Total number of individuals	Influenza-like illnesses	
			No.	%
		1951		
1950	Yes	53	3	5.7
	No	192	46	24.0
		1953		
1951	Yes	69	4	5.8
	No	161	33	20.5

Occurrence of illness in epidemic spans Total number and Influenza-like illnesses columns.

illnesses in 1953; in contrast, 20% of persons not in contact with
the virus in 1951 suffered influenza-like illnesses in 1953. Thus,
prior familial contact with the virus effected an approximate 70%
reduction in rates of influenza-like disease after an interval of either
1 or 2 years.

Of other tabulations done to measure immunity, one utilized the
antibody responses described subsequently. Individuals who developed four-fold or greater increases in titer as a result of the 1951
epidemic experienced a 50% reduction in development of such
increases during the 1953 epidemic. Of 39 individuals who had such
a rise in titer in 1951, 7 (18%) also had a rise in 1953. In contrast,
of 99 individuals who failed to show a rise in titer in 1951, 40 (40%)
showed rises in 1953—differences which are significant ($P=.02$).
Tabulations similar to those in table 63 and comparable analyses of
antibody responses showed that families and individuals who had
had influenza in 1950 did not have a reduced attack rate in 1953.
Thus, when influenza-like illnesses in the families were used as the
criterion for immunity, individuals in families infected in 1950 had
significantly less influenza in 1951, and individuals in families infected in 1951 had less influenza in 1953. Some degree of immunity,
then, persisted for 1 or 2 years, but not for three.

SEROLOGICAL STUDIES

Table 64 shows the increases and decreases in titer of antibodies
against influenza viruses A and B demonstrated in serum specimens

TABLE 64

Relative frequency of fourfold changes in influenza antibody titer during consecutive 6-month intervals

Time interval*	A antigens**			B antigens***		
	No. tested	Increase %	Decrease %	No. tested	Increase %	Decrease %
F47-S48	33	15.2	12.1	31	3.2	16.1
S48-F48	128	17.2	7.0	123	9.8	8.1
F48-S49	171	16.4	12.3	162	7.4	10.5
S49-F49	162	15.4	12.3	154	9.1	7.8
F49-S50	188	14.9	11.7	180	17.2	11.7
S50-F50	202	6.4	7.9	192	10.9	10.3
F50-S51	189	23.8	7.9	178	5.6	11.2
S51-F51	172	6.4	12.2	167	11.4	9.6
F51-S52	211	10.0	11.8	205	26.8	12.7
S52-F52	228	5.7	7.0	228†	4.8	7.0
F52-S53	244	26.6	5.7	244†	4.9	2.9
S53-F53	219	6.4	8.2	219†	1.4	2.3

*In this table S designates spring and F designates fall.
**PR8, FM1, FW1/53 viruses.
***Lee and WRU/53/50 viruses.
†Lee antigen was omitted for these series of tests.

collected approximately every 6 months. Although not shown in this summary table, the majority of these rises were measured with antigens closely related to the current strain. FM1 (1947) virus was a more sensitive antigen than PR8 (1934); A/FW1/53 was, in turn a better antigen than FM1; WRU/53/50 was a more sensitive B antigen than Lee (1940).

The data indicate that infections with influenza viruses were constantly occurring. During epidemic periods 15 to 25% of individuals showed significant increases in titer to the prevalent viruses, both A and B in 1950, A in 1951 and 1953, and B in 1952. During each endemic period, rises in titer were found. The majority of increases in the endemic periods were measured with antigens closely related to the current strain, and when examined for a single antigen, FM1 virus, 17 to 60% of significant increases were eight-fold or greater. These facts support the conclusion that the titer increases were, indeed, induced by endemic infections.

In addition to plotting median antibody levels for segments of the population, two other methods were used to illustrate fluctuations in the antibody profile of the population over the 6-year period. Both methods represent attempts to illustrate net changes in antibody levels in reference to the susceptibility of the population and

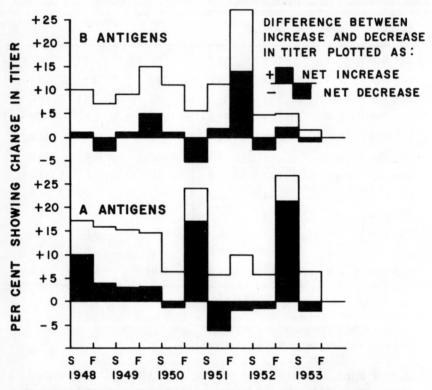

Fig. 45   Influenza "antibody balance": changes in antibody titer during consecutive 6-month intervals plotted so as to show net percentage of individuals who showed four-fold or greater increases or decreases in titer

the occurrence of epidemic disease. Figure 45 illustrates the first approach. Here the percentage of individuals showing 4-fold or greater increase in titer (table 64) is plotted up from the zero point. Then the percentage of individuals showing decreases in titer is plotted down from the increase point. The shaded areas show the difference between the two and represent a kind of "antibody balance" for the population. Figure 46 was constructed to show average changes in titer plotted as fractions of a two-fold dilution. The curves do not reflect absolute mean antibody levels, but rather indicate again the balance between increases and decreases in titer. The occurrence of influenza A1 infections in the spring of 1950 is

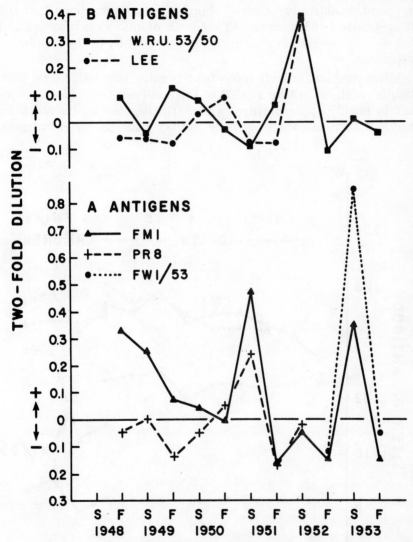

AVERAGE CHANGE IN ANTIBODY TITER

Fig. 46 "Antibody balance": Average changes in antibody titer
at successive 6-month intervals

not reflected by either method for these infections apparently did
not interrupt the downward trend of change that began after the
occurrence of similar infections in 1949. The 1951 and 1953 A1
epidemics are strikingly shown, as is the 1952 B epidemic. Figure

45 shows that before the influenza A epidemics of 1951 and 1953 and the influenza B epidemics of 1950 and 1952, the population showed more falls than rises and thus, in a sense, had developed a "negative antibody balance." Similarly, figure 46 shows that the B epidemic of 1952 and the A1 epidemic of 1953 were preceded and followed by periods during which the average titer of the population decreased.

When median antibody levels for the entire population were plotted, fluctuations in titer related to the occurrence of epidemics were not so readily apparent (figures 47-50). Only the adults and older children had significant levels of antibody for the older antigens,

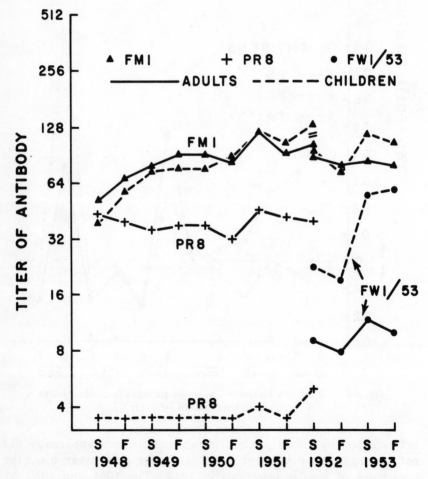

Fig. 47   *Median levels of antibody to influenza A virus antigens at successive 6-month intervals*

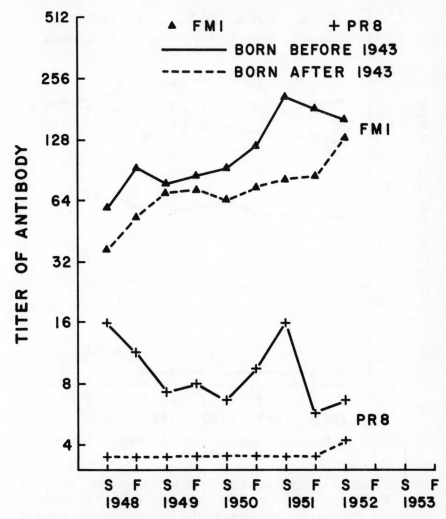

Fig. 48   Median levels of antibody to influenza A virus antigens in children
of different ages

PR8 (A) and Lee (B). The median FM1 titers for adults and
children were similar and ran parallel (figure 47), and the response
of the children to the more recent A/FW1/53 antigen started at a
higher level and was greater. However, the levels of median titers
to more recent antigens, such as FM1 and B/WRU/53-50, were not
influenced significantly by the presence or absence of antibody to
the older antigens. Only those children with prior PR8 or Lee antibodies (figures 48 and 50) developed increases in titer of these antibodies when exposed to the more recent antigens.

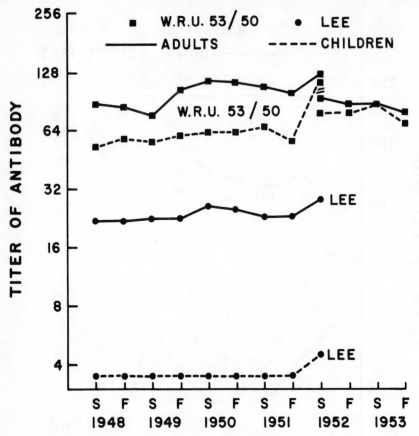

*Fig. 49   Median levels of antibody to influenza B virus antigens in
children and adults*

By utilizing the virus isolation data it was possible to derive
curves for median antibody titers which did reflect the epidemic
occurrence of influenza. In figure 51 the median antibody titers of
the three groups of individuals from whom influenza A1 viruses
were isolated in 1950, 1951, and 1953 are plotted. The median
FM1 titer of those individuals from whom virus was isolated in 1950
more than doubled in the spring of that year, and increased four-
fold by fall. There was an accompanying change in PR8 antibody
level. This group had a low level of antibody for the new A1 strain
of 1953, but showed no response to this antigen. In marked contrast,
the median FM1 titer of those individuals from whom virus was
isolated in 1951 remained constant in 1950, only to increase six-fold
in 1951. Again there was an accompanying change in the median
PR8 antibody level. This group already had a respectable level of

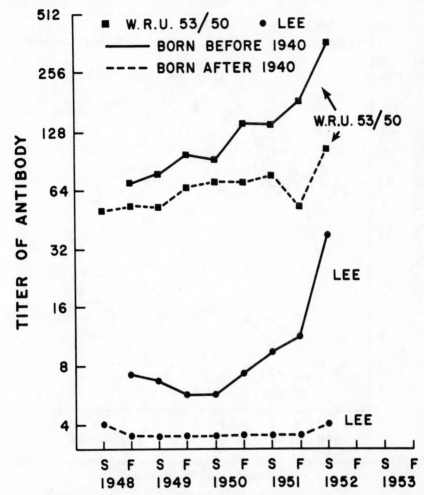

Fig. 50   Median levels of antibody to influenza B virus antigens in
children of different ages

antibody for the 1953 virus in sera drawn in the spring of 1952, and
the level actually decreased during the 1953 epidemic. By 1952,
all components of the population had good levels of FM1 antibody,
and infections with A1 viruses might have smouldered along except
for the appearance of an antigenic variant within the A1 set of
viruses, represented by A/FW1/53. Those individuals in the groups
infected in either 1950 or 1951 had antibody which inhibited this
strain, the median titers being 12 and 64, respectively, but those
individuals from whom influenza viruses were isolated in 1953 had
a median A/FW1/53 titer of only slightly more than 4 (figure

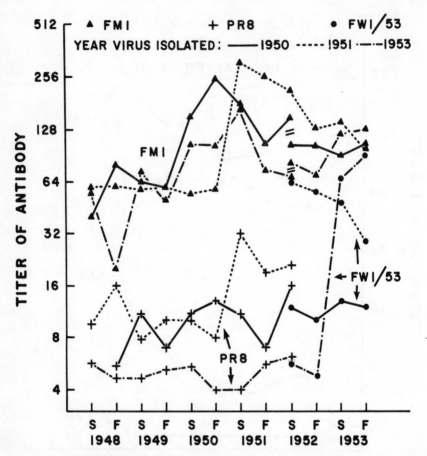

Fig. 51　Median antibody levels of individuals from whom influenza A viruses
were isolated in 3 different years

51). This group showed a striking increase in the level of antibody
to this new antigen, and was the only group to show an increase
of FM1 antibody. Thus, when correlated with the virus isolation
data, the serologic studies further demonstrated that recurrent influenza A1 infections involved different individuals in different years.

It is clear that studies during the 6-year period, 1948-1953, provided information particularly regarding the occurrence of infection
with members of the A1 family of viruses. In the 2 years following
the appearance of the FM1 strain in 1947, 15% of individuals developed increases in titers of antibodies in each 6-month interval, and
A1 viruses were isolated from influenza-like illnesses in 1949 and
1950. During endemic intervals when influenza was not recognized
clinically, 5 to 10% of individuals developed significant increases in

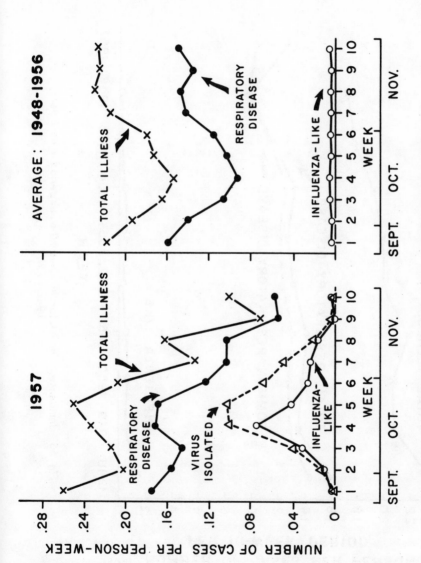

Fig. 52   Incidence of illness by week during comparable 10-week periods, 1948-1956 and 1957

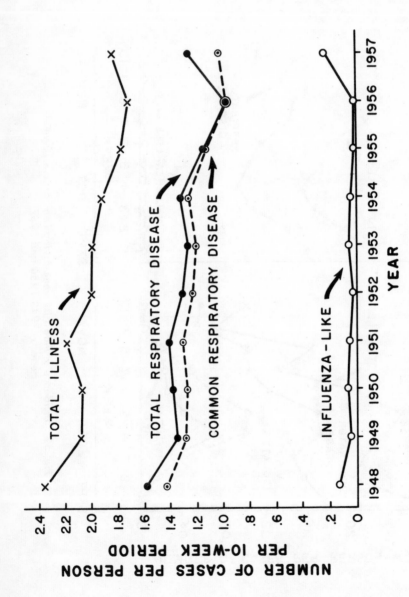

Fig. 53   *Incidence of illness, for the same 10-week period in each year, 1948-1957*

titer of antibodies. With the occurrence of A1 epidemics in 1951 and
1953, approximately 25% of the population demonstrated serologic
evidence of infection. As measured by virus isolation also, approximately one-fourth of the families were infected in each of the three
A1 epidemic years, and one-half to three-quarters of the individuals
in these families suffered respiratory illnesses at that time. The
illness, virus isolation, and serologic attack rates recorded seemed
high when first measured, but these rates were quite low compared
to those observed with the appearance of the Asian influenza (A2)
virus.

ASIAN INFLUENZA

As already mentioned, detailed study of the families had been
discontinued in the spring of 1957. In anticipation of the Asian
influenza epidemic the study was reactivated in September, 1957
when the 60 remaining families agreed to participate again in the
collection of detailed clinical and epidemiological data. A2 virus was
first isolated in Cleveland in June, 1957, and two other sporadic
infections were documented in July and August. The first known
case in the study population occurred on September 2; Cleve-

TABLE 65

The occurrence of illness and testing of illnesses for influenza A2
virus, September 22—November 30, 1957

Clinical category	Total illnesses during period		Illnesses tested for virus		Virus isolated from illness	
	No.	Percent*	No.	Percent**	No.	Percent†
Respiratory disease						
Influenza-like	71	12.5 ⎫	71	100.0 ⎫	65	91.5 ⎫
Other common R.D.	314	55.1 ⎬ 68.2	211	67.2 ⎬ 73.3	56	26.5 ⎬ 42.5
Specific R.D.	4	0.7 ⎭	3	75.0 ⎭	0	0.0 ⎭
Gastroenteritis	100	17.5	29 (10)‡	29.0	5 (3)‡	17.2
All other illnesses	81	14.2	11 (2)‡	13.6	0	0.0
Totals	570	100.0	325 ‡	57.0	126 ‡	38.8

*Percent of total illnesses.   **Percent of illnesses in clinical category.
†Percent of illnesses tested for viruses.
‡Twelve persons each had 2 illnesses with simultaneous onsets. In 10 instances, a respiratory
  disease and a gastroenteritis began at the same time and were tested by the same swab.
  Virus was recovered in 3 such instances. Thus virus was isolated from 123 persons at the
  time of 126 illnesses.

land schools opened on September 9; the next two cases occurred on September 19 and 20 at the beginning of the epidemic.

PATTERN OF ILLNESS

As in previous years, respiratory disease rates had risen after the opening of schools and were already high by the week of September 22, which is Week 1 in figure 52. For the next 2 weeks, nearly all of the respiratory illnesses resembled the common cold and its variants. Then more severe, influenza-like illnesses increased in frequency, reaching a peak during the week of October 13, the fourth week of the study. In 8 weeks the epidemic was over. Unlike previous years, the rates for both total illness and respiratory disease were low at the end of the 10-week period. When curves were constructed for comparable 10-week periods in each of the preceding 9 years, it was seen that the epidemic of Asian influenza almost completely reversed the earlier curves. Despite this marked alteration in the pattern of occurrence of illness, there was surprisingly little change in the total amount of illness experienced by the population (figure 53). In 1957, the total respiratory disease rate was boosted just enough by the occurrence of influenza-like illnesses to return almost to the level of 1954. Further, despite the epidemic, the distribution of illness by broad diagnostic categories (table 65) resembled the stable figures for this same population in previous years (table 2). Respiratory infections accounted for two-thirds of all illnesses; 18% of all illnesses were classified as gastroenteritis. Twelve percent of all illnesses were classified as influenza-like.

TABLE 66

Incidence of influenza A2 by age, 1957

Age group (years)	Measure of infection	
	Virus isolation %	Antibody increase* %
0-4	43	50
5-9	58	67
10-14	59	78
15+	47	71
Adults	19	24
Total	41	55

*In unvaccinated persons

VIRUS ISOLATIONS AND SEROLOGICAL STUDIES

Approximately 73% of all respiratory illnesses were sampled for viruses; A2 virus was recovered from 42.5% (table 65). Virus was isolated from 92% of those thought clinically to be influenza and 27% of milder illnesses classified clinically as common respiratory diseases. A2 viruses were isolated from 52 (86.7%) of the 60 families and from 126 (40.9%) of the 308 members of these families. The combined results of the complement-fixation and hemagglutination-inhibition tests showed that 93% of persons from whom virus was isolated showed four-fold or greater increases in antibody titer.

All told, 60% of the population developed increases in antibody titer during the epidemic. This rate, however, was not the true serologic attack rate, for a number of the titer increases measured by the hemagglutination-inhibition test could be attributed to vaccination. For this reason, only unvaccinated individuals were considered when calculating serologic attack rates by age (table 66), and by

TABLE 67

Incidence of influenza A2 by class of individual, 1957

Family status	Measure of infection	
	Virus isolation %	Antibody increase* %
Father	13	16
Mother	24	32
School child	57	73
Preschool child	44	30
Total	41	55

*In unvaccinated persons

family status (table 67). Attack rates for children were much higher than for adults and were maximum in the 5 to 15+ year old groups. The pattern of attack rates in the family resembled that of the common respiratory diseases, being lowest in the fathers and highest in the school children. The importance of the school was emphasized by further examination of the data. Considering the first virus-positive case as the index case, influenza was introduced into the 52 households as follows: 43 times by a school child (83% of all intro-

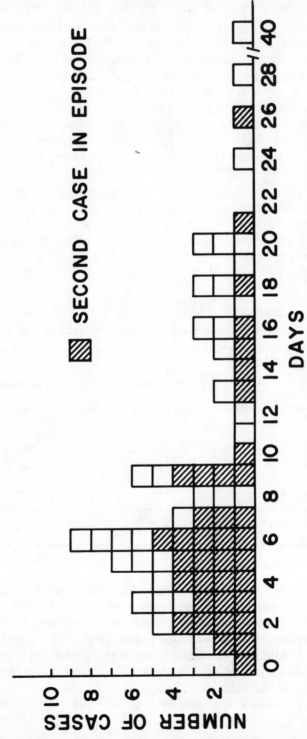

Fig. 54   Intervals between onsets of first and subsequent virus-positive
cases of influenza in families

ductions), once simultaneously by a school child and mother, 3 times by a mother and pre-school child, and only twice by a father.

The virus obviously spread within the home, but an unexpected observation was the length of intervals between the onsets of virus-positive cases. As measured by virus isolation, the secondary attack rate was 35%; as measured by antibody response, the secondary attack rate in 21 unvaccinated families was 36.5%. However, the length of the intervals between the onsets of virus-positive cases suggested that many secondary infections were not acquired in the home (figure 54). Considering all multiple cases, the average of the intervals between the first and all subsequent cases was 9.4 days; the median interval was 7.4 days. The average of the intervals between successive cases was 5.3 days; the median interval was 3.8 days.

CLINICAL ASPECTS

Adequate clinical data were recorded for 125 virus-positive cases of Asian influenza in 1957. A few cases of influenza A1 infection had been recognized in 1956, and these added to those from the three other epidemic years provided 73 cases of influenza A1 infection diagnosed by virus isolation. These two groups were then compared to determine whether or not the A2 cases differed clinically from those previously seen. Ninety-five (76%) of the cases of Asian influenza were less than 15 years of age, and 30 were 15 years or older. Forty-five (62%) of the previous cases were less than 15 years of age, and 28 were 15 years or older. The occurrence of various symptoms and clinical signs in 1957 and in previous years is shown in tables 68 and 69. The symptoms and signs of Asian influenza were similar to those of previous influenza A infections and this new variant, therefore, was not associated in this population with any distinctive clinical features when contrasted with previous influenza A infections.

THE EFFECT ON BACTERIAL FLORA

When all laboratory measurements of infection were combined, the data showed that 146 of the 308 adults and children had been infected, an individual attack rate of 47.4%; 54 of the 60 families were infected, a family attack rate of 90%. Despite the very high attack rate with a new influenza virus, which experienced similar success throughout the world, the virus had very little effect on the pharyngeal bacterial flora of the adults and children in this population. When pre- and post-epidemic surveys for bacteria were compared, the post-epidemic increase in the numbers of streptococci was insignificant, and the increase of pneumococci was no greater than that which could be attributed to season (table 70). Further,

TABLE 68

Occurrence of various symptoms in proved cases of Asian (A2) influenza (1957) and in previous cases of influenza A1 (1950, 1951, 1953, 1956)

Symptoms	Asian influenza, 1957			Influenza A1, 1950, 1951, 1953, 1956		
	0-14 yrs. (95 cases)	15+ yrs. (30 cases)	Total (125 cases)	0-14 yrs. (45 cases)	15+ yrs. (28 cases)	Total (73 cases)
	Percent showing symptoms*					
Sudden onset	65.2	46.4	61.0	66.6	32.1	53.4
Chilliness	37.2	64.3	43.4	54.5	78.6	63.9
Feverishness	92.6	71.4	87.8	91.1	78.6	86.3
Headache	80.6	72.4	78.7	59.5	82.1	68.6
Myalgia	32.9	62.1	39.8	17.7	78.6	44.1
Irritable	17.0	22.2	18.2	33.3	42.9	37.0
Listless	68.0	66.6	67.8	73.3	71.4	72.6
Sneezing	37.8	66.6	44.3	40.0	50.0	56.2
Nasal discharge	67.3	82.1	70.7	73.3	92.9	80.8
Obstructed nose	54.2	51.8	57.9	46.6	71.4	56.2
Sore throat	62.3	62.1	62.3	42.8	75.0	55.7
Hoarseness	22.3	37.0	25.6	28.8	32.1	30.1
Cough	86.3	89.7	87.1	75.5	92.9	82.2
Sputum	19.1	40.7	24.0	22.2	55.6	34.7
Anorexia	69.1	37.0	62.0	71.1	64.3	68.5
Nausea	23.4	3.7	19.0	†	†	†
Vomiting	26.3	7.4	22.1	24.4	3.7	16.7
Diarrhea	2.1	0.0	1.7	11.1	11.1	11.1
Abdominal pain	31.1	0.0	24.2	†	†	†

*Percentages represent the proportion showing a given symptom of those cases in which presence or absence was specifically recorded.

†Data not available.

TABLE 69

Occurrence of various physical signs in proved cases of Asian (A2) influenza (1957) and in previous cases of influenza A1 (1950, 1951, 1953, 1956)

Physical signs	Asian influenza, 1957			Influenza A1, 1950, 1951, 1953, 1956		
	0-14 yrs. (95 cases)	15+yrs. (30 cases)	Total (125 cases)	0-14 yrs. (45 cases)	15+yrs. (28 cases)	Total (73 cases)
	Percent showing physical signs*					
Moderately severe illness	44.5	20.8	41.0	57.5	43.5	52.4
Flushed face	28.4	24.0	28.2	37.5	8.7	27.0
Conjunctival abnormalities	61.1	56.0	60.2	40.4	13.0	30.2
Nasal discharge	38.0	20.0	34.2	47.5	30.4	41.3
Nasal injection	50.4	64.0	55.2	46.0	28.6	40.0
Nasal edema	33.5	4.0	28.4	15.3	14.3	15.0
Tonsillar exudate	2.5	0.0	2.2	11.1	0.0	10.0
Palatal injection	39.0	44.0	40.2	17.9	13.6	16.4
Pharyngeal injection	60.0	68.0	60.9	50.0	73.9	58.7
Pharyngeal lymphoid hyperplasia	45.0	32.0	42.4	17.5	39.1	25.4
Pharyngeal exudate	1.0	0.0	0.9	0.0	0.0	0.0
Cervical adenopathy	37.7	8.0	29.1	45.0	8.7	31.7
Tender cervical nodes	5.4	0.0	4.3	12.8	8.7	11.3
Pulmonary abnormalities	2.2	0.0	2.2	0.0	0.0	0.0
Complications	10.8	4.0	9.3	12.5	16.7	14.1
Maximum temperature: (F)						
100°	10.9	12.5	11.3	4.7	13.1	7.7
100−101.9°	38.5	58.3	34.8	16.6	47.8	27.7
102°+	60.4	29.2	53.9	78.5	39.1	64.6

*Percentages represent the proportion showing a given sign of those cases in which presence or absence was specifically recorded.

TABLE 70

Pharyngeal flora before and after Asian influenza epidemic

| Organisms present in pharynx | Pre-epidemic surveys | | | | Post-epidemic survey | |
| | First | | Second* | | | |
	No.	Percent	No.	Percent	No.	Percent
No. cultured	303†	100.0	278	100.0	307	100.0
Streptococci	3	1.0	1	0.4	10	3.3
Staphylococci	35	11.6	18	6.5	30	9.8
Pneumococci	10	3.3	16	5.8	37	12.1
H. influenzae	4†	1.7	12	4.3	7	2.3

*Individuals with respiratory illnesses excluded.
†238 persons tested for H. influenzae in this period.

TABLE 71

The influence of influenza A2 virus on the pharyngeal flora at time of respiratory illness

Organisms in pharynx	Present at time of illness				Acquired* at time of illness			
	Virus+		Virus—		Virus+		Virus—	
	No.	Percent	No.	Percent	No.	Percent	No.	Percent
No. cultured	118	100.0	159	100.0	116		155	
Streptococci	5	4.2	5	3.1		3.4		2.6
Staphylococci	15	12.7	15	9.4	108	12.0	142	8.5
Pneumococci	10	8.5	16	10.1	106	8.5	147	8.2
H. influenzae	7	5.9	17	10.7	104	2.9	140	7.9

*Organism considered as acquired if absent at time of preceding culture.

the bacterial flora present or acquired at the time of those respiratory illnesses from which viruses were recovered differed little from that of illnesses which were negative for influenza virus (table 71). When the results of the pre-epidemic and post-epidemic cultures from individuals designated as "influenza-positive" were compared, insignifiicant changes occurred with streptococci and *H. influenzae*. As regards staphylococci, the proportion of individuals who acquired the organism following influenza was exactly balanced by the proportion of such individuals who lost this organism during the epidemic period. For pneumococci, acquisition was actually higher for those individuals who did not have influenza, and for all individuals the yield was comparable to carrier rates expected at this time of year. Thus, the passage of A2 influenza virus through this particular population produced no significant change in the pharyngeal flora of its members.

COMMENTS

The observations reported contributed in a small way to the growing understanding of the epidemiologic mechanisms responsible for the recurrence and periodicity of epidemics and pandemics of influenza (122). Although the factors responsible for the emergence of variant strains remain a mystery, data were obtained regarding the behavior of members of the last two sets, or families, of influenza A viruses to appear. The behavior of A1 viruses was recorded during the 6-year period following their appearance; the initial epidemic due to A2 virus was studied in detail. Less extensive data were collected regarding the behavior of influenza B virus infections.

In addition to the documentation of epidemic disease, the longitudinal study demonstrated that both influenza A1 and B infections occurred throughout the 6-year period, 1948-1953. The fact that 5 to 10% of individuals developed significant increases in titer of antibodies for A or B viruses during successive 6-month intervals, although the disease was not recognized clinically, confirms the notion that these viruses persist in the population in interepidemic periods. What triggered the A1 and B epidemics in the late winters and springs during the first half of the 1950's is unknown, but observation of the same individuals and families showed that epidemics occurred following periods during which more decreases than increases in antibody titer had occurred in the population and that members of families infected in 1 year had significantly less influenza the next. With members of the A1 set of influenza viruses, then, the occurrence of influenza could be related to at least three factors: chance, persistence of immunity for 2 years, and the emergence of minor antigenic variants.

When A2 virus appeared, few, if any, members of the population had specific antibody. In contrast to serological attack rates of 15 to 25% observed with the A1 strains, the serological attack rate in unvaccinated persons was 55% for the A2 virus. In comparison with the earlier A1 epidemics, Asian virus infected more than three times as many families and two to three times as many persons. Despite this high attack rate, the clinical disease produced resembled that caused by the A1 strains; no significant alterations in the bacterial pharyngeal flora in the population accompanied or followed the virus infections, and no complications occurred. There were no individuals over 60 years of age in the particular population under study, and this may account for the fact that no complications were observed, for in the greater Cleveland area, as throughout the United States and the world, the Asian influenza epidemic was associated with an excess number of deaths from influenza and pneumonia (58, 103). The morbidity rates and the pattern of spread in the Cleveland population was consistent with that reported for the rest of the United States (132). In particular, the importance of the school is emphasized by the Cleveland data. The attack rate was highest in the 5 to 15+ year old age group, and school children were responsible for more than four-fifths of the introductions of virus into the homes. Further, the length of the intervals between the onsets of the index and subsequent virus-positive cases in the families suggests that many of the secondary infections were acquired at school rather than in the home. The median interval of 7.4 days between the first and all subsequent cases is very similar to the interval observed in outbreaks in two other cities (56). These data suggest that during the initial wave of Asian influenza community spread of the virus was greater than intra-family spread. There is no ready explanation for this apparently paradoxical behavior of a highly infectious agent, but one explanation which may be offered is that it was the result of a combination of the greater susceptibility of children plus the opportunity for greater multiplicity of contact within the school. Virus had been present in the community for more than 3 months before the epidemic, and in Cleveland, as elsewhere, the opening of schools seems to have been one of the provocations that triggered the epidemic (84). A2 infections have continued to occur in Cleveland, as elsewhere, and it will be interesting to learn whether members of the A2 set of viruses dominate the next decade and behave as did members of the A1 family.

Chapter XI

GASTROINTESTINAL ILLNESSES

Infectious gastroenteritis ranked second in frequency of occurrence in the study; approximately 16% of all illnesses recorded were placed in this diagnostic category. The contents of this chapter are divided into three major sections. The first shows the incidence of infectious gastroenteritis, or acute nonbacterial gastroenteritis, as well as its introduction into and spread within families; the second presents a description of the clinical characteristics of the syndrome; and the third concerns etiology and includes data derived from transmission studies in volunteers.

INCIDENCE

As in the case of respiratory disease, staff members relied heavily on clinical judgement in identifying and classifying gastrointestinal illnesses. There were, for example, many instances in which gastrointestinal symptoms occurred, but seemed, in the opinion of the clinician, to be secondary to another illness or due to some cause other than illness. Such cases were not classified as infectious gastroenteritis. A detailed discussion of the methods used to identify and classify gastrointestinal illnesses is included in Appendix 19.

A total of 4057 cases of infectious gastroenteritis occurred in the study, an incidence rate of 1.52 cases per person-year. The variation in total incidence of these illnesses from year to year is shown in table 4. In distinction to the incidence of respiratory disease which decreased with the passage of time, the incidence of infectious gastroenteritis fluctuated from year to year but showed no overall trend. The seasonal pattern of occurrence is shown in figure 3.

INCIDENCE BY AGE AND SEX

The incidence of infectious gastroenteritis was lower in both male and female infants under 1 year of age than in children during the next several years of life (figure 55). From age one through age 9 or 10 years the incidence was relatively constant for both sexes and slightly higher for boys than for girls. Above age 13 years the rates for females were somewhat higher than for males. The person-years of observation in this age group were, however, based on a small number of individuals. The incidence among mothers was slightly higher than that among fathers through age 41; above this age the reverse was true (table 72).

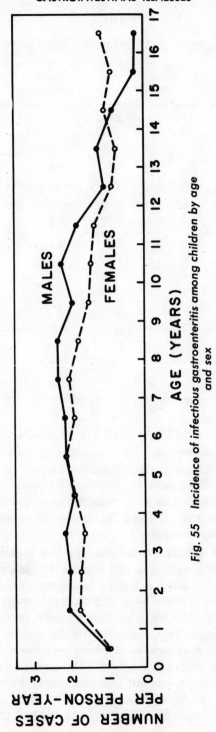

Fig. 55 *Incidence of infectious gastroenteritis among children by age and sex*

TABLE 72

Incidence of infectious gastroenteritis among parents by sex and age

Age group in years	Number of illnesses	Number of person-days	Cases per person-year
A. Males			
22-31	57	26,722	0.78
32-41	412	146,177	1.03
42-51	71	29,264	0.89
B. Females			
22-31	207	62,935	1.20
32-41	475	125,678	1.38
42-51	25	14,342	0.64
C. Total			
22-31	264	89,657	1.07
32-41	887	271,855	1.19
42-51	96	43,606	0.80

INCIDENCE IN RELATION TO SCHOOL ATTENDANCE

The use of the two variables, school attendance and family size, as measures of the effect of "adequate contact" on the incidence of illness has been discussed in Chapter VI in relation to the common respiratory diseases. The same reasoning presumably applies to consideration of the role of these factors in determining the incidence of infectious gastroenteritis.

The effect of school attendance on the incidence of infectious gastroenteritis (figure 56) is not completely definitive. School children, however, did have a higher incidence at ages 3 and 5 years than did children not in school, and the rates were, in general, higher among preschool children who had siblings in school than among preschool children of the same age who did not. When the incidence among these three groups of children was examined separately for that part of the year when school was in session (September-May) and that part when it was not (June-August) a consistent difference in rates among the three groups was seen to occur only during the school months (figure 57). These facts suggest that school attend-

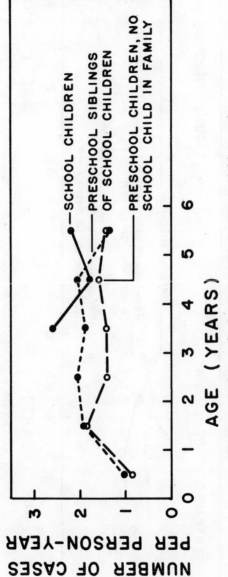

Fig. 56 Incidence of infectious gastroenteritis in children under 6 years of age, by age and school status

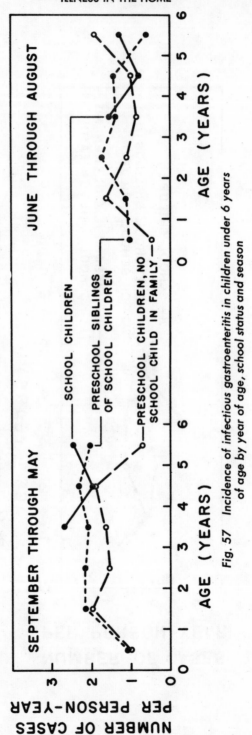

Fig. 57 Incidence of infectious gastroenteritis in children under 6 years of age by year of age, school status and season

ance and intra-familial contact with children attending school may have been of some importance in determining the incidence among children. The role of school attendance in the introduction of infectious gastroenteritis into the family is considered in a later section.

INCIDENCE IN RELATION TO FAMILY SIZE

The number of cases per family per year increased with increasing family size (table 73); this would be expected, since in larger fami-

TABLE 73

Incidence of infectious gastroenteritis by family size

Family size	Person-days	Family days	Number of illnesses	Illnesses per family-year	Illnesses per person-year
3	38,991	12,997	104	2.92	0.97
4	269,604	67,401	869	4.71	1.18
5	399,450	79,890	1671	7.63	1.53
6	201,396	33,566	1044	11.35	1.89
7	36,491	5,213	189	13.23	1.89
8	31,104	3,888	180	16.90	2.11
Total	977,036	202,955	4057	7.30	1.52

lies there are more persons to become ill. The incidence of these illnesses among individual family members also became progressively higher with increased family size, presumably as a result of a greater number of introductions of illness and a greater number of intra-familial exposures in larger families. Mothers, fathers, and children all showed an increase in frequency with increase in family size (table 74).

DETAILED STUDY OF GASTROINTESTINAL SYMPTOMS
1948-1950

In the classification of illnesses as infectious gastroenteritis, those cases with gastrointestinal symptoms which were considered to be secondary to other illnesses or to be due to causes other than illness were excluded, as has already been indicated. To obtain information about all occurrences of gastrointestinal symptoms, regardless of whether they were considered to be primary or secondary, a detailed study of the original records was made for the 3-year period 1948-1950. This study was undertaken for two reasons. First, in describing the spread of infectious gastroenteritis in families, as well as the

TABLE 74

Incidence of infectious gastroenteritis in male adults, female adults and children by family size

Family size	Male adults			Female adults			Children		
	Person-days	No. of illnesses	Illnesses per person-year	Person-days	No. of illnesses	Illnesses per person-year	Person-days	No. of illnesses	Illnesses per person-year
3	12,997	18	0.51	12,997	31	0.87	12,997	55	1.54
4	66,913	133	0.73	67,401	174	0.94	135,290	562	1.52
5	79,586	221	1.01	79,890	295	1.35	239,974	1155	1.76
6	33,566	137	1.49	33,566	159	1.73	134,264	748	2.03
7	5,213	22	1.54	5,213	23	1.61	26,065	144	2.02
8	3,888	9	0.84	3,888	25	2.35	23,328	146	2.28
7+8	9,101	31	1.24	9,101	48	1.93	49,393	290	2.14
Total	202,163	540	0.97	202,955	707	1.27	571,918	2810	1.79

clinical characteristics of this syndrome, it seemed desirable to be able to state precisely how many occurrences of gastrointestinal symptoms had been excluded as being secondary to other causes and to give the reasons for their exclusion. Second, the investigation of the association between respiratory and gastrointestinal symptoms described in the following section required an accurate count of all instances in which the two groups of symptoms occurred together in the same individual. In the routine diagnosing of illnesses, this concurrence was frequently considered to represent gastrointestinal symptoms occurring secondarily to another illness, e.g., common respiratory disease.

The methods used to select and classify gastrointestinal illnesses in this study differed somewhat (see Appendix 19) from methods used in the routine diagnosis of those illnesses. Briefly, though both sets of methods depended largely on clinical judgment in determining which gastrointestinal symptoms should be considered secondary to other causes, these major features distinguish the techniques used in the 1948-1950 study:

1) All occurrences of gastrointestinal symptoms were listed (see Appendix 19 for definition).

2) The illness records were carefully searched for notes by mothers, field workers, and visiting physicians suggesting possible explanations for the occurrence of gastrointestinal symptoms. These explanations were listed and evaluated. From them was compiled a roster of explanations that were considered adequate causes for gastrointestinal symptoms and each such cause was then consistently accepted.

3) The presence of a common respiratory disease in an individual was not considered to be the cause of gastrointestinal symptoms unless some specific mechanism (e.g., vomiting caused by hard coughing) was noted.

4) All otherwise unexplained occurrences of gastrointestinal symptoms were classified as cases of infectious gastroenteritis.

By these criteria, 1466 occurrences of gastrointestinal symptoms were identified during 1948-1950. Of these, 362 were accompanied by circumstances included on the list of acceptable explanations and were thus considered to be due to causes other than infectious gastroenteritis (Appendix 19, table 1). For the purpose of computing incidence and studying intra-familial spread of infection, the remaining 1104 occurrences of gastrointestinal symptoms were considered together as infectious gastroenteritis. The association of certain of these illnesses with common respiratory symptoms in the same individual and the evidence that this association may sometimes represent a separate syndrome are discussed in a later section.

The total incidence of infectious gastroenteritis during 1948-1950, based on 1104 cases, was 1.64 cases per person-year. This is quite similar to the 10-year incidence of cases classified as infectious gastroenteritis by routine methods of diagnosis. In general, the various specific incidence rates for the two periods are also similar and therefore those for 1948-1950 (11) are not presented here.

INTRODUCTION AND SPREAD OF INFECTIOUS GASTRO-ENTERITIS IN THE FAMILY

The measurement of the relative importance of various family members in introducing an infectious illness into a family and the use of secondary attack rates to describe the spread of such an illness within the family have been discussed in Chapter VI with respect to the common respiratory diseases. The discussion of the rationale for employing these methods, as well as their limitations, applies also to their use in the study of infectious gastroenteritis. The family episodes upon which these analyses were carried out were defined as follows:

An episode began with the onset of infectious gastroenteritis in a member of a family in which no similar illness had begun during the prior 19 days. That illness represented the index case for that particular episode. If a second case occurred in a family on the same calendar day, it was also considered an index case for the same episode. Included in the episode were all other cases beginning in the family during the next nine days. These were designated as secondary cases. Omitted as episodes were all instances which fulfilled these criteria but in which one or more cases of gastrointestinal symptoms were associated with a specific acute infectious disease other than a common respiratory infection, or in which a

TABLE 75

Ratios showing the relative frequency with which five classes of individuals introduced infectious gastroenteritis into the home (1948-1950)

Class of Individual	Ratio
Fathers	1.00
Mothers	1.10
School children 6 years of age and over	1.74
Preschool children	1.93
School children under 6 years of age	2.17

person had a gastrointestinal illness more than once within the defined limit of the episode.

As in comparable analyses presented for the common respiratory diseases (Chapter VI), the choice of intervals for these episodes was largely arbitrary. The intent, however, was to include as episodes only those sets of cases in which it seemed most likely that the index case was not acquired as a result of intra-familial exposure and that the secondary cases were acquired as a result of such exposure.

The relative frequency with which various classes of family members introduced infectious gastroenteritis into the home is shown in table 75 as a series of ratios. These ratios relate the number of times that illnesses among individuals of each class were index cases in family episodes of infectious gastroenteritis to the number of times that illnesses among fathers in such families were index cases. Appropriate measures were employed to take into account the variation in family size and composition. The ratios are, therefore, interpreted as the average relative risk to individuals of each class of acquiring the infection outside the home.

TABLE 76

Secondary attack rates from infectious gastroenteritis
by age of contact (1948-1950)

Age of contact (years)	No. of secondary cases	No. of exposures	Secondary cases per exposure
<1	13	76	.17
1	17	90	.19
2	15	98	.15
3	13	75	.17
4	17	85	.20
5	17	84	.20
6	12	71	.17
7	11	46	.24
8	4	44	.09
9	4	36	.11
10+	5	66	.08
Mothers	44	337	.13
Fathers	34	345	.10

Fathers introduced the fewest gastrointestinal infections into the homes, but mothers introduced such infections with only slighly greater frequency. Preschool children and school children 6 years of age and older brought home more than one and one-half times as many gastrointestinal infections as did their fathers; school children under six brought home more than twice as many.

Secondary attack rates, computed by dividing the number of secondary cases in family episodes by the number of individuals exposed to the index case or cases, are shown in table 76 for various age groups. From infancy through age seven, the rates varied somewhat but no trend was discernible. Among these young children approximately one in every five or six intra-familial exposures to gastroenteritis resulted in recognizable illness. Children 8 years of age and older and adults had secondary attack rates which were about one-half as great as those of younger children.

There was considerable variation in secondary attack rates depending on the number of major gastrointestinal symptoms (vomiting, diarrhea, and abdominal pain) present in the index case (table

TABLE 77

Secondary attack rates from infectious gastroenteritis by number of gastrointestinal symptoms present in index case (1948-1950)

Number of GI symptoms	Number of secondary cases	Number of exposures	Secondary cases per exposure
1	97	927	.10
2	61	376	.16
3	48	150	.32

77). Thus, only 1 out of every 10 exposures to an index case with a single gastrointestinal symptom resulted in a secondary case. When two gastrointestinal symptoms were recorded in the index case, about one in every six exposures resulted in illness, and when the index case exhibited all three gastrointestinal symptoms, this rate rose to one case for every three exposures. Although the data are not shown, the secondary attack rates were similiar following index cases with a single gastrointestinal symptom regardless of which symptom was present. Similarly, the presence or absence of fever and of respiratory symptoms in the index case did not appear to alter the subsequent secondary attack rate. Because of the small number of cases, more detailed analyses of secondary attack rates by age of index case, season, and symptomatology, did not seem warranted.

The various specific incidence rates for infectious gastroenteritis, as well as the introduction and spread of illness in the family, showed a pattern similar in many respects to that observed for the common respiratory diseases. For both, the age-specific incidence rates increased from a low level in infants under 1 year of age to a higher level in childhood. In addition, the rates during childhood were generally higher among males for both kinds of illness. A major difference was that for infectious gastroenteritis the attack rates were very nearly the same among adult males and females, while for the common respiratory diseases adult females had a considerably higher incidence than did males.

School attendance also seemed to be related to the incidence of both gastrointestinal and respiratory illnesses. Thus, for both kinds of illness, rates at comparable ages were higher among school than among preschool children. They were also higher among preschool children with school siblings than among preschool children without school siblings through age 4 years; after this age the experience was too small to warrant conclusions. When the introduction of illness into the family was examined, young school children, as a group, were the most frequent source of both gastrointestinal and respiratory illnesses.

The resemblance between the specific incidence of infectious gastroenteritis and respiratory disease may be due in part to the fact that the rates among certain of the subgroups were based on relatively few individuals. In such instances the incidence of both gastrointestinal and respiratory disease may have been greatly affected by the experience of the same one or two individuals even though the rates presented are averages based on a large number of person-days of experience.

There were also similarities as well as certain differences in the seasonal variation in occurrence of the two disease groups (figure 3). Both occurred more frequently in winter than in summer. While the incidence of the common respiratory diseases was usually low through June, July, and August, however, that of infectious gastroenteritis showed a small, sharp, recurring mid-summer increase in July or August. This was followed in most years by another short period of low incidence before the rate rose to higher winter levels. The marked increase in the incidence of respiratory disease that takes place in September and is associated with the opening of school was not as prominent in the case of gastrointestinal illness. Furthermore, after a wintertime peak, the incidence of infectious gastroenteritis decreased much more rapidly than did the incidence of the common respiratory diseases.

CLINICAL CHARACTERISTICS

In reviewing the records of the 1104 cases of infectious gastroenteritis subjected to detailed epidemiological analysis, the impression was gained that there was an excessive occurrence of these cases at or about the time of onset of respiratory disease. To eliminate symptoms possibly due to dual infections, the clinical characteristics of the 683 cases of infectious gastroenteritis with onsets more than 5 days removed from the onset of respiratory symptoms are first described (13). Then, the association of gastrointestinal and respiratory symptoms in all of the cases is described. Finally, an estimate is made regarding the symptomatology of a postulated "respiratory-gastrointestinal" syndrome.

Infectious gastroenteritis.—The clinical description of infectious gastroenteritis is based on the frequency of occurrence, severity and duration of the three major gastrointestinal symptoms (vomiting, diarrhea and abdominal pain), the occurrence of certain nonspecific symptoms, and the duration of illness in the 683 cases. The methods and definitions are summarized in Appendix 20.

There was considerable variation in the occurrence of the major symptoms (table 78). Afebrile illnesses with only one major gastrointestinal symptom made up almost one-half of the total; among these, diarrhea was the most frequent. Illnesses involving various combinations of two gastrointestinal symptoms occurred with approx-

TABLE 78

The occurrence of major symptoms and fever in 683 cases of infectious gastroenteritis (1948-1950)

Major symptom	With fever (% of all cases)		Without fever (% of all cases)		Total (% of all cases)	
Vomiting only	4.7		15.4		20.1	
Diarrhea only	1.8	8.8	19.6	47.3	21.4	56.1
Abdominal pain only	2.3		12.3		14.6	
Vomiting and diarrhea	2.8		9.2		12.0	
Vomiting and abdominal pain	1.8	6.5	7.9	25.9	9.7	32.4
Diarrhea and abdominal pain	1.9		8.8		10.7	
All three	3.2		8.3		11.5	
Total	18.4		81.6		100.0	

imately the same frequency as those in which all three were present. Though not shown directly in table 78, the proportion of illnesses that were febrile varied from 8% of the cases with diarrhea only, to 28% of the cases in which all three gastrointestinal symptoms were present.

TABLE 79

The occurrence of major symptoms in 683 cases of infectious gastroenteritis, by age (1948-1950)

| Age group | Number of cases | Percent of cases in the age group in which symptom was present | | | |
		Vomiting	Diarrhea	Abdominal pain	Fever
<1	21	52.4	66.7	9.5	19.0
1-3	161	60.9	62.7	21.7	25.5
4+	258	63.2	33.3	58.5	22.1
Mothers	131	45.8	74.0	52.7	11.6
Fathers	112	28.6	73.2	54.5	8.4
Totals	683	53.3	55.6	46.6	18.4

The percentage of cases which manifested each of these symptoms is shown in table 79 separately for three groups of children and for mothers and fathers. The relative frequency of vomiting was fairly constant throughout childhood, but was lower for adults. Diarrhea was recorded in approximately two-thirds of the cases in infants and young children. This symptom, however, was recorded in only one-third of such illnesses among children 4 years of age or older. Diarrhea was present in about 74% of cases in adults. The most likely explanation for the difference in the frequency of occurrence of diarrhea in the various age groups is the failure of toilet-trained children to report the event. The relative frequency of abdominal pain increased progressively with age through early childhood, probably reflecting the increasing ability of the child to describe this symptom. Fever occurred less often among adults than among children. The illnesses of mothers and fathers were quite similar except for greater frequency of vomiting among mothers. The explanation for this difference is not apparent.

A detailed analysis of the minor symptoms is not shown. Anorexia occurred most often, being reported in 58% of illnesses. In decreasing frequency were listlessness (40%), feverishness (21%) and irritability (19%). Anorexia and listlessness showed little variation

TABLE 80

The day of onset of symptoms in 683 cases of infectious
gastroenteritis (1948-1950)

Symptom	Number of cases with symptoms present	Day of illness on which symptom began*					
		Before GI symptoms	1st day	2nd day	3rd day	4th or later day	Symptom present, date of onset unknown
		Percent of cases with symptom present					
Vomiting	364	.....*	92.0	3.6	2.7	1.6	0
Diarrhea	380	.....*	84.7	9.7	2.9	2.6	0
Abdominal pain	318	.....*	96.2	2.2	0	0.6	0.6
Fever	126	8.7	65.9	19.8	5.6	.....**	0

*The onset of each illness was the day of appearance of the first major gastrointestinal symptom even though non-specific symptoms were present prior to this.

**Symptoms other than major gastrointestinal symptoms which began after the third day of illness were considered to be absent for that illness.

TABLE 81

The severity of symptoms in 683 cases of infectious gastroenteritis (1948-1950)

Fever

Maximum temperature during illness*	Illnesses	
	No.	%
<100°F	557	81.6
100 - 100.9°F	58	8.5
101 - 101.9°F	27	4.0
102 - 102.9°F	18	2.6
103°F or more	23	3.4
Totals	683	100.0

Vomiting

Maximum number of times in 24 hours	Illnesses	
	No.	%
0	318	46.6
1	144	21.1
2	84	12.3
3	34	5.0
4	23	3.4
5	11	1.6
6	17	2.5
7+	30	4.4
Present, max. no. unknown	21	3.1
Unknown whether present or absent	1	.1
Totals	683	100.0

Diarrhea

Maximum number of stools in 24 hours	Illnesses	
	No.	%
0	302	44.2
1	78	11.4
2	63	9.2
3	62	9.1
4	52	7.6
5	28	4.1
6	27	4.0
7+	34	5.0
Present, max. no. unknown	36	5.3
Unknown whether present or absent	1	.1
Totals	683	100.0

*From the day before through the second day after the day of onset of gastrointestinal symptoms.

with age; irritability and feverishness were more common in young children. Because information regarding the occurrence of nausea, constipation, flatulence, dizziness, etc., was not specifically requested on the check sheet kept by the mothers, the relative frequency of these symptoms could not be determined.

The onset of infectious gastroenteritis was usually abrupt. In only about 8% of the illnesses were nonspecific symptoms, such as anorexia and listlessness, present for one or more days prior to the onset of major gastrointestinal symptoms. Table 80 relates the onset of each of the three major gastrointestinal symptoms and fever to the onset of the first gastrointestinal symptom. If vomiting or abdominal pain occurred during an illness, it usually began on the first day of gastrointestinal symptoms, while diarrhea began on the second day or later in approximately 15% of all illnesses during which it was present. Fever of 100° F. or more was first recorded on the day after the onset of gastrointestinal symptoms, or later, in about 25% of the cases in which it occurred.

Most of the cases of infectious gastroenteritis that occurred in this group of families were not severe illnesses (table 81). About 12% consisted of a single episode of vomiting or one diarrheal stool. In only 6% of cases was the temperature 102° F. or higher. This degree of fever was less common in older children than in those under 5 years of age, and was quite unusual in adults, being present in less than 2% of their illnesses. In only 12% of cases did the individuals vomit four or more times in a single day; there was no consistent relation to age. Four or more stools occurred in a single day in about 21% of all cases. This degree of diarrhea was more common in children under 2 years and in adults than in older children.

The duration of infectious gastroenteritis was short in most instances. Fifty-nine percent of illnesses lasted 1 calendar day or less, and in only 12% did symptoms last more than 3 days. In over half of the cases in this latter group the individual had one or more days of freedom from gastrointestinal symptoms in the course of the illness. Similarly, the duration of each of the major gastrointestinal symptoms was brief (table 82). Vomiting was present for more than 2 days in less than 8% of the cases in which it occurred. Diarrhea and abdominal pain persisted more than 2 days in 20 and 16%, respectively, of cases in which they occurred. Vomiting tended to last somewhat longer in young children than in older individuals; otherwise, there was little to suggest a trend in duration of the major gastrointestinal symptoms with age.

In summary, when the 683 cases of infectious gastroenteritis were considered as a group, the clinical picture was that of a mild illness

TABLE 82

Duration of symptoms in 683 cases of infectious gastroenteritis
(1948-1950)

Duration of symptom (days)	Vomiting		Diarrhea		Abdominal pain	
	No.	%	No.	%	No.	%
1	306	84.1	225	59.2	206	64.8
2	30	8.2	78	20.5	54	17.0
3	13	3.6	28	7.4	30	9.4
4	5	1.4	13	3.4	7	2.2
5	7	1.9	12	3.2	3	.9
6	3	.8	11	2.9	1	.3
7+	0	0.0	11	2.9	9	2.8
Present, duration unknown	0	0.0	2	.5	8	2.5
Number of cases with symptom present	364	100.0	380	100.0	318	100.0

of abrupt onset and short duration. Almost half the cases were
afebrile illnesses consisting of only one major gastrointestinal symptom. It was unusual for an individual to vomit repeatedly, to have
a large number of diarrheal stools in a single day, or to have high
fever. Although not comparable in detail with any other report,
these findings are in general agreement with the usual description
of infectious gastroenteritis.

The characterization of this syndrome presents considerable difficulty. It is recognized that these cases may represent not one,
but a group of diseases. There is, in fact, evidence from volunteer
studies (page 214) indicating the existence of more than one agent
as a cause of acute infectious nonbacterial gastroenteritis. In those
studies two inocula were used. One inoculum produced mild afebrile
gastrointestinal illnesses in which watery stools were a feature.
More severe illnesses resulted from the other inoculum, and were
usually febrile, without marked diarrhea, but with rather persistent
abdominal pain. Other differences, as well as similarities, were also
noted. Some of the cases in the present study met the criteria of
the two types of illnesses produced in volunteers. However, on the
basis of clinical records, it was not possible to identify the two types
of illnesses with sufficient clarity to warrant descriptions of their
epidemiological characteristics.

The Association of Respiratory and Gastrointestinal Symptoms.
Data from several sources describe the simultaneous occurrence of
respiratory and gastrointestinal symptoms in the same individual
(49, 81, 109, 110, 111, 118). In the present study the two
groups of symptoms were observed together in the same individual on numerous occasions. Since both gastrointestinal and common respiratory diseases occur in the general population with considerable frequency, it is to be expected that, in some instances,
individuals would be affected by both simultaneously. That is, a
number of what might be called "double infections" would be expected to occur. Data will be shown, however, to indicate that the
concurrence of these two groups of symptoms is considerably greater
than would be expected from chance double infections alone and
that in many cases the two may be presumed to be causally related.
For the analyses of this section (12), the 1466 occurrences of gastrointestinal symptoms during 1948-1950 were divided into four groups.
The first three of these groups were formed by the subdivision of
the 362 cases of gastrointestinal symptoms which had been attributed to some specific recorded cause other than infectious gastroenteritis, as follows:

a. Those which occurred in association with, and have been taken
to be manifestations of, one of the specific acute infectious diseases:
116 cases.

b. Those which were attributed to coughing or gagging, or occurred following the administration of an antibiotic or other medication that might result in gastrointestinal symptoms: 104 cases.

c. Those for which a variety of other explanatory circumstances,
not related to respiratory illness, were noted: 142 cases. Included
are 63 cases in which the gastrointestinal symptoms were attributed
to food or drink and 18 cases in which nervous or emotional factors
were present.

d. Those for which no acceptable explanation was noted, termed
infectious gastroenteritis: 1104 cases.

Incidence rates at various intervals from the diagnosed onset of
respiratory disease will be presented separately for these four groups.
The method used to determine incidence rates is shown in Appendix 21.

Figure 58 shows the incidence of each of the four classes of
gastrointestinal symptoms according to the interval to the nearest
case of common respiratory disease. Infectious gastroenteritis (figure
58d) showed an excessive incidence at the onset of common respiratory disease and for 5 days thereafter; from the +6th through the
+19th day there was a general downward trend in incidence. From
the −6th through the −19th day the incidence of gastroenteritis

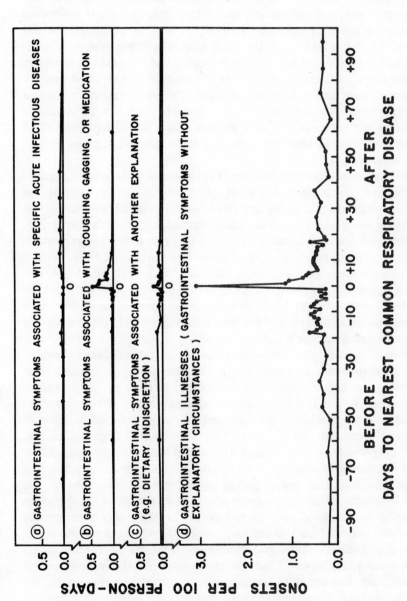

Fig. 58 Incidence of four classes of gastrointestinal symptoms according to
the interval to the nearest common respiratory disease in the same individual

showed day-by-day variation but on the whole was quite constant. At times further removed from respiratory illnesses, a slightly lower incidence obtained, due in part to the fact that a large proportion of the person-days at long intervals from respiratory disease was made up of summer experience, and attack rates for gastrointestinal illness were lower in summer than in winter. In addition, the decreased incidence reflected the fact that there were certain individuals who rarely had either respiratory or gastrointestinal illnesses. These people contributed a greater proportion of the total person-days experience at periods remote from common respiratory disease than they did at other times. As a result, their low incidence of infectious gastroenteritis had a greater effect in lowering the total rate at long than at short intervals from the nearest common respiratory disease.

The incidence of gastrointestinal symptoms associated with coughing, gagging or medication (figure 58b) was relatively high at the onset of respiratory disease and for about 10 days thereafter.

Neither the gastrointestinal symptoms associated with the variety of miscellaneous explanations (figure 58c), nor those accompanying specific acute infectious diseases (figure 58a) appeared to be related to the occurrence of respiratory disease. The slight peak on day zero in figure 58c represents a total of eight cases of gastrointestinal symptoms and is most likely the result of attributing a few such illnesses to accompanying circumstances with which they were not truly associated except in time.

In cases of infectious gastroenteritis where gastrointestinal symptoms were in some way related to the respiratory symptoms, the respiratory symptoms appeared at the same time as, or preceded, but did not follow the gastrointestinal symptoms. For this reason, estimates were made of the amount of excessive concurrence of these two forms of illness during the 6-day period from the day of onset of respiratory symptoms through the fifth day thereafter. The magnitude of the excess was determined by comparing the incidence during this 6-day period with that considered to be the usual incidence of acute gastroenteritis. On the basis of the rates presented in figure 58, the period from the sixth day through the nineteenth day before the nearest common respiratory disease was selected to indicate the usual incidence. The choice of this period has several advantages. First, by choosing a relatively brief period of time near the onset of each common respiratory disease in the same individual, the seasonal variation in the incidence of infectious gastroenteritis was largely taken into account. Second, the low rates of the few individuals who rarely had any recorded illness did not unduly influence the incidence of infectious gastroenteritis during this time period. Finally, the rates during this period were relatively constant and were based on a large number of person-days of experience. The 5 days immediately preceding respiratory disease were not included in establishing the expected rate of occurence of gastrointestinal symptoms, although their inclusion would not have influenced the results by more than a fraction of a case.

On the basis of the attack rates observed from the sixth through the nineteenth day before respiratory disease, 110 cases of infectious gastroenteritis would have been expected during the 6-day period beginning with the onset of respiratory disease. There were 326 cases of gastrointestinal symptoms without apparent explanation observed during this 6-day period. Thus, it was estimated that there were 216 more cases diagnosed as infectious gastroenteritis accompanying common respiratory disease than would be anticipated. These 216 instances are considered to be different from the remainder of the 1,104 cases of infectious gastroenteritis and for convenience will be referred to as 216 cases of "respiratory-gastrointestinal" syndrome. Presumably in these cases the gastrointestinal and respiratory symptoms are causally related.

The excessive association of gastrointestinal and respiratory symptoms was found in both summer and winter, and among both adults and children.

The "respiratory-gastrointestinal" syndrome made up about 20% of all gastrointestinal illnesses (216/1078)* and about 5% of the cases of common respiratory disease (216/4245).

Unlike the 362 cases of gastrointestinal symptoms attributed to causes other than respiratory disease, these 216 cases of "respiratory-gastrointestinal" syndrome could not be identified and excluded from descriptions of acute gastroenteritis. To be sure, there were specific cases that could be explained, on clinical grounds, as gastrointestinal manifestations of the constitutional component of respiratory disease. Preliminary attempts made along these lines were unsuccessful, however, and it was concluded that acceptable clinical criteria could not be formulated that would identify these 216 cases.

The inability to specify which of the concurrent gastrointestinal and respiratory illnesses represented independent double infections means that any analysis of infectious gastroenteritis in this study can, at best, lead to only an approximate description. Arbitrary decisions dictated which cases were included and which were excluded from such analyses. Cases of infectious gastroenteritis occur-

---

*Although there were 1104 occurrences of gastrointestinal symptoms that were unexplained and therefore classified as gastroenteritis, for 26 of these it was not possible to determine exactly the interval to the nearest common respiratory disease.

ring at the same time as respiratory illness in the same person have been included in the episode analyses used to describe introduction of infectious gastroenteritis into the family and to determine secondary attack rates. In the clinical description of infectious gastroenteritis, on the other hand, all such cases of concurrent gastrointestinal and respiratory illness were omitted. Furthermore, since it was not possible to indicate the particular 216 cases in which the gastrointestinal and respiratory symptoms might be causally related, it was not possible to describe directly the symptoms present in this group of illnesses. It was possible, however, if certain assumptions were made, to estimate their symptoms. Such an estimate of the specific respiratory and gastrointestinal symptoms present in cases of "respiratory-gastrointestinal syndrome" might help to explain the excessive association of these two groups of symptoms.

Estimate of symptoms of associated gastrointestinal and common respiratory diseases.—The estimates to be presented (14) were based on the assumption that of the 326 cases of infectious gastroenteritis and of common respiratory disease which occurred together, 110 did so by chance alone. It was further assumed that, in these 110 instances, the concurring infections were typical in symptomatology of the other cases of infectious gastroenteritis and of the common respiratory diseases observed in the same population. The number of times each gastrointestinal symptom would be expected in the 110 concurrent but unrelated illnesses was estimated from the frequency with which it was recorded in the 683 cases of infectious gastroenteritis which were not associated with the common respiratory diseases. The symptoms present in these cases were described earlier in this section (table 79). Similarly, the expected respiratory symptomatology was calculated from cases of the common respiratory diseases which were not associated with gastrointestinal symptoms. The difference between the number of times each symptom was expected from these estimates and the number of times it was observed in the 326 cases of concurrent respiratory and gastrointestinal illnesses was taken to represent the occurrence of that symptom in the 216 cases of "respiratory-gastrointestinal" syndrome.

Table 83 shows the estimated symptomatology of the "respiratory-gastrointestinal" syndrome. Details of the calculation by which these percentages were derived are not presented, but the method employed is described and all the data necessary for the calculations are presented in Appendix 22. For ease of comparison, the symptomatology of independently occurring common respiratory diseases and infectious gastroenteritis is repeated in table 83. As far as symptoms referable to the respiratory tract are concerned, there was no great difference between the occurrence of symptoms of common respira-

TABLE 83

Comparison of symptoms present in common respiratory diseases, infectious gastroenteritis and the "respiratory-gastrointestinal" syndrome (1948-1950)

Symptoms	Percentage of cases with each symptom or with indicated number of symptoms		
	"Respiratory-gastro-intestinal" sydrome (estimated)	Common respiratory diseases	Infectious gastroenteritis
Sneezing	60	62	
Watery nasal discharge	61	67	
Thick nasal discharge	41	47	
Obstructed nose	54	54	
Sore or irritated throat	37	34	
Hoarseness	31	23	
Cough	63	51	
Fever or feverishness	62	23*	25*
Vomiting	42		53
Diarrhea	52		56
Abdominal pain	30		47
No. of gastrointestinal symptoms**: 1	95		56
2	5		32
3	0		12

*Would expect 43% of simultaneously occurring independent infections to have fever or feverishness (see text).
**Includes vomiting, diarrhea and abdominal pain.

tory disease and the estimated symptoms of "respiratory-gastrointestinal" syndrome. Nasal symptoms occurred with about the same or a slightly lower frequency in cases of "respiratory-gastrointestinal" syndrome than in cases of the common respiratory diseases unassociated with gastrointestinal symptoms. Throat symptoms, hoarseness and cough, however, occurred in a somewhat greater proportion of cases of the "respiratory-gastrointestinal" syndrome than in the common respiratory diseases. The presence of these latter symptoms is usually considered to indicate a more severe respiratory illness.

Considering the estimated gastrointestinal symptomatology, the differences between the "respiratory-gastrointestinal" syndrome and cases of gastroenteritis not associated with respiratory disease are relatively great. Only 5% of cases of "respiratory-gastrointestinal" syndrome were estimated to consist of more than one major gastrointestinal symptom as compared to 44% of cases of infectious gastroenteritis. Each individual gastrointestinal symptom was estimated to have occurred less frequently in the "respiratory-gastrointestinal" syndrome. This difference was not, however, as great for diarrhea as for vomiting and abdominal pain. The occurrence of gastrointestinal symptoms other than vomiting, diarrhea and abdominal pain could not be estimated.

Fever or feverishness occurred in about 62% of cases of "respiratory-gastrointestinal" syndrome. Fever and feverishness tended to be associated with symptoms of the lower respiratory tract in cases of the common respiratory diseases (Chapter VI). In cases of infectious gastroenteritis, however, fever occurred least frequently in those cases with one major gastrointestinal symptom and most frequently in cases with all three major gastrointestinal symptoms.

Tabulations of these symptoms by age were examined but are not included in this report. The differences found were of the nature of those shown in table 83 and the latter were not due to differences in age distributions.

The estimated symptomatology of the "respiratory-gastrointestinal" syndrome, then, can be summarized as follows:

1. The respiratory component tends to be at least as severe in terms of the type of symptoms present, as is the case in the usual common respiratory diseases. The slightly increased frequency of sore or irritated throat, hoarseness and cough suggests that, if anything, the respiratory symptoms of the "respiratory-gastrointestinal" syndrome are more severe.

2. The gastrointestinal component of the "respiratory-gastrointestinal" syndrome, however, appears to be less severe than in infectious gastroenteritis. In almost all cases of the syndrome only a single gastrointestinal symptom occurred.

3. Fever or feverishness occurred in a relatively large proportion of cases.

It has been shown that in the "respiratory-gastrointestinal" syndrome respiratory symptoms began at the same time as or before gastrointestinal symptoms. This fact, together with the estimated symptomatology, indicates that the sydrome is primarily and principally one of respiratory tract involvement.

Several possible explanations for the associated gastrointestinal symptoms might be mentioned. Quantitative measurements appear to rule out the possibility that all the associated respiratory and gastrointestinal symptoms were unrelated and occurred together by coincidence. Explanations which seem consistent with the time relations and the symptoms present in the "respiratory-gastrointestinal" syndrome are: (a) that gastrointestinal symptoms occur with some (possibly the more severe) cases of the common respiratory diseases in much the same way that such symptoms occur with some cases of various acute infectious diseases; (b) that the "respiratory-gastrointestinal" syndrome is a disease entity or group of entities in which specific etiological agents as, for example, certain of the reoviruses (111, 116) or ECHO viruses (49, 118) give rise to both gastrointestinal and respiratory manifestations; and (c) that a gastrointestinal symptom is more likely to be noticed and recorded at a time when symptoms of a common respiratory disease are present. The findings of the present study do not permit the choice of one of these explanations in preference to the others. Indeed, it is probable that the group of cases referred to as "respiratory-gastrointestinal" syndrome is a heterogeneous one.

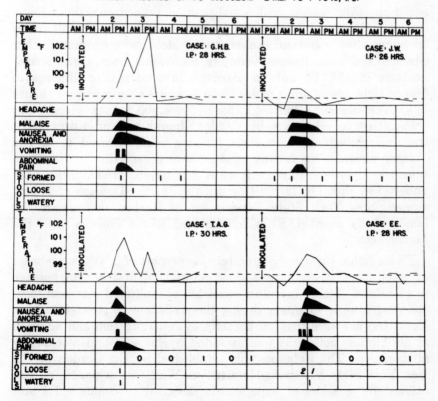

Fig. 59   Graphic representation of the illnesses induced in 4 of 8 volunteers by feeding 2 ml. of stool supernate from a patient with febrile gastroenteritis

ETIOLOGY

Since gastroenteritis obviously was an important cause of illness and behaved as an infectious disease, attempts were made to identify possible etiologic agents. During the last 6 months of 1950, 70 rectal swabs and 7 stool specimens from individuals considered clinically to have this syndrome were cultured; no *Shigella* or *Salmonella* organisms were isolated (11). Although enteropathogenic *E. coli* (102) were not excluded, it was presumed that the majority of the acute gastrointestinal illnesses, particularly those occurring in the winter months, represented virus infections. No viruses etiologically related to gastroenteritis were identified with the rather primitive culture systems then in use. Accordingly, in January and February 1951, stool specimens were collected and processed (7) with the view to reproducing the naturally occurring disease in volunteers.

Early observations had suggested that at least two types of gastroenteritis—afebrile and febrile—were occurring in the population. Bacteria-free supernate of a stool from a mother who experienced anorexia, nausea, abdominal pain, and diarrhea without feverishness induced mild symptoms in one of seven young adult males 56 hours after ingestion. Supernate of stool from another mother who had headache, nausea, vomiting, abdominal cramps, and a temperature of 101° F., but no diarrhea, induced similar illnesses in four of eight young adult males 26 to 30 hours after ingestion (figure 59). The afebrile, diarrheal disease resembled that successfully transmitted to volunteers by Gordon, Ingraham, and Korns (68), the unidentified agent in stool filtrates being referred to as the "Marcy strain." No further studies were done with the inoculum from the afebrile family study case, but collaborative studies were undertaken with Dr. Irving Gordon, then at the Division of Laboratories, New York State Department of Health, to compare the family study agent (FS) which induced febrile illnesses with the Marcy agent.

FS inoculum consisted of unfiltered supernate of a 20% suspension of three loose stools from a case induced on first human passage in Cleveland. Marcy inoculum consisted of unfiltered diarrheal feces collected from a volunteer during the sixth human passage in New York. Inocula were freed of bacteria by centrifugation and addition of antibiotics; poliovirus was excluded by intracerebral inoculation of monkeys. The isolation unit established by Dr. Gordon at the New York State Vocational Institution, West Coxsackie, N. Y., was utilized for a series of experiments designed to compare FS and Marcy strains. In a cross-immunity experiment (figure 60) two groups of volunteers in individual isolation were fed FS and Marcy

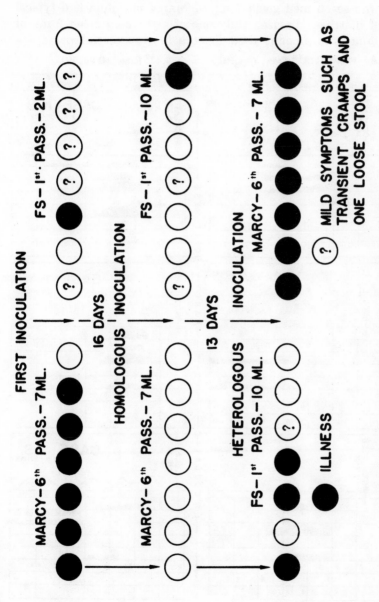

Fig. 60 Results of inoculation of homologous and heterologous stool supernates from cases of afebrile (Marcy) and febrile (FS) gastroenteritis. Each circle represents a volunteer; the sequence of events for each man is indicated by a single vertical column of circles.

inocula, respectively. Each group was reinoculated twice at approximately 2-week intervals, first with homologous, then with heterologous inocula.

Six of the seven men given 7 ml. of Marcy inoculum had typical attacks of diarrheal disease. Only one of eight men given 2 ml. of FS inoculum—the amount used for the first successful passage—

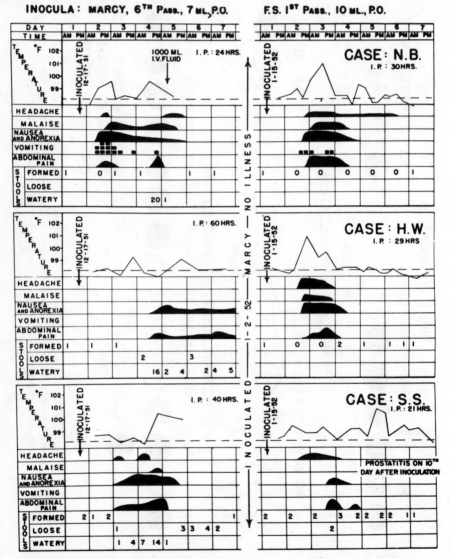

Fig. 61   *Graphic representation of the responses of the same individuals to two different gastroenteritis inocula. Volunteers who initially responded to Marcy inoculum had no symptoms when fed the same type of inoculum 16 days later. They did become ill following the ingestion of FS inoculum.*

had a definite illness; he developed a temperature of 101.8° F., nausea, anorexia, and headache after an interval of 24 hours. Sixteen days later the men ingested the same inocula, but 10 ml. instead of 2 ml. of FS were given. The Marcy group remained well, but one of the FS group became ill. Cross-immunity was tested 13 days after the second inoculation. Marcy inoculum induced diarrhea in seven of eight men, including two previously sick following FS inoculum. FS inoculum induced febrile disease in three of seven men, all convalescent from experimental Marcy gastroenteritis. Figure 61 illustrates the responses of three volunteers to the two different gastroenteritis inocula.

Illnesses induced with the FS inoculum differed from the afebrile Marcy disease (table 84). The average incubation period of experimental Marcy illness was 60 hours, whereas that of the FS type was 27 hours. Fever was characteristic of the FS illness, and constitutional symptoms were more marked; the watery diarrhea

TABLE 84

Characteristics of illnesses induced by two different
gastroenteritis inocula

	Inoculum	
	Marcy	FS
Incubation period:		
Range, hrs.	24 - 120	20 - 30
Average, hrs.	60	27
Duration: Average, hrs.	96	24
Fever	Usually absent; late with dehydration, below 101°F.	Usually present; often relatively high
Constitutional symptoms	Usually mild	Usually marked
Headache	Mild or absent	Moderate or severe
Nausea and anorexia	Common; moderate or severe	Common; moderate or severe
Abdominal pain	Hyperactive peristalsis; cramps of moderate intensity preceding diarrheal stools	Persistent pain and cramps, often severe, associated with desire to vomit or move bowels
Vomiting	Often occurs in bouts early in illness	Often occurs in bouts early in illness
Stools	Frequent; watery	Infrequent; normal or loose

of Marcy disease was lacking. It was believed that FS illness, like Marcy disease, represented an infection, since the feeding of 10 ml. of autoclaved supernate prepared from stools from five individuals to each of 18 volunteers and the ingestion of 10 ml. of autogenous stool supernate by eight subjects failed to produce such symptoms. Thus, evidence was obtained that a least two agents were responsible for nonbacterial gastroenteritis. Neither disease could be associated serologically with ECHO viruses, types 7, 8, 9, 11 and 12, or reovirus, type 1.

COMMENTS

Several years after these experiments were conducted, Gordon (67) reviewed the status of etiologic studies, pointing out that the Niigata strain passed in volunteers by Japanese investigators (90) produced an illness similar to Marcy infections. Tateno et al. (131), using human embryonic skin-muscle cell cultures, subsequently isolated an agent with the general characteristics of an ECHO virus from diarrheal stools provoked by Niigata inoculum. No cytopathic agent was isolated from two Marcy specimens. The ECHO-like virus did not induce illness when given by duodenal tubes to three volunteers without neutralizing antibody, and was considered to be a "fellow traveller."

In recent years, a number of investigators (59, 89, 108, 128) have related many different ECHO virus types to acute gastroenteritis, while others (94) have reported the virtual absence of detectable viruses from stools of children during epidemics of gastroenteritis. That more than one agent may be responsible for acute gastroenteritis now seems clear. At present, however, the agents present in FS and Marcy inocula remain unidentified, and it is believed that those responsible for the majority of gastrointestinal illnesses observed in the family study population are in the same category.

Chapter XII
POLIOMYELITIS

During the summer and fall of 1952 the Cleveland metropolitan area (Cuyahoga County)* experienced the highest incidence of poliomyelitis in its history. There were 590 cases (48.5/100,000) and 30 deaths. As shown in figure 62 a few cases were reported in June, but the highest incidence occurred between mid-July and late September. Cases declined sharply in number during October and were sporadic during November and December (29).

Reports from other areas of the country (34,136) as well as

TABLE 85

Poliovirus isolations from selected patients admitted to University Hospitals of Cleveland and their contacts (1952 epidemic)

	Number of isolations*		Total tested
	Type 1	Type 2	
Patients	19	5	66
Contacts	4	1	86
Total	23	6	152

*Both stool specimens and throat swabs were examined. Virus was present in the stools of 17 patients and in both stools and throat swabs of 7 patients. Among the contacts, three had virus in their stools and two in their throats.

isolation studies conducted at this laboratory (table 85), indicated that during the 1952 season type 1 poliovirus was the one most frequently associated with clinical disease.

Although there are many reports in the literature to document the occurrence of subclinical infections with polioviruses, they are primarily concerned with infections in which contact with an overt case (usually from the same household) had been definitely established. Much of these data support the view expressed by Brown et al (38) that subclinical infections are characteristically grouped around definite cases and not scattered at random. The experience with type 1 poliovirus during the post-epidemic season of 1954 among families with illnesses in which the only symptomatology was respiratory (Chapter IX), provided evidence that subclinical poliomyelitis

*1950 census showed a total population of 1,378,225 persons.

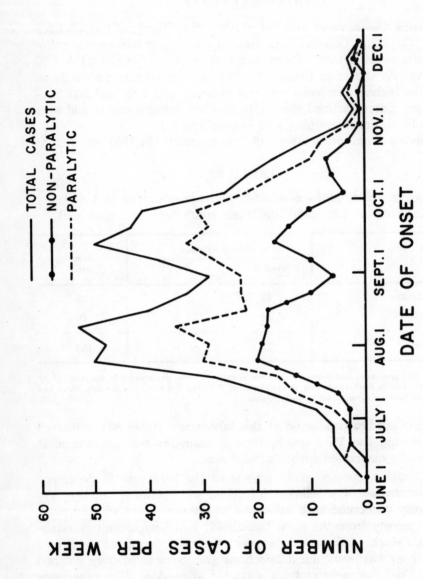

Fig. 62 Occurrence of poliomyelitis, Cuyahoga County,
June 1-December 31, 1952

may arise without known association with a clinical case. Similar findings have been reported by others (62, 69, 77, 98).

Certain aspects of poliomyelitis as it occurred in the families were studied during the 1952 epidemic. The study included determination of the incidence and distribution of subclinical infections as revealed by serological methods and virus isolation, the significance of seroimmune status in relation to the occurrence of subclinical infection, and the influence of subclinical infection on the development or enhancement of heterotypic antibody. In addition, the use of the pharyngeal swab for the detection of virus carriers was investigated.

The availability of serum specimens from the same individuals over a period of years permitted the study of antibody development during years both preceding and following the 1952 epidemic season.

DEFINITION AND INTERPRETATION OF LABORATORY DATA

An individual without detectable neutralizing antibody in a 1:5 (final) dilution of serum was considered to be susceptible to infection with the homologous virus. Demonstration of antibody in a subsequent specimen was considered to indicate that infection or experience with the homologous virus had taken place in the interval between the paired specimens. Evidence of infection was also provided by the isolation of virus. When paired serum specimens were not available, virus isolation was the sole means of establishing infection.

OCCURRENCE OF CLINICAL POLIOMYELITIS

The only illness clinically diagnosed as poliomyelitis occurred in a a 13-year-old boy who gave a history of having had poliomyelitis at 6 years of age.

The onset was gradual with anorexia without fever for 2 days. On the third day he complained of headache, feverishness, stomach-ache, pain in the legs, cough, nausea, and dizziness and had a temperature of 101° F. There was no vomiting or diarrhea. Physical examination at this time revealed a moderately ill boy with slight stiffness of neck and back as the only abnormal finding. The symptoms and fever of approximately 100° F. persisted and on the fifth day he was lethargic and his hands and arms shook so that he could not hold a paper still enough to read. The following day he had difficulty in swallowing and was hospitalized. He was lethargic and nauseated, and vomited. In addition to stiffness in the neck and back, he had generally hyperactive reflexes, with increased tonus in muscles of the upper extremities, fine tremors in both hands and wrists and occasional gross involuntary movements of both pectoral and deltoid muscles. His voice sounded nasal in character. The abdominal and cremasteric reflexes were present and equal and no definitive muscle weakness could be detected. The Kernig sign was positive. Examination of the cerbrospinal fluid revealed 140 cells (25% polymorph-

TABLE 86

Illnesses occuring during July-October for years 1948
through 1956 by diagnosis

Diagnostic category	Percentage of total illness for each season								
	1948	1949	1950	1951	1952	1953	1954	1955	1956
Common respiratory diseases	57.6	60.9	60.4	54.9	56.8	50.2	57.5	51.7	53.9
Specific respiratory diseases	7.1	1.5	2.4	3.6	5.5	1.1	2.6	3.2	1.6
Gastrointestinal illnesses	16.2	16.5	16.3	16.7	15.2	17.9	16.7	14.1	17.9
Other infections	6.2	9.1	7.6	8.3	7.4	6.7	7.2	8.9	5.8
Other illnesses	12.9	12.1	13.3	16.5	15.1	24.0	16.1	22.1	20.9
Total number of illnesses	649	662	669	823	973	878	739	813	765
Person-years of observation	87.9	104.3	106.0	113.4	138.7	133.3	136.5	133.5	129.3
Number illnesses per person-year	7.4	6.3	6.3	7.3	7.0	6.6	5.4	6.1	5.9

onuclear leucocytes and 75% lymphocytes), protein 70 mg. %, chlorides 402 mg. %, and sugar 71.3 mg. %. Cultures revealed no growth. Urine and blood examinations were normal. He improved during the next 4 days and was discharged on the twelfth day of illness, at which time muscle evaluation demonstrated normal function throughout. Evaluation a year later revealed no abnormalities.

Laboratory investigation of this case confirmed the diagnosis. Neutralization tests on paired sera revealed antibody acquisition to type 1 poliovirus with a convalescent titer of 512. Type 1 poliovirus was isolated from pharyngeal swabs taken on the third and fourth days of illness, but not from swabs obtained 4 days prior to and 9 days following onset. No antibodies to mumps were demonstrated by hemagglutination-inhibition. Type 1 poliovirus was also isolated from the throat of a 3-year-old sibling and serological evidence of infection with type 1 was established in a 9-year old sibling.

COMPARISON OF ILLNESSES OCCURRING DURING EPIDEMIC PERIOD (1952) WITH THOSE OF OTHER YEARS

The percentage distribution of various illness categories during the epidemic period July through October of 1952 is shown in table 86, along with distributions in similar periods for 4 years preceding and 4 years following 1952. The number of illnesses per person-year for 1952 (7.0) was comparable to the rates for 1948 and 1951, but was greater than any during the other 7 years of observation when the rates varied between 5.4 and 6.6. The distributions of the various illness categories were remarkably similar during all these periods, excess illness being noted only for "specific respiratory disease" in 1948 and 1952, with percentages of 7.1 and 5.5, respectively. In 1948, 5.7% and in 1952, 4.5% of all illnesses were diagnosed as "nonbacterial tonsillitis and pharyngitis" and were thus included in the broader diagnostic category of "specific respiratory diseases." In retrospect, these were probably chiefly adenovirus infections, although the possibility existed that many of these illnesses, as well as other illnesses classified as "minor," were due to the polioviruses.

An attempt was therefore made to characterize the illnesses that occurred in each person during the period of 7 days preceding through 7 days following the date of the first isolation of poliovirus from his throat. The isolation (type 1) from the patient who had clinical poliomyelitis was excluded, as were the three isolations from the stool only (two were type 2 and one was type 3). Of the remaining 48 primary isolations from the throat, 35 were found to be related to 40 illnesses by the above criteria (five persons had two illnesses each). Eight of the isolates were type 1 and 40 were type 2. No illnesses were related to 13 isolations (four were type 1 and nine were type 2). These 40 illnesses were termed Group I.

The Group I illnesses were compared with three other groups of of illnesses:

Group II comprised 41 illnesses occurring in the period July 1 to October 31, 1951, among the same 48 individuals in Group I. For each person, the illness closest to the date corresponding to the poliovirus isolation in 1952 was selected. If two illnesses in an individual had been included in the Group I list, an attempt was made to select two illnesses for that person in the Group II list. In only two instances was this possible. Of the remaining 46 persons, 9 had no illnesses.

Group III consisted of 39 illnesses occurring in the period July 1 to October 31, 1952, among members of families in which there was no evidence, either by isolation of virus or serologically, of infection with poliovirus. Insofar as possible these illnesses were matched by age and date with the illnesses of persons included in Group I. Four had two illnesses each.

Group IV consisted of 40 illnesses occurring in the period July 1 to October 31, 1951, in the same families of Group III, selected in the same fashion. Four persons had two illnesses each.

The clinical characteristics of the illnesses in the four Groups are presented in tables 87 and 88 and Appendix 23, tables 1, 2 and 3. The figures given in the tables were not converted to percentages since the number of illnesses in each Group were approximately the same.

The illnesses in Group I, namely those associated with isolations of polioviruses from the throat, differed from those in the three comparison Groups in several outstanding respects, while those in the latter three Groups were similar. In general, the illnesses in Group I were more acute and in three-fourths of them the onset was sudden. Fever or feverishness or both were noted in 38 of 40 illnesses (95%) but in only one-quarter of the illnesses in the comparison Groups. Of those who had fever, the maximum temperatures of those in Group I were higher (Appendix 23, table 1).

Illnesses associated with constitutional symptoms (headache, listlessness, feverishness, irritability, loss of appetite, and chilliness) were twice as frequent in Group I, and the number of constitutional symptoms per illness was greater (table 88). Symptoms referable to the throat (sore or irritated throat) were approximately twice as frequent. Muscular aches and pains occurred in 7 of the 40 illnesses in Group I but in only 1 illness in the 3 comparison Groups. The

TABLE 87

Comparison of the clinical characteristics of illnesses which occurred at the time poliovirus was first isolated from throat swabs in 1952 with those of three other groups

Clinical characteristic[1]	Poloivirus isolated in 1952		No evidence of infection in 1952	
	1952 illnesses Group I	1951 illnesses Group II	1952 illnesses Group III	1951 illnesses Group IV
Onset				
Sudden	30	22	23	22
Gradual	9	15	13	14
Indeterminate	1	4	3	4
Fever or feverishness	38	12	10	9
Symptoms				
Constitutional[2]	36	19	17	19
Nasal	16	22	21	20
Throat	21	8	9	15
Cough	10	11	14	18
Gastrointestinal[3]	8	8	10	9
Aches and pains (muscular)	7	0	1	0
Other[4]	4	5	4	8
Duration (days)				
<4	25	11	14	16
4 or more	14	28	22	21
Indeterminate	1	2	3	3
Total illnesses	40	41	39	40

[1]Figures in the table refer to number of cases presenting the indicated characteristic.
[2]Headache, listlessness, feverishness, irritability, loss of appetite, chilliness.
[3]Nausea, vomiting, diarrhea.
[4]Dizziness, photophobia, pain in eyes, conjunctivitis, earache, epistaxis, wheezing, stomach-ache.

duration of the illnesses was shorter, approximately 60% lasting less than 4 days (table 87 and Appendix 23, table 2).

Although the data regarding physical findings were limited to only a portion of the cases (Appendix 23, table 3) for reasons beyond

TABLE 88

Number of constitutional symptoms per illness in 4 groups of cases

No. of constitutional symptoms	Poliovirus isolated in 1952		No evidence of infection in 1952	
	1952 illnesses Group I	1951 illnesses Group II	1952 illnesses Group III	1951 illnesses Group IV
0	4	22	22	21
1	4	5	10	8
2	6	4	4	4
3	7	5	1	5
4	12	5	2	2
5	5			
6	2			
Total	40	41	39	40

our control, signs referable to involvement of the throat were prominent in Group I illnesses; this was compatible with the symptomatology of these cases.

The gastrointestinal symptoms of nausea, diarrhea and vomiting were similar in all four Groups, a finding which seems rather surprising and for which there is no apparent explanation.

Because of the nature of the illnesses in Group I, it seems reasonable that most of them were infections with polioviruses. The prominence of symptoms and signs relating to involvement of the throat confirms Sabin's suggestion (117) that many of those cases termed "summer sore throat" may in actuality be due to infection with polioviruses.

ANTIBODY STATUS PRECEDING THE 1952 EPIDEMIC

The antibody status of the population prior to the 1952 epidemic was utilized for an estimate of the susceptibility and resistance to infection with the three types of polioviruses. As already stated, absence of detectable antibody in a serum dilution of 1:5 was considered to indicate susceptibility and presence of antibody to indicate resistance or immunity. This analysis was limited to 227 persons from whom both pre-epidemic and post-epidemic sera were available since this was the only group in which changes in antibody status could be determined.

One hundred fifty-eight persons (70%) were found to be susceptible to type 1, 154 (68%) to type 2 and 160 (70%) to type 3 (table 89). As was expected, the proportion of the population

TABLE 89

Susceptibility of 227 persons to 3 types of poliovirus as judged by antibody status before the 1952 epidemic

Age	Total number of individuals	Susceptible					
		Type 1		Type 2		Type 3	
		No.	%	No.	%	No.	%
0 - 2	11	10	91	11	100	9	82
3 - 5	32	28	87	29	91	29	91
6 - 8	32	23	72	22	69	26	81
9 - 11	19	12	63	15	79	13	68
12+	7	6	86	6	86	4	57
Total children	101	79	78	83	82	81	80
Mothers	63	39	62	42	67	37	59
Fathers	63	40	63	29	46	42	67
Total	227	158	70	154	68	160	70

susceptible to each of the types decreased with increasing age. Without exception, children up to 5 years of age demonstrated the highest percentage of susceptibility to each type. Children as a group, as well as mothers, displayed similar susceptibilities for each of the three types. Fathers were comparable to mothers in susceptibility to types 1 and 3 but demonstrated the lowest susceptibility (46%) of all age groups to type 2.

The broader antibody spectrum of parents preceding the epidemic of 1952 is illustrated by the occurrence of antibodies to more than one type of virus. Seventy-six percent of both mothers and fathers possessed antibody to at least one type, as compared to 46% of children. Antibodies to at least two types were found in 35% of both mothers and fathers and in 13% of children. Antibodies to all three types occurred in only one child (1.0%), one mother (1.6%) and six fathers (11%).

It is thus apparent that in general the population was highly susceptible to the polioviruses as judged by antibody status. In part, at least, such susceptibility was a reflection of the economic status of the families.

OCCURRENCE OF INFECTION
SEROLOGICAL EVIDENCE

Table 90 shows the frequency with which antibodies to polio-viruses were acquired during the epidemic period. Of the 158 persons without antibody to type 1 in their pre-epidemic specimens, 11, or 7.0%, acquired this antibody. For type 2 there were 34 acquisitions, or 22%, among 154 susceptibles. For type 3 there was only one acquisition among 160 susceptibles.

TABLE 90

Incidence of infection with polioviruses as determined by antibody acquisition (1952)

	Type of poliovirus		
	1	2	3
Number of persons susceptible	158	154	160
Number of antibody acquisitions	11	34	1
% of antibody acquisitions	7.0	22.0	0.6

It is evident from these data that during the 1952 season, sub-clinical or nonparalytic infections with polioviruses in this population were predominantly due to the type 2 strain. This is of interest in view of the fact that type 1 virus was the type most frequently isolated from clinical cases, not only in the Cleveland area (table 85) but also in studies conducted elsewhere (34, 98, 136).

QUANTITATION OF ANTIBODY ACQUIRED AND ITS RELATION TO VIRUS RECOVERY

Quantitation of antibody response for 40 of the 46 instances of acquisition detected by the 1:5 screen is shown in Appendix 23, table 4. Post-epidemic titers were found to vary from 18 to greater than 1024. Eight (20%) demonstrated titers of 100 or less, 16 (40%) demonstrated titers of 280-400, 6 (15%) demonstrated titers of 512-768, and there were 10 (25%) with titers of 1024 or greater. Among this group there appeared to be no relation between age and antibody response.

In correlating virus recovery and antibody titer, it was found that virus was isolated from 5 of 8, or 62%, of persons with antibody titers of 100 or less, from 12 of 16, or 75%, with titers of 280 to 400, from 3 of 6, or 50% with titers of 512 to 768, and from 9 of 10, or 90%, with titers of 1024 or greater. The isolation of virus from persons who demonstrated a wide range of post-infection antibody titers indicates that the level of antibody response was not necessarily related to the ability to recover virus.

Although not quantitated, antibody acquired during the 1952 season was still detectable in a 1:5 dilution of sera drawn from the same persons during 1955. Since the majority of these individuals received vaccine after 1955, persistence of antibody beyond this time could obviously not exclude the booster or an anamnestic effect of the vaccine.

HETEROTYPIC ANTIBODY RESPONSE

There were no persons who demonstrated acquisition of antibody to more than one type during the 1952 epidemic season. Of 18 instances, however, in which antibody acquisition occurred in the presence of heterotypic antibody, there was a heterotypic rise in 17. Of the four instances in which type 1 was the infecting virus, there were two heterotypic rises each for types 2 and 3. Of the 13 instances in which type 2 was the infecting virus, there were seven rises to type 1 and six rises to type 3. There were no infections with type 3 virus in the presence of heterotypic antibody. Twelve of the heterotypic rises were fourfold or greater, three were twofold and two were less than twofold. There were four infected persons (all adults) with antecedent antibody to both heterologous types; antibody rises occurred in every instance. These data indicated that subclinical infections with types 1 and 2 evoked a rise in the heterotypic antibody already present.

TABLE 91

Serological status of persons tested for poliovirus

Serological evidence of infection	No. of persons examined	Number of virus isolations			
		Type 1	Type 2	Type 3	All types
A. Present (antibody acquistion)	46	7	27	1	35
B. Absent 1. Associated with family infection	19	0	0	0	0
2. Not associated with family infection	24	0	0	0	0
C. Unknown	58	2	15	0	17
Totals	147	9	42	1	52

CORRELATION OF VIRUS ISOLATIONS WITH SEROLOGICAL EVIDENCE OF INFECTION

Data from attempts to isolate polioviruses from 147 persons provided information that was both confirmatory and supplementary to the serological findings. These persons were classified as follows:

A. Those with serological evidence of infection

B. Those with no serological evidence of infection

C. Those whose serological status was unknown

The results are presented in table 91. Viruses were isolated from 35 of 46 persons (Group A) who showed serological evidence of infection during the outbreak, thus confirming 76% of the infections indicated by antibody acquisitions. Polioviruses were not isolated from any of 43 persons who had no serological evidence of infection. Nine of 19 persons in infected families had pre- and post-outbreak antibodies to the family-infecting type without a rise in titer; the remaining 10 did not. Although this group was small, the opportunity for contact with virus was presumably optimal. Failure to obtain viruses from those persons would seem to indicate that isolation would not be likely when homotypic antibody was either present in pre-epidemic sera or absent in post-epidemic sera. Polioviruses were isolated from 17 of 58 persons whose serological status was unkown. On the basis of the results obtained from group B, no further search for virus was made from the balance of the population that had demonstrated no evidence of infection in the serological screening.

Thus of 147 persons tested for virus, there was a total of 52 isolations. As with the serological data, type 2 was most frequently encountered, 42 strains being isolated. There were nine isolations of type 1 and one isolation of type 3. Since virus isolation yielded 17 additional infections not detected by serological means, combined methods indicated infection in a total of 63 persons or about 20% of the population.

Since the data showed no evidence of infection in the presence of homotypic antibody, an evaluation of age as a factor in infection was made in the "susceptible" portion of the population. Table 92 shows the age distribution of infections determined by serological methods. Six of the nine children with type 1 antibody acquisitions were 9 years of age or older. In contrast, 18 of the 19 children who showed serological evidence of infection with type 2 poliovirus were less than 9 years of age. Type 1 infections were relatively more frequent among children (9 of 79 or 11%) than among parents (2 of 79 or 3%). The incidence of infection with type 2 virus was similar for parents and children.

TABLE 92

Antibody acquisitions in persons in whom antibody to polio-viruses was absent* in pre-epidemic sera

Age (years)	Type 1			Type 2			Type 3		
	No. susceptible	Antibody acquisition No.	%	No. susceptible	Antibody acquisition No.	%	No. susceptible	Antibody acquisition No.	%
0 - 2	10	1	10	11	7	64	9	0	0
3 - 5	28	2	7	29	5	17	29	0	0
6 - 8	23	0	0	22	6	27	26	0	0
9 - 11	12	3	25	15	1	7	13	0	0
12 - 15+	6	3	50	6	0	0	4	0	0
Total children	79	9	11	83	19	23	81	0	0
Mother	39	1	3	42	10	24	37	0	0
Father	40	1	2	29	5	17	42	1	2
Total parents	79	2	3	71	15	21	79	1	1
Total	158	11	7	154	34	22	160	1	1

*No detectable antibody in a 1-5 dilution of serum.

TABLE 93

Relationship between susceptibility and infection in 67 families as determined by combined methods of serology and virus isolation

	Known number persons susceptible per family*							Total no. of families with 1 or more susceptibles
	0	1	2	3	4	5	6	
Type 1								
Number of families	6	11	22	11	13	4	0	61
Number of families infected	0	0	0	1	1	2	0	4
Number of persons infected per family	0	0	0	2	3	3,5	0	13
Type 2								
Number of families	5	13	16	17	10	5	1	62
Number of families infected	0	2	2	3	5	4	0	16
Number of persons infected per family	0	1,1	2,2	1,2,3	4,4,4, 4,4	3,4,5, 5	0	49
Type 3								
Number of families	8	15	10	15	14	5	0	59
Number of families infected	0	1	0	0	0	0	0	1
Number of persons infected per family	0	1	0	0	0	0	0	1

*Assumes susceptibility in 15 instances in which infection was established by virus isolation in absence of paired sera.

Virus isolations were too few in number to warrant detailed analysis by age.

FAMILIAL OCCURRENCE
DISTRIBUTION OF INFECTIONS

If the assumption is made that the absence of detectable antibody in pre-epidemic sera represents susceptibility, then both antibody acquisition and isolation of virus may be presumed to represent infection.

On the basis of this assumption, there were 61 (91%) of 67 families (table 93) in which at least one person was susceptible to type 1, 62 (93%) with susceptibility to type 2, and 59 (88%) with susceptibility to type 3. Evidence of infection with type 1 was demonstrated by at least one member in four of the 61 susceptible families (7%), with type 2 by 16 (26%) of the 62 susceptible families, and with type 3 by one (2%) of the 59 susceptible families. As would be expected, the more susceptible members a family contained, the greater was the likelihood of the family becoming infected.

PERIOD OF TIME FOR SPREAD OF VIRUS IN FAMILY

Estimation of the period of time involved in the spread of virus through a family, as measured by the number of days between the initial isolation from any member of the family and subsequent isolations from familial associates, is shown in table 94. In all but seven instances virus was isolated from the throat. Since throat cultures were obtained at weekly intervals, the virus acquisition could have occurred any time between the last negative and the first positive culture—a period of 7 days.

Of the 21 households infected there were 15 in which more than 1 member showed detectable virus. In one household all four infected members demonstrated virus on the same day. Thus there remained a total of 14 families demonstrating isolations subsequent to the primary. Six families demonstrated their first subsequent isolation between the first and sixth days, and eight between the seventh and twelfth days. There were seven families with second subsequent isolations; one between the first and sixth days, four between the seventh and twelfth days, and two between the thirteenth and eighteenth days. There were four families with third subsequent isolations: one each for the 7-12 and the 13-18 day periods and two for the 19-31 day period.

Of the 27 persons harboring virus subsequent to the initial family isolation, 8 isolations were from specimens taken between the first and sixth days, 14 between the seventh and twelfth days, 3 between the thirteenth and eighteenth days, and 2 between the nineteenth

TABLE 94

Intervals between initial and subsequent isolations of polioviruses within families

Number days following initial family isolation*	Subsequent Isolations						Total number of persons
	First		Second		Third		
	Families No.	Persons No.	Families No.	Persons No.	Families No.	Persons No.	
1 - 6	6	7	1	1	0	0	8
7 - 12	8	9	4	4	1	1	14
13 - 18	0	0	2	2	1	1	3
19 - 31	0	0	0	0	2	2	2**
Total	14	16	7	7	4	4	27

*Number of days subsequent to index isolation date.

**One of these represents isolation from the stool on the 31st day.

and thirty-first days. Thus, 81% of the subsequent isolations occurred by the twelfth day. All five isolations occurring after the twelfth day were preceded by two or three isolations from familial associates. The large number of isolations occurring after the seventh day suggests that a considerable number of subclinical infections arose as secondary infections from infected familial associates.

RELATION OF AGE TO SEQUENCE OF INFECTION AS JUDGED BY VIRUS ISOLATIONS

Of the 14 families with secondary isolations, all index isolations occurred in children under 10 years of age, 10 of them being in children 4 years of age or younger. In families in which virus was isolated from parents, the parents were the last members of their respective households to demonstrate virus.

VIRUS ISOLATIONS
BY MONTH

The months in which isolations were made from 52 different persons are tabulated in table 95. All nine of the type 1 isolations

TABLE 95

Number of isolations of polioviruses, by month

Month	. Type Isolated			All Types
	1	2	3	
July	0	8	0	8
August	0	23	1	24
September	0	10	0	10
October	9	1	0	10
Total	9	42	1	52

were confined to October. This was of interest in view of the fact that clinical cases in the Cleveland area occurred during July through October. Forty-two type 2 isolations were spread over July through October with a concentration of 23 during August. The single type 3 isolation occurred during August.

IMMUNE STATUS AND SECONDARY INFECTION RATE AS DETERMINED BY PHARYNGEAL SWAB

There were 74 persons exposed to an index infection in 21 families and from 29 of these the infecting type of poliovirus was isolated

TABLE 96

Distribution of 74 persons in 21 families exposed to infection* within the home, according to pre-epidemic immune status and whether or not poliovirus was isolated from their throats

Pre-epidemic immune status	Throat isolation result	Number of persons
Susceptible	+	23
(45)	0	22
	unknown	0
Unknown	+	6
(17)	0	9
	unknown	2
Immune	+	0
(12)	0	9
	unknown	3
Total		74

*Index infections as determined by first virus isolation: throat—15; stool—5; both throat and stool on same day—1. These persons are excluded from the above analysis.

from the throat (table 96). Of 45 persons susceptible to the infecting type of poliovirus, 23 or one-half acquired the virus. In contrast, none of nine individuals having detectable antibodies were found to harbor virus. These data suggest a high degree of parasitism in persons exposed within the family and who were immunologically susceptible, and high resistance in those presumably immune. Although not directly comparable, the results are similar to those reported by Brown *et al.* (38) and Bhatt *et al.* (33) based on recovery of virus from stools of family associates of clinical cases of poliomyelitis.

PERSISTENCE OF VIRUS IN THE THROAT

Perisistence of polioviruses in the throat as determined by weekly assay is shown in table 97. Of the 49 persons demonstrating virus in their throats, 41, or 84%, were positive only during the first week of detection. The remaining eight, or 16%, harbored virus from 8 to 14 days after first dectection. These data show that polioviruses are infrequently recovered from the throats of subclinical cases beyond the first week of detection.

TABLE 97

Persistence of poliovirus in the throat

Number of days between first and last isolation*	Number of persons	%
1 - 7	41	84
8 - 14	8	16

*In six instances the first negative swab tested preceding the first positive swab was in excess of 7 days. In 13 instances the first negative swab tested following the last positive swab was in excess of 7 days.

THE USE OF THE PHARYNGEAL SWAB FOR THE ISOLATION OF POLIVIRUSES

The recovery of polioviruses from the pharynx of symptomatic and asymptomatic contacts of clinical cases has been reported by several investigators (37, 39, 41, 74, 88, 97, 120, 138, 139). Where comparison has been made with stool specimens, superiority of the latter has been demonstrated. As has been shown with clinical cases and their contacts (39, 41, 74, 88, 97, 120, 138), the recovery of virus from the throat is limited to a brief period early in the course of the disease. The present investigation, dealing with asymptomatic persons, has consequently utilized the assay of pharyngeal swabs collected at frequent intervals during the epidemic season, in order to determine the frequency of detecting virus at this site. This regimen may have afforded a more thorough evalution of the frequency of occurrence of poliovirus in the throat than has been heretofore reported.

COMPARISON OF THE PHARYNGEAL SWAB WITH THE STOOL SPECIMEN

Throat and stool specimens were examined from 45 persons who had demonstrated experience with virus, either by serological evidence or by virus isolation, and from whom both types of specimens were available. Comparison of virus isolation from the two sources is shown in table 98. Virus was recovered from both the stool and the throat of 21 (47%) of the 45 persons. Nine (20%) demonstrated virus in the throat but not in the stool. Three (7%) had virus in the stool but not in the throat. Twelve (27%) persons failed to yield virus from either source although serological evidence of experience with virus was present.

These data are not interpreted to imply that the pharyngeal swab *per se* is a source more likely to yield virus than the stool. The

TABLE 98

The frequency with which polioviruses were isolated from pharyngeal swabs and from stool specimens in 45 persons

Stool	Pharyngeal Swab		Totals
	Positive	Negative	
Positive	21 (47%)	3 (7%)	24
Negative	9 (20%)	12 (27%)	21
Total	30	15	45

greater number of throat swabs (14.6 per person) than stool specimens (2.0 per person) examined has undoubtedly contributed to the higher isolation rate obtained with the former. The relative ease both in procuring and examining multiple pharyngeal swabs would, however, recommend their use.

QUANTITATION OF VIRUS FROM PHARYNGEAL SWABS

Quantitation of virus was performed on the pharyngeal swabs of 39 persons. The original swab suspension was diluted serially in tenfold increments through 10^{-4}. One-tenth ml. of each dilution was inoculated into each of four tissue culture tubes. The cell cultures were observed for cytopathic change for 6 to 8 days. Pairs of tubes of a given dilution without typical degeneration were pooled and 0.1 ml. inoculated into fresh tubes. Frequently cytopathic change was not manifest until the second passage. The titer was considered to be the highest dilution of the original swab suspension showing the presence of virus in either the first or the second HeLa culture passage. Results are tabulated in table 99.

TABLE 99

Titer of poliovirus isolated from the throats of 39 individuals

Virus titer	Number of individuals	% of total tested
Undiluted	4	10
10^{-1}	11	28
10^{-2}	13	33
10^{-3}	6	15
10^{-4}	5	13
Total	39	100

More than 60% of the swabs yielded virus in concentrations of 10^2 or greater. Since the results were based on single positive swabs, the titers expressed do not necessarily represent the maximum attained by an individual in the course of his infection. The magnitude of titers obtained suggested that the respiratory tract may be a more important focus in the spread of infection than has heretofore been conceded by many students of the disease.

Chapter XIII
COMMUNICABLE DISEASES AND OTHER INFECTIONS

Most of the common communicable diseases occurred and recurred in this population during the period of the study, with the exception of smallpox, diphtheria and pertussis. The children all received the regular courses of immunization from their pediatricians which included, as a minimum, smallpox and pertussis vaccines and diphtheria and tetanus toxoids. The absence of smallpox and diphtheria was not surprising in view of the immunization program and the lack of opportunity to acquire these infections in Cleveland during the period of the study. The absence of pertussis, however, may be a reflection of the efficacy of pertussis vaccine, since whooping cough occurred in Cleveland each year of the study (table 100) (29).

TABLE 100

Number of reported cases of 6 communicable diseases in Cleveland, 1948-1957

Year	Chicken-pox	German measles	Diphtheria	Measles	Mumps	Whooping cough
1948	4151	117	5	547	600	389
1949	1533	317	8	7698	1746	408
1950	2852	78	2	321	807	2190
1951	2280	207	0	2487	961	285
1952	2403	381	5	6016	611	390
1953	1811	347	3	893	1434	1095
1954	928	740	6	6741	417	720
1955	1440	90	7	1586	531	653
1956	946	423	1	3513	1153	247
1957	988	90	1*	534	432	485

*A questionable case. This case was not confirmed by diagnostic procedures.

The diseases of chief importance are shown in table 101. Diseases which occurred less frequently or were of less importance may be found in Appendix 5, table 1.

TABLE 101

Number of cases of communicable diseases and other infections as diagnosed clinically

Disease	Number of cases	Number of persons	Number of outbreaks
Chickenpox	165	165	71
Measles	156	150	76
Mumps	114	113	64
Rubella	66	63	44
Roseola infantum	54	50	54
Conjunctivitis	188	141	....
Herpes simplex	172	50	....
Furunculosis	136	76	....
Cervical adenitis	55	46	....
Warts	27	25	....
Impetigo	25	22	....
Worm infestations	23	15	....

CHICKENPOX

During the course of the study 165 cases of chickenpox occurred in 71 outbreaks involving 62 families. One case occurred while the patient was hospitalized for another reason and as a result the family was not exposed. The analyses are, therefore, based on 164 cases and 70 outbreaks. Two outbreaks were experienced by each of eight families.

ANNUAL AND SEASONAL OCCURRENCE

Chickenpox is ordinarily endemic in large populations and usually shows a peak in the late winter and spring. In general, this seasonal occurrence is shown by our data (figure 63). In 2 years, 1951 and 1952, moderate peaks occurred in June. Examination of the data, however, showed that these peaks were concentrated in a few family outbreaks — six cases in four families in June, 1951, and four cases in three families in 1952. This variation probably reflects little more than the small number of cases involved. During the winter of 1952-1953, there was a high occurrence of chickenpox which might account for the absence of the disease from May, 1953 until January, 1955 and might thus represent an exhaustion of susceptibles. That such was probably not the case, however, is indicated by the fact that approximately 30% of the

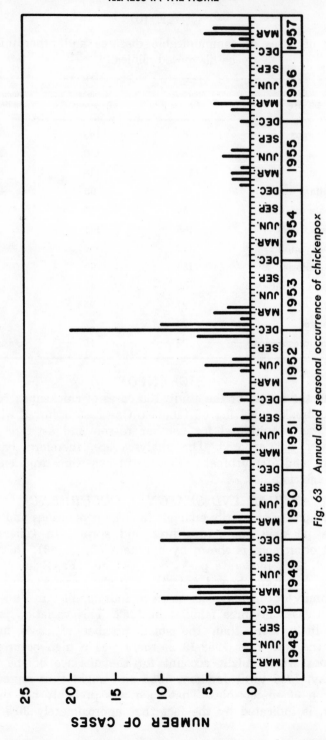

Fig. 63   Annual and seasonal occurrence of chickenpox

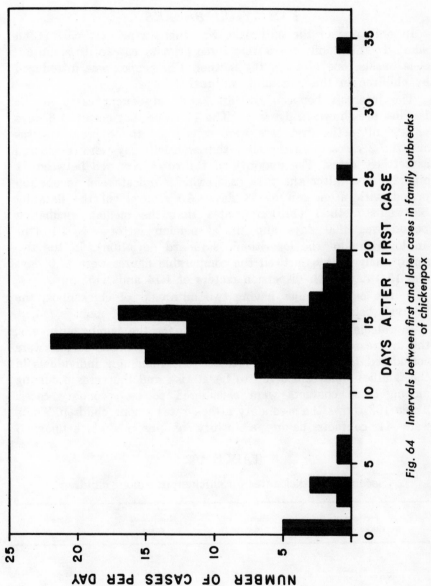

Fig. 64 Intervals between first and later cases in family outbreaks
of chickenpox

study population was still susceptible in 1954. A more likely explanation is that the risk of exposure in the community was low. This is borne out by the data for reported cases in Cleveland (table 100) which show that 1954 was a year of low occurrence.

FAMILY OUTBREAKS

In only one of the outbreaks was there a primary case in an adult. In this family there were three primary cases with simultaneous onsets, one of them the mother. Chickenpox was introduced by children in the remaining outbreaks.

The intervals between the first and subsequent cases in the families are shown in figure 64. The 11 cases that occurred 6 days or less after the first case were considered to be primary cases and the 2 cases occurring after the twentieth day were considered as tertiary cases. The majority of the cases occurred between 11 and 20 days after the first case, which indicates an incubation period with a median of 13 days. An analysis of the data by Sartwell's method (119) indicates that the median incubation period was 13.0 days and the dispersion factor was 1.1 (the antilogarithm of the logarithmic standard deviation). In the two series analyzed by Sartwell the comparable figures were 14.0 days and 15.0 days with dispersion factors of 1.14 and 1.15.

In the eight families having two outbreaks of chickenpox, the intervals between the outbreaks varied from 6 to 87 months.

In calculating secondary attack rates for the family outbreaks, the first case, or cases in the event of simultaneous onsets, were considered to be the primary cases. The remaining individuals in the families were considered to be at risk and the cases occurring among these contacts were considered to be secondary cases. Table 102 shows the secondary attack rates among children. There were 41 contacts having a history of previous chickenpox; 3

TABLE 102

Secondary attack rates for chickenpox among children

Previous chickenpox	Number of contacts	Number of cases	Rate %
Yes	41	3	7
No	85	78	92
Unknown	1	1	100
Total	127	82	65

developed the disease, an attack rate of 7%. Among the 85 contacts who had no history of previous chickenpox, 78 cases occurred, a secondary attack rate of 92%. There were no cases among 115 adults who had a history of previous chickenpox and there was 1 case among the 21 who had no such history, an attack rate of 5% (table 103).

TABLE 103

Secondary attack rates for chickenpox among parents

Previous chickenpox	Number of contacts	Number of cases	Rate %
Yes	115	0	0
No	21	1	5
Unknown	3	0	0
Total	139	1	1

There were three children in the study who had two illnesses diagnosed as chickenpox. One of these had a history of chickenpox prior to entering the study but developed the disease later while under observation. In the other two children, the first illnesses were atypical and occurred in a nonepidemic season (August and September), but the most likely diagnosis was considered to be "probable" chickenpox. The second illnesses in all three children were clinically and epidemiologically typical of chickenpox so that doubt must remain about the true nature of the first illnesses.

INTERESTING FAMILY EPISODE

In this family of five members, both parents had had chickenpox in childhood but none of their three children had experienced the disease. The mother developed herpes zoster and all three children became sick simultaneously with classical chickenpox 17 days later, an occurrence similar to those described by others relating herpes zoster and chickenpox epidemiologically.

Case I: Age 35 years, mother.—Five days prior to the onset of symptoms specifically referable to herpes zoster, this mother developed slight irritation of the throat and mild cough. One day later she had headache as well. For 3 days prior to the onset of herpes zoster, she complained of feeling miserable and developed a fever blister on her lower lip. The respiratory symptoms remained the same. On the next day, the first symptom suggestive of herpes zoster appeared as intermittent shooting pains in the left side of her head and ear. This day was considered to be the day of onset of zoster. On the next day shooting pains extended into the left arm which became tender to touch. The following day her left arm was still uncomfortable and a rash appeared on the left side of her face. On the fourth day her arm felt better but the rash extended from her ear to beneath her chin. The lymph nodes on the left side of her neck and under her chin were swollen. Her neck felt stiff and sore. On the fifth day the neck was more comfortable but the left side of her face was covered with clusters of vesicles. Her throat still felt irritated and she was coughing, mostly at night. On the sixth day her face was very painful and the vesicles extended from the ear to the neck and under the chin; the eye was not involved. For the next 4 days she experienced a great deal of pain in her face. She continued to cough at night. On the eleventh day of illness the pain began to subside. By the eighteenth day the lesions on her face had completely dried and she felt perfectly well. During the subsequent week the lesions cleared gradually; at no time was there evidence of secondary infection.

Case II: Age 3 years, male.—Sixteen days after the onset of herpes zoster in the mother, this youngster complained of being tired and asked to be put to bed. He felt slightly warm. The mother noted two or three little "red spots" on his body. On the next day the lesions of chickenpox were evident. During the next 3 days he had a great deal of itching and discomfort without fever. He was fully recovered by the twelfth day.

Cases III and IV: Ages 5 and 8 years, females.—Both of these girls developed chickenpox lesions on the same day, 17 days after the onset of herpes zoster in their mother. Neither one had fever, but both of them experienced considerable itching and discomfort. The disease lasted 10 days in each instance.

MEASLES

During the study there were 156 cases diagnosed as measles in 76 family outbreaks involving 62 families. Clinically the illnesses were typical of measles with the exception of three cases. In the latter cases no rash was present, the diagnosis of measles being based on respiratory and constitutional symptoms and the history of exposure. All three children had received gamma globulin after exposure. No secondary cases developed in two of the families and the occurrence of secondary cases in the third family was unknown since the family left the study on the sixth day after the onset of the case under consideration. These three cases have been omitted from most of the subsequent tabulations because of reasonable doubt that they were measles. Sera from one of the cases failed

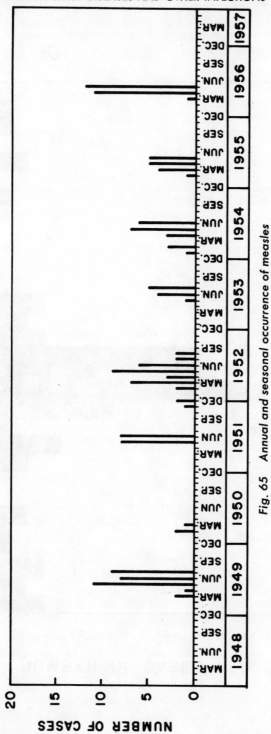

Fig. 65   Annual and seasonal occurrence of measles

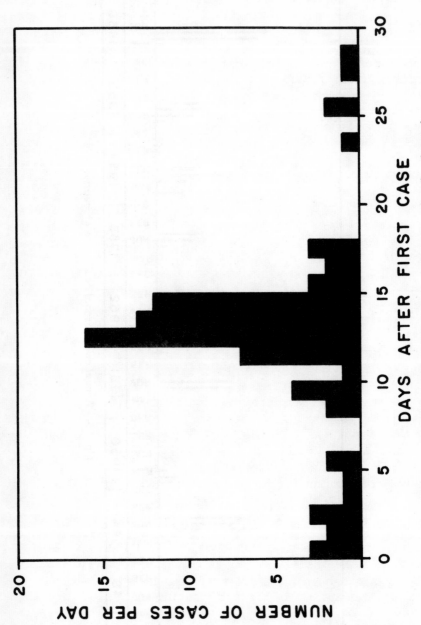

Fig. 66   Intervals between first and later cases in family outbreaks of measles

to confirm the diagnosis of measles. In the second instance, sera were not available after the illness, but the child developed characteristic clinical measles with an antibody response at a later date. No sera were available from the child whose family left the study. Most of the analyses, then, are based on 153 cases occurring in 73 outbreaks in 61 families. Each of 14 families had two outbreaks diagnosed as measles. In two of these families, however, there was a question as to whether or not the first outbreaks were actually measles, as indicated above.

The annual and seasonal occurrence of measles is shown in figure 65. As is generally true, measles occurred predominantly in the spring of the year. In 1949 to 1952, a 3-year cycle was apparent and thereafter there was a suggestion of 2-year cycles, although measles occurred each year except 1948 and 1957.

A study of family outbreaks provided considerable information regarding the incubation period, secondary attack rates, and multiple outbreaks. The intervals between the first cases and later cases in the families are plotted in figure 66. These intervals were based on the dates on which the rash appeared in most instances. In three outbreaks where the dates of rash in one or more of the cases were not known, the interval was based on dates of onset as determined from the clinical record. Somewhat arbitrarily, 12 cases which occurred five or less days after the first case in the family were considered as primary cases. Sixty-three cases which occurred between 8 and 17 days after the first case were considered as secondary cases and the remaining five cases occurring in the 23 to 28 day period were considered as tertiary cases. If the 63 secondary cases are analyzed in accordance with Sartwell's method (119), the median incubation period was 12.0 days and the dispersion factor was 1.2. Thus the data were very comparable to those in other series analyzed by Sartwell.

In 72 of the family outbreaks a child was the first case and in only one was an adult the first case. Secondary attack rates among the children are shown in table 104. There were two cases occurring among 32 contacts who had a history of having had measles previously, a secondary attack rate of 6%. There were 63 cases of measles among the 100 children who had no history of measles, an attack rate of 63%. This figure seems to be somewhat low in view of the reputed infectiousness of measles.

Antibody studies (complement fixation) were carried out on 20 children with a history of measles whose families had two outbreaks of measles while under observation, so that it was known that they had at least two exposures. Sera from the remaining 12 children were not tested. The two children who developed measles

TABLE 104

Secondary attack rates for measles among children

History of measles	Number of contacts	Number of cases	Rate (%)
Yes	32	2*	6
No	100	63	63
Total	132	65	49

*These children are also included among the 63 cases of measles which developed among the 100 contacts with no history of measles. The sequence of events is described in detail later in the text (Family 2, page 253).

had no detectable antibody in their sera prior to the family outbreaks; both developed antibody after their illnesses. Seventeen of the remaining 18 children had antibody prior to the outbreaks; 1 was considered to be unknown because the pre-outbreak serum was anticomplementary. None of these 18 children developed illnesses and none showed a significant or "booster" increase in titer of antibody in post-outbreak sera. It is thus apparent that there was an excellent correlation between the presence of antibody and resistance to infection.

Of the 63 children (table 104) who had no history of measles and who developed clinically diagnosed disease, antibody data were available for 10. Seven of these had no detectable antibody in their pre-outbreak sera; all developed antibody after the outbreak. One had a pre-outbreak titer of 4 and a post-outbreak titer of 64. The other two children received gamma globulin and were considered to have had "modified" measles. Neither of them had antibody before or after the outbreak and both later developed measles with antibody responses. Sera from the remaining 53 children who developed measles were not tested.

There were 37 children who had no history of measles and failed to develop the disease as the result of exposure in the family outbreaks. Eight children (three less than 6 months of age) had detectable antibody in their pre-outbreak sera and thus were probably immune. In 19 instances, the pre-outbreak sera showed no antibody. Two of these were children less than 6 months of age who may have been resistant to infection as the result of persistent but undetectable antibody. Three children developed antibody in their post-outbreak sera and thus represented inapparent infections. Two of the other 16 children later developed measles. For 10 children, pre-outbreak sera were anticomplementary or not available; thus their pre-outbreak immune status was considered as "unknown." Four of these children had antibody in post-outbreak sera. Two others later developed measles. Thus, of the 37 children, 10 probably failed to develop measles because of immunity, 7 may represent inapparent infection and 20 escaped infection.

TABLE 105

Secondary attack rates for measles among parents

Previous measles	Number of contacts	Number of cases	Rate (%)
Yes	124	0	0
No	14	3*	21
Unknown	7	0	0
Total	145	3	2

*Confirmed serologically.

Secondary attack rates among the parents are shown in table 105. No cases developed among the 124 contacts who had histories of measles. There were three cases among the 14 contacts who had no history of measles, an attack rate of 21%. Serological studies on 22 of the 124 parents who gave a history of measles showed that all 22 had detectable antibody. The remaining 102 were not tested. Examination of the sera from the 14 persons who did not give a history of measles showed that six had antibody and thus were presumably immune. Of the eight contacts (seven parents) who had no pre-outbreak antibody, three developed measles as secondary cases. Thus the secondary attack rate in the non-antibody group was 3/8 or 38%.* Six of the seven persons who did not know whether they had had measles previously had antibody in pre-outbreak sera. One did not but developed a titer of 32 after the family outbreak. He had no illness and presumably represented a subclinical infection or an anamnestic response from an undetectable level. Thus, a definite history of measles was a reliable indication of immunity to the disease, although the converse was not the case.

There were 12 families in which two outbreaks of measles occurred. The shortest interval between the first and second outbreaks was 9 months and the longest was 84 months. A number of

*At a later date two additional parents in this group developed measles. One parent without antibody had neither clinical illness nor antibody after two household exposures.

interesting variations in the behavior of measles was noted in these families. Events in two of the families are summarized below.

MEASLES IN FAMILY 1

This family had outbreaks in 1949 and 1952. Both parents had had measles but none of the four children had a history of measles. During the first episode all four children were given gamma globulin and two of them subsequently developed measles in modified form. During the second outbreak the index case had a classical attack of measles while the second case had a modified infection after receiving gamma globulin. The two children previously infected remained well.

First outbreak, Case I: Age 6 years, female.—This child was given gamma globulin on July 5, 1949, one day after being exposed to measles. On the 11th day (July 16) after injection her mother observed that the child was cranky and she remained so for 3 more days. She developed anorexia as well on the 4th day (July 19). On the next day she developed a temperature of 101.2°F., a scattered morbilliform rash, vomiting and diarrhea. Two Koplik spots were seen on the anterior tonsillar pillars. During the remainder of her illness there were no respiratory or gastrointestinal symptoms, and she was fully recovered by the 11th day (July 26). The antibody titer of her pre-outbreak serum was 8; that of the post-outbreak serum was 32.

Case II: Age 10 years, male.—This child was given gamma globulin on June 27, 1949, after exposure to measles. On the 23rd day (July 20) after injection and on the day of appearance of rash in the sister, he developed anorexia, followed on the next day by a temperature of 102°F., headache and malaise. On the third day of illness his temperature rose to 103°F. and a faint rash was seen on his back and face. Also there were two suspicious Koplik spots. This illness proved to be very mild with no respiratory symptoms and he had fully recovered by the seventh day. The pre-outbreak serum showed no detectable antibody; the titer of the post-outbreak serum was 64.

Second outbreak, Case I: Age 6 years, female.—The illness in this child began on April 26, 1952, with a temperature of 100°F., watery nasal discharge and throat cough that continued on the second day without fever. On the third day she had a temperature of 103°F. with continued respiratory symptoms. On the fourth day the temperature rose to 105°F., Koplik spots were evident and the rash emerged. The nasal discharge and cough continued but the course of her illness was uncomplicated with full recovery by the 12th day. No antibody was detectable in a serum obtained on

October 27, 1950, between the two outbreaks; the titer of the post-outbreak serum was 32.

Case II: Age 4 years, male.—This child became abruptly and acutely ill on the 9th day (May 8, 1952) after the onset of rash in his older sister. He had received gamma globulin on the day after the sister's rash appeared. On the first day he had a temperature of 102.3°F. and an irritated throat. A throat culture taken on the day prior to onset revealed normal flora. On the second day he had a sore throat, exudative tonsillitis, an injected pharynx and enlarged and slightly tender anterior cervical lymph nodes. Again, the throat culture showed no pathogenic bacteria. He was given an injection of penicillin on the second day (after the culture) and oral penicillin on the third and fourth days, but remained acutely ill. On the fourth day his temperature was 102.3°F. and he developed a cough but the sore throat was no longer present. On the fifth day he had a temperature of 105.2°F. and a rash. The cough continued. The rash was considered to be modified and he was fully recovered by the twelfth day. His pre-outbreak serum was anticomplementary; the post-outbreak serum had a titer of 64.

MEASLES IN FAMILY 2

This family had outbreaks in 1950 and 1951. The mother and all three children had not had measles historically. During the first episode all four susceptible members received gamma globulin. The mother escaped infection but the three children were believed to have had modified illnesses. Two of them, however, were such mild cases that they might have passed unnoticed. During the second family episode the mother was the index case and the two children who had mild illnesses during the first outbreak were given gamma globulin again and again experienced modified rashes that were, however, more definite than the first time. The child who had the more certain case of modified measles during the first outbreak was not given gamma globulin but escaped infection in the second outbreak.

First outbreak, Case I: Age 5 years, female.—On the seventh day (February 8, 1950) after exposure to measles this child was given gamma globulin. During the following 2 days she complained that her eyes felt tired. She appeared to be normal during the next 3 days. On the sixth day (February 14) after gamma globulin and the 13th day after exposure she developed a nasal discharge and her temperature was 100.4°F. Her temperature rose to 102.2°F. on the next day and she complained that her eyes hurt. She was a little better on the following day. Finally, on February 17 a rash appeared accompanied by temperature of 102°F., continued nasal discharge and an irritated throat. There were no complications and she was fully recovered on the 7th day after the onset of the rash. No antibody was detectable in the pre-outbreak serum; the titer of the post-outbreak serum was 64.

Case II: Age 3 years, female.—This child was given gamma globulin on the day after her older sister developed a rash. On the tenth day, February 28, after injection she seemed irritable and her temperature was 100.3°F. On the following day her mother said that she had a slight throat cough and her temperature was 100.2°F. No rash was evident. On the third day (March 2) a public health nurse stated that a rash was present. The patient was examined by a family study physician on the fourth day. He found a questionable rash on the left thorax. The mother then stated that there was a slight rash that persisted over the next 9 days. It was never described specifically. The child had no respiratory symptoms or any other complaints during the period when the rash in question appeared. Antibodies were not detectable in either pre-outbreak or post-outbreak sera.

Case III: Age 1 year, male.—This infant was given gamma globulin on Feb. 18, the day after his older sister's rash appeared. On the day following injection he experienced a watery nasal discharge which persisted through March 7. On the 10th day (March 1) after injection, the mother remarked that he was a "little off his feed" and seemed slightly irritable and he continued to be this way for the next 4 days. He was seen by the public health nurse on March 2 who declared that he too had a rash. On the following day a family study physician described a measles-like rash on this thorax but also noted that he had had a papular rash on his hands and forearms for several weeks. On the next day his temperature was 100°F. and the mother noted that he was "pulling" at his ear. He was not examined again and the slight fever was present for just one day. Antibody was not detected in either the pre-outbreak or post-outbreak sera.

Second outbreak, Case I: Age 30 years, mother.—The mother became chilly on November 22, 1951, and her temperature proved to be 100.4°F. On the next day she had generalized malaise and a temperature of 102°F. She remained about the same on the third day. On the fourth day, her temperature rose to 103.2°F. accompanied by sneezing, irritated throat and cough; she remained unchanged throughout the next day. Finally, on the sixth day a rash appeared accompanied by continued fever and respiratory symptoms. Koplik spots were also seen. The course of her illness was uncomplicated and she was fully recovered by the 20th day after onset. Antibody was not found in the pre-outbreak serum; the titer of the post-outbreak serum was 128.

Case II: Age 5 years, female.—This child was given gamma globulin on the day after her mother's rash appeared. On the 13th day after injection and 14 days after the mother's rash she complained of a headache and it was noted that she had a nasal discharge and that her temperature was 102° F. She had the same temperature on the following day and her throat felt irritated. Examination revealed injection of the nasal mucosa, tonsils, soft palate and pharynx but no Koplik spots. The fever and respiratory symptoms continued on the third day together with diarrhea. On the fourth day she developed a blotchy rash that disappeared within four days. Fever (102.3°F.) was still present the day the rash appeared but was absent during the subsequent three days. She was fully recovered by the eighth day. Antibody was not found in the pre-outbreak serum; the titer of the post-outbreak serum was 128.

Case III: Age 3 years, male.—This boy was given gamma globulin on the day following the appearance of the rash in his mother. On the 16th day after injection he had a rash and anorexia but no fever or respiratory symptoms. He was away from the family and was not examined. He felt feverish on the fourth day and the rash was gone by the sixth day. There were no other symptoms. Antibody was not found in the pre-outbreak serum; the titer of the post-outbreak serum was 16.

A summary of the occurrence of measles in the children and parents in the 12 families which experienced two outbreaks is

TABLE 106

The occurrence of measles in children in the 12 families with multiple outbreaks of measles

Measles previous to first outbreak	Ill in first outbreak	Ill in second outbreak	
		Yes	No
Yes	Yes	....	....
Yes	No	....	....
No	Yes	4	18
No	No	11	2
	Not born	2	2

TABLE 107

The occurrence of measles in parents in the 12 families
with multiple outbreaks of measles

Measles previous to first outbreak	Ill in first outbreak	Ill in second outbreak	
		Yes	No
Yes	Yes	....	....
Yes	No	....	21
No	Yes	....	....
No	No	1	2

given in tables 106 and 107. There were four children who had had no previous history of measles but who were ill in both the first and second episodes. The experience of two of these children (Family 2) has been presented above. The third child's pre-outbreak serum showed no detectable antibody. After both outbreaks his antibody titer was 32. The fourth child had two illnesses approximately 4 years apart. No antibody was demonstrable in two sera collected between these outbreaks. After the second outbreak his antibody titer became 16.

There were 18 children who had no previous history of measles, developed illness in the first outbreak, and were subsequently immune. There were 11 children who had no history of measles and who did not become ill during the first outbreak in the family but did become ill during the second. In addition, there were two children who apparently experienced two outbreaks of measles in their families without acquiring the clinical disease. The family outbreaks in one instance occurred when the child was 1 month of age (cord blood titer of 32) and 10 months of age. His antibody titer was 8 approximately 1 year after the second outbreak. The second child experienced the first outbreak at 1 month of age. The cord blood showed no detectable antibody despite a titer of 32 in the mother's serum. No detectable antibody was present 1 year after birth, nor was it present 2 years later, before the second outbreak. No apparent illness occurred but the antibody titer after the second family outbreak was 16. Both of these children may be examples of inapparent infection.

In contrast, none of the 21 adults who had a previous history of measles developed measles during the first or second outbreaks and only one of three who had no history of measles developed the disease. Interestingly enough, this occurred during the second outbreak. Antibody studies showed no detectable antibody before or after the first outbreak or before the second outbreak, but the titer was 128 after the clinical illness in the second outbreak. Of the two others who had no history of measles and did not develop measles in either outbreak, one had antibody before the first outbreak and the other had no antibody either before or after the two outbreaks.

THE EFFECT OF GAMMA GLOBULIN ON SECONDARY ATTACK RATES

One of the questions that arose during analysis of the data on measles concerned the effect of gamma globulin on secondary attack rates. Since most of these families had their own pediatricians, gamma globulin was very extensively employed. No specific plans had been made in advance to collect such data, so that there was no routine questioning regarding the use of gamma globulin. Our confidence in the data is therefore quite limited and we present the analyses that have been made only to show the difficulties in interpreting data that were obtained in part retrospectively. In general, if no comment was made on the record, the child was considered not to have received gamma globulin. Table 108 presents

TABLE 108

Secondary attack rates among children 6 months of age or older who had not had measles, according to whether or not they were given gamma globulin

Gamma globulin	Number of contacts	Number of cases	Rate (%)
Yes	61	45*	74
No	30	17	57
Total	91	62	68

*Of these, 38 notes regarding gamma globulin were made by the mothers at the time when the children were given the injection; 1 was made by the visiting nurse at the time when the primary case in the family developed; 1 was made by the examining physician on the day following gamma globulin, but before the case was actually diagnosed as measles; 5 were made at the time when the children actually developed measles.

the secondary attack rates in terms of the use of gamma globulin for the 91 children 6 months of age or older who had not had measles previously. Three cases of measles, two of whom had received gamma globulin 13 days after exposure and one of whom had received gamma globulin 18 days after onset of the first case were considered not to have received gamma globulin. Table 108 shows that the clinical attack rate among the 61 contacts who received gamma globulin was 74% and among the 30 who had not, was 57%. This result was scarcely what would have been expected in view of the presumed efficacy of gamma globulin in preventing or modifying measles.

Accordingly, it was decided to restrict the analysis to those cases for which specific information regarding the use of gamma globulin was available in the records prior to the onset of each secondary case. On this basis, 40 of the 56 contacts who had received gamma globulin became ill, as did 22 of the 35 contacts who had presumably not received gamma globulin. That these figures are not reliable, however, is indicated by the fact that 5 of the 22 cases (23%) were known to have received gamma globulin, but a record of this fact was made only because they developed measles. If this same proportion of all 35 contacts had received gamma globulin, 8 of those recorded as not having received gamma globulin actually had received it. On this basis, the occurrences may be estimated to be as follows: 70% of those receiving gamma globulin developed measles, as did 63% of those who did not receive it (table 109), a difference which is not statistically significant.

TABLE 109

Secondary attack rates among children 6 months of age or older who had not had measles, adjusted for estimated deficiencies in recording the use of gamma globulin

Gamma globulin	Number of contacts	Number of cases	Rate (%)
Yes	64	45	70
No	27	17	63
Total	91	62	68

An attempt was then made to determine whether or not the secondary attack rate varied according to the interval between time of the rash of the primary case and the time of administering gamma globulin to the contact. This comparison was not possible because too few contacts were given gamma globulin more than 3 days after the onset of the index case. Apparently gamma globulin was given to prevent rather than to modify measles in most cases.

If any credence at all can be given to these data, there is an indication that gamma globulin may not be as effective as generally thought in preventing or modifying measles.

SECOND ATTACKS OF MEASLES

Second attacks of measles were reported as having occurred in six persons during the study and all six had had gamma globulin preceding their first illnesses, which were recorded as "modified measles". These include two cases whose first illnesses were omitted from most of the analyses because no rash developed. One additional child who developed measles while in the study gave a history of measles prior to entering. The diagnosis could not be confirmed serologically in five of the persons after the first "clinical" attack; two were unknown because sera were not available. Serological confirmation was obtained in all seven children after their second attacks.

AN INTERESTING FAMILY OUTBREAK

An interesting outbreak of measles occurred in a family of six members, none of whom had a history of the disease. On April 12, 1955, the mother delivered her fourth baby. On April 24, 12 days later, her second oldest child developed measles. On May 6 and 7, the oldest child and the mother acquired the disease. The mother's rash appeared on May 11; she was very sick with constitutional symptoms and a temperature of 105.2°F. On May 23 the newborn baby, then 41 days old, developed measles with characteristic signs of conjunctivitis, rash and fever (100.2°F.). The illness was mild; no gamma globulin was given to the baby. The child had not been nursed by the mother.

The father escaped infection. A daughter, aged 3 years, was given gamma globulin on the third day (May 2) after the onset of rash in the index case. She, too, did not develop measles. Furthermore, on the eighth day (May 10) after receiving gamma globulin and on the fourth day after the onset of prodromal symptoms in the second case in the family, she was sent away and did not return until after the recovery of the last individual.

Case I: Age 6 years, male.—On April 24 this child developed a temperature of 101°F. and generalized malaise for one day. He then went to school for 2 days during which time he appeared to be well. On the fourth day he developed nasal discharge and a croupy cough that persisted another day prior to the appearance of the rash on April 29. His temperature was not taken during the illness but it was noted that he was feverish. A slight acute catarrhal otitis media was observed on the day the rash appeared but the child never complained of an earache during the illness. He was fully recovered by the thirteenth day.

Case II: Age 7 years, male.—On the seventh day, May 6, after the onset of rash in Case I, this boy complained of aches and pains and appeared to be listless. His malaise persisted for 3 more days and on the fifth day he developed a temperature of 104°F. and a dry cough. On the sixth day, May 11, the rash appeared and his temperature remained at 104°F., accompanied by continued coughing. There were no complications and recovery was complete by the 14th day.

Case III: Age 28 years, mother.—On the eighth day (May 7) after the onset of rash in the index case, the mother began to feel dizzy and tired. These symptoms lasted through the next day. On the third day she had headache, discomfort in her eyes, generalized aching and cough. On the next day her temperature was 102°F. On the fifth day the rash appeared and her temperature rose to 105.2°F. accompanied by continued coughing and marked prostration. No complications developed, however, and she was fully recovered by the 15th day.

Case IV: Age 41 days, female.—On the twelfth day (May 23) following the onset of rash in the mother, the baby developed watery eyes and her temperature was 100.2°F. On the next day she had a generalized rash that receded rapidly on the following day and there was no sign of illness on the fourth day. The baby had no respiratory symptoms. Although the course of this baby's illness was unusual, it is reasonable to believe that this truly was a case of measles.

Antibody studies confirmed the diagnosis of measles in the 4 persons who had clinical illnesses. Antibody developed in the 3-year-old daughter who was not ill and thus probably had an inapparent infection. The father's pre-outbreak serum showed the presence of antibody.

MUMPS

There were 113 cases of clinically diagnosed mumps in 64 outbreaks in 55 families. Two outbreaks occurred in seven families and three outbreaks in one family. A child was the first case in all of the family outbreaks.

ANNUAL AND SEASONAL OCCURRENCE

As shown in figure 67, mumps occurred in each of the 9 years after 1948 although there was only one case in each of 4 years. Multiple cases occurred in 5 years, the biggest year being 1953 in which there were 37 cases. No cyclical occurrence is apparent either in these cases or in the reported cases in the City of

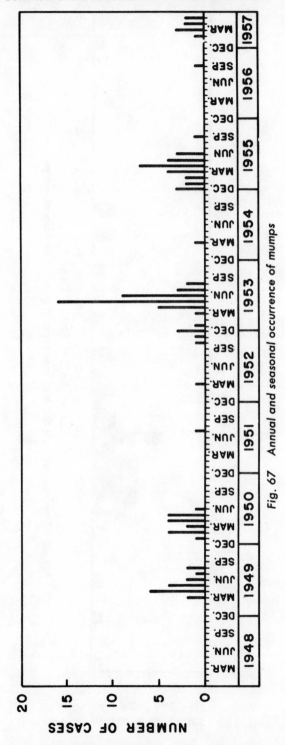

Fig. 67   Annual and seasonal occurrence of mumps

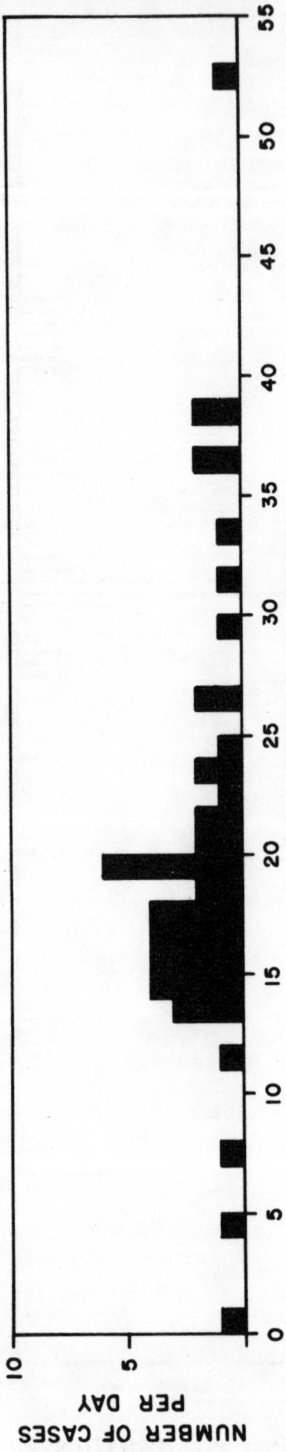

Fig. 68 Intervals between first and later cases in family outbreaks of mumps

Cleveland (table 100). The peak seasonal occurrence was between March and August.

FAMILY OUTBREAKS

The intervals between the first and subsequent cases in the family outbreaks are shown in figure 68. Assuming that cases which occurred at an interval of less than 12 days after the first case were primary cases, the most likely incubation period is from 13 to 26 days; the median incubation period determined by Sartwell's method (119) was 16.9 days with a dispersion factor of 1.24. There were eight cases that occurred more than 26 days after the first cases. In each of these families there were intervening cases at periods varying from 17 to 24 days, so that in all likelihood, the cases appearing more than 26 days after the first case represent tertiary cases.

TABLE 110

Secondary attack rates for mumps among children

History of mumps	Number of contacts	Number of cases	Rate (%)
Yes	19	0	0
No	94	38	40
Unknown	1	0	0
Total	114	38	33

Secondary attack rates among 114 children are shown in table 110. No cases occurred among those who had a history of mumps nor did the one child whose history was unknown develop the disease. All 38 cases occurred among the 94 children who had no history of mumps, an attack rate of 40%.

Data regarding the presence of complement-fixing antibody prior to exposure within the family were available for 99 of these 114 children, and post-outbreak antibody was determined for 92 of the 99 (Appendix 24, table 1). Two of the 19 children with a history of mumps had no detectable pre-outbreak antibody; one of these showed a post-outbreak rise in antibody titer, suggesting an inapparent infection or anamnestic response. There were 94 children who had no history of mumps. Sixteen of these had detectable pre-outbreak antibody, of whom four developed mumps; three of these four showed post-outbreak rises in antibody titer. Of the 12 remaining children who did not develop mumps, 3 had increases in antibody titer in the post-outbreak sera. No pre-outbreak antibody could be detected in 63 children, 28 of whom developed clinical mumps. Twenty-six of these 28 for whom sera were available showed confirmatory increases in antibody titer. Among the 35 children in this category who did not develop mumps, 12 showed rises in post-outbreak antibody titers, suggesting subclinical infections. Examination of the data without reference to the history of

TABLE 111

Secondary attack rates for mumps among parents

History of mumps	Number of contacts	Number of cases	Rate (%)
Yes	87	0	0
No	37	7	19
Unknown	4	0	0
Total	128	7	5

mumps showed that 4 of 33 children having detectable pre-outbreak antibodies developed mumps (12%), whereas 28 of 66 children (43%) without pre-outbreak antibody developed the disease.

Secondary attack rates among parents are shown in table 111. As was the case with children, no one of the 87 contacts who had a history of mumps developed the disease nor was there illness among the 4 whose history was unknown. All 7 cases occurred among the 37 individuals who had no history of mumps, an attack rate of 19%.

Of the seven parents who developed clinical mumps, six had no pre-outbreak antibody (Appendix 24, table 2). A rise in antibody titer was found in five of the six. There were 20 persons who apparently had inapparent infections or anamnestic responses as judged by the antibody studies.

These data indicate that a history of mumps provides the best index of resistance to the disease. In general, the presence of complement-fixing antibody against the mumps virus confirms these histories. A history of not having had mumps, however, does not have the same reliability, regardless of the presence or absence of antibody. There are enough inconsistencies to show that complete reliance cannot be placed on the presence or absence of antibody as an index of resistance or susceptibility to the disease. It is further apparent from these data that infection may occur without manifestations of disease, but be evident by changes in antibody status. Further study is necessary to demonstrate the role of such "inapparent infections" in the maintenance and spread of mumps.

Multiple outbreaks of mumps occurred in eight families. The intervals between the outbreaks varied from 98 days to 82 months and each episode was distinct. A number of unusual incidents occurred. For example, in one family two children escaped the disease during the first outbreak but developed it in the second. Neither child had antibody before or after the first outbreak. After the second outbreak both had antibody. There were two cases in which a clinical diagnosis of mumps was made but no antibody response was found serologically. In another family, one child was the only case of mumps in two outbreaks. He developed antibody following the first illness, lost it before the second outbreak, but developed it after the second outbreak. He did not become ill in the third family outbreak.

RUBELLA (GERMAN MEASLES)

Rubella or German measles is a mild communicable disease generally characterized by fever, catarrhal inflammation of the mucous membranes of the upper respiratory tract, enlargement of the posterior cervical, suboccipital, and postauricular lymph nodes, and a light, macular or pinpoint exanthem occurring on the face, chest, abdomen, thighs, and upper extremities. The clinical picture may be produced by one or more viruses, but a specific rubella virus thus far has not been isolated in the laboratory, so that serological tests for confirmation of the diagnosis are not available.*

During the study there were 66 cases which occurred in 44 outbreaks in 35 families. Two outbreaks occurred in each of seven families; three outbreaks occurred in one family.

CLINICAL DESCRIPTION

The diagnosis of rubella was based on the clinical features of the illnesses since laboratory methods for confirmation of the diagnosis were not available. In general, the illnesses corresponded quite closely to the classical textbook picture. The diagnosis was not made in the absence of a rash despite the fact that rubella has been reported to occur without a rash (91). A number of family contacts were suspected of having the infection without a rash but

---

*Since this section was written, an apparently specific rubella virus has been isolated by two groups of investigators (Parkman, P.D., Buescher, E. L. and Artenstein, M.S. Recovery of Rubella Virus from Army recruits. Proc. Soc. Exper. Biol. and Med., 111:225-230, 1962; Weller, T. H. and Neva, F. A. Propagation in Tissue Culture of Cytopathic Agents from Patients with Rubella-like Illness. Proc. Soc. Exper. Biol. and Med., 111:215-225, 1962). Practical laboratory procedures for the determination of antibody levels are in the process of development.

were excluded for purposes of this analysis. The onset was sudden in approximately two-thirds of the cases, a rash and fever varying from 99 to 103.5°F. appearing on the first day of illness. In these patients symptoms of feverishness, listlessness, anorexia, headache, irritability, chilliness, vomiting and abdominal pain were more apt to occur than in the cases where the onset was gradual. In the latter group the prodromal symptoms in general consisted of nasal discharge and obstruction, sneezing, sore or irritated throat, hoarseness, and cough (usually dry in character and rarely associated with production of sputum); nausea, diarrhea and photophobia occurred rarely.

Despite fever and other symptoms, most of the children appeared to be well and showed little evidence of discomfort from the illness. The rash was maculopapular or morbilliform in nature in the majority of instances and varied in color from pink to red. Generally it appeared on the face and the trunk and less frequently on the arms and legs, often disappearing from one area as it appeared in another. In a few instances it was diffuse, covering the entire body, and in some instances it was erythematous and scarlatiniform in nature. In some patients there was a blotchy injection of the soft palate, but in none were typical Koplik spots observed. In six patients the rash was associated with itching. Other findings were conjunctivitis, nasal injection or edema, nasal discharge and injection of the pharynx with lymphoid hyperplasia. Adenopathy in the posterior cervical chain or in the anterior cervical region was found in almost all of the cases. In only five patients was there no adenopathy. The spleen was palpable in one patient.

Joint involvement occurred in seven of the cases, five of whom were mothers; the other two were children, 11 and 8 years of age. One of the children was a boy and the other a girl. The involvement of the joints was principally in the fingers, wrists, ankles and toes, although in some patients the knees, the neck and the arms were also affected. In general, the joints were swollen and painful and in some instances stiff. Joint involvement varied in duration from 6 to 14 days.

The only complication that occurred in this series was catarrhal otitis media in one patient. Although five mothers had rubella while in the study, none of them was pregnant at the time of the illness.

ANNUAL AND SEASONAL OCCURRENCE

Cases of rubella occurred in each year of the study with 1952 and 1956 being the years of peak occurrence (figure 69). These data do not follow the pattern of the reported cases in Cleveland

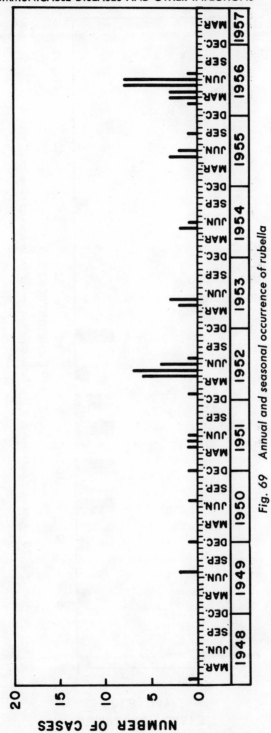

Fig. 69   Annual and seasonal occurrence of rubella

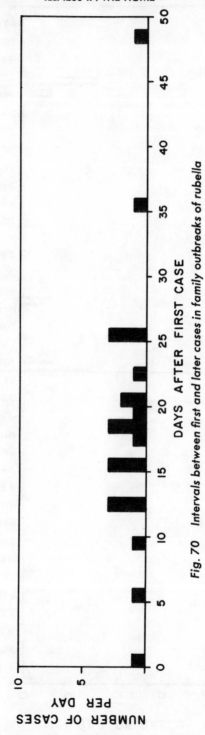

Fig. 70   Intervals between first and later cases in family outbreaks of rubella

(table 100), but that is not surprising in view of the small size and selective nature of our population and the fact that many mild cases of rubella are not reported.

Seasonal occurrence of the disease was characteristic, since 53 of the 66 cases occurred during the months from April to June. Analyses of larger series have shown that approximately two-thirds of the reported cases occur in this time interval (76).

FAMILY OUTBREAKS

As with the other communicable diseases of childhood, the interval between the occurrence of the first case and subsequent cases in the families provided an indication of the probable incubation period. This interval varied from 1 to 48 days (figure 70). In each family in which there were multiple cases and the interval between the first case and a subsequent case exceeded 25 days, there were intervening secondary cases. For example, in one family a case occurred 35 days after the index case but 18 days after a previous secondary case. In another family in which the interval was 48 days, there had been a previous case 23 days after the index case. It seems reasonable to accept these cases as tertiary cases rather than secondary. If the two cases which occurred 5 days or less after the first case are considered as multiple primary cases, the incubation period, then, would appear to vary from 9 to 25 days with a median of 18 days. The incubation period following inoculation of susceptible persons ranged from 9 to 16 days in one series (91) and from 13 to 20 days in another (27).

The index cases in the family outbreaks were children in 43 of the episodes and a mother in one. Persons without illness or with onset of illness more than 5 days after the first case were considered to be contacts at risk and the illnesses occurring among these persons were considered to be secondary cases for the purpose of calculating attack rates.

TABLE 112

Secondary attack rates for rubella among children

Previous rubella	Number of contacts	Number of cases	Rate %
Yes	18	2	11
No	82	14	17
Unknown	2	0	0
Total	102	16	16

Secondary attack rates among children are shown in table 112. The overall attack rate was 16%. The rate among the contacts who had a history of rubella was 11% and among those with no history of rubella it was 17%. Although the number of cases is small, these data suggest that one attack may not necessarily provide immunity, although serological data would be needed to confirm the diagnosis since illnesses due to certain viruses in the ECHO and Coxsackie groups may present similar characteristics.

The secondary attack rates among parents are shown in table 113. The total attack rate was 5%. Three of the 47 contacts who had a history of rubella developed the disease, an attack rate of 6%. One of the 27 persons with no history of rubella became ill, an attack rate of 4%.

TABLE 113

Secondary attack rates for rubella among parents

Previous rubella	Number of contacts	Number of cases	Rate %
Yes	47	3	6
No	27	1	4
Unknown	13	0	0
Total	87	4	5

Second attacks of rubella presumably occurred in 10 persons; 3 of these were children, both of whose illnesses were observed while the study was in progress. The other seven persons had a history of rubella before entry into the study and had their second attacks while under observation; four of these were adults and three were children. The second attacks did not aggregate in time so that there was no indication of the epidemic occurrence of another disease.

With two exceptions, the shortest interval between outbreaks in the families was 241 days. In one family, a case which developed 86 days after the onset of the initial case and 38 days after a final secondary case of the first outbreak, was considered to be the primary case of a new outbreak. In another family, a case which occurred more than 30 days after the onset of the primary case of the first outbreak was considered to be the primary case of a new outbreak. The exact number of days between primary cases could not be determined. In neither outbreak was there a secondary case.

INTERESTING CASE

Four illnesses that occurred in one child are described because they illustrate the difficulties in the diagnosis and differential diagnosis of rubella.

The patient, a boy, was aged 1 year and 7 months when the first of these illnesses occurred. It was diagnosed as a streptococcal infection with a rash. The onset was sudden with a temperature of 101°F., feverishness, irritability, anorexia, nasal discharge, cough, and a "blotchy" complexion. Physical examination on the second day of illness revealed slight injection of the pharynx and tonsils and enlarged posterior cervical nodes, but no enanthem or changes in the tongue. The rash at this time was described as brownish and papular without erythema, occurring almost exclusively on the trunk. No rash was apparent in the axillary or anticubital folds. The patient was treated with oral penicillin and recovered gradually, with a low grade temperature between 99 and 100°F. persisting for approximately 14 days. The rash disappeared on the eighth day of the illness. No desquamation occurred. Cultures of the throat on the first day of illness revealed a group A, type 4 streptococcus. Cultures taken after penicillin therapy was begun showed no streptococci. For a period of approximately 6 months before this illness and for a year afterward, this boy carried a group G streptococcus in his throat.

The second illness occurred 4 years later and was again diagnosed as a streptococcal illness with a rash. This time the onset was gradual with watery nasal discharge and obstruction, sneezing, feverishness, anorexia, headache and cough. Temperature was 100°F. A rash appeared on the second day of illness on the face spreading to the neck and trunk. At this time the patient appeared to be well with mild conjunctivitis, injection of the nasal mucosa with slight watery discharge, but with no injection of the tonsils or pharnyx, although slight lymphoid hyperplasia was present. The anterior cervical and submental nodes were enlarged. The rash appeared as a fiery red scarlatiniform eruption. Circumoral pallor was present. He was treated by his family physician with sulfonamides. A low grade fever persisted for 9 days. He was completely well on the tenth day of illness. Cultures of the throat at this time revealed no beta-hemolytic streptococci.

Fourteen months later, following exposure at school, he developed a third illness diagnosed as modified measles. The onset was sudden, with nasal discharge, sneezing, cough, headache, and a slight earache. The temperature was 102.4° F. and remained elevated for a period of 6 days. A blotchy red maculopapular rash appeared on the face and trunk on the fourth day of illness. Other physical findings were conjunctivitis, left catarrhal otitis media, injection of the nasal mucosa and anterior and posterior cervical adenopathy. Cultures of the throat revealed no pathogenic bacteria. With the exception of continuing slight nasal discharge, he was well on the eighth day of illness. His sister developed characteristic measles 18 days later.

Approximately 18 days after the onset of the above illness, the boy developed a fourth illness which presented a diagnostic problem. The onset was gradual with feverishness, chilliness, nasal discharge, irritated and sore throat, hoarseness, cough, anorexia, and vomiting on one occasion. His temperature ranged from 99° to 102°F. for 4 days. At the time of examination on the second day of illness the patient appeared to be listless. There was slight injection of the nasal mucous membranes and watery discharge. The uvula was slightly edematous and the pharnyx was slightly injected with lymphoid hyperplasia. The posterior and anterior cervical nodes were enlarged and firm, but not tender. Later that day a rash appeared. The patient was seen again on the fourth day of illness at which time he appeared to be only slightly ill, but a fine papular rash was present associated with a diffuse "scarlet" erythema of the face, trunk, arms and the popliteal areas. There were also conjunctival injection, injection of the nasal mucous membranes with watery discharge, injection of the soft palate, slight injection of the pharnyx, and adenopathy as noted above. The temperature persisted for 4 days at levels varying from 99° to 102°F. and the rash lasted a total of 5 days. Desquamation of the skin did not occur. Cultures of the throat on the second and fourth days of illness revealed the presence of group A, type 4, streptococci. No specific treatment was given. The course of this illness resembled rubella, but the appearance of the rash suggested scarlatina. No other cases of rubella occurred in the family.

It seems clear that this boy's third illness was measles, but the exact nature of the other 3 illnesses is more difficult to determine, and any one of them might have been rubella. It was finally decided on clinical grounds that the illness (his fourth) following the attack of measles was probably rubella.

Antistreptolysin 0 titers were determined in an attempt to clarify the nature of these illnesses (table 114). Three serum specimens before the first illness had titers of less than 12 (the lowest dilution employed). The titer 3½ months after the illness was 50, and declined during the subsequent 3 years to undetectable levels. These changes in titer and the cultural results provide probable confirmation of the clinical diagnosis.

TABLE 114

Four illnesses that occurred in one child, illustrating the difficulties in the diagnosis of rubella

No. Illness	Onset of illness	ASO Titer Date	ASO Titer Titer	Throat culture	Clinical diagnosis	Probable final diagnosis
1	1/21/51	9/5/49	<12	Streptococcus, Group A type 4	Streptococcal infection	Streptococcal infection
		5/1/50	<12			
		10/4/50	<12			
		5/7/51	50			
		10/11/52	12			
		4/2/53	12			
		9/3/53	<12			
		10/24/54	<12			
2	1/20/55	4/2/55	<12	No β hemolytic streptococci	Streptococcal illness	? Rubella
		10/20/55	<12			
		4/2/56	<12			
3	4/19/56			No pathogenic bacteria	Measles	Measles
4	5/7/56	10/28/56	166	Streptococcus, Group A type 4	Rubella	Streptococcal infection
		4/28/57	166			

The laboratory results did not confirm a diagnosis of streptococcal infection in the second illness, which may well have been rubella. In contrast, the cultural and serological findings indicated a diagnosis of streptococcal infection, rather than rubella, in the fourth illness.

It is of interest that this child apparently had two illnesses due to the same type of group A streptococcus, which is unusual. It is possible that treatment with penicillin in the first illness inhibited the immune response to a degree sufficient to allow a return of susceptibility.

ROSEOLA INFANTUM

Roseola infantum (exanthem subitum) has been considered to be the most common febrile exanthem in infants and children under 3 years of age (32, 35). The classical clinical picture consists of a febrile illness lasting from 3 to 5 days with a paucity of other symptoms and the appearance of a morbilliform rash coincident with the return of the temperature to normal, or shortly thereafter. It is considered by most authorities, however, that the disease may occur in a variety of modified forms and it has been estimated that while the disease is recognizable in only 15 to 30% of children, possibly all children have been exposed to the etiological agent by the age of 5 years.

In this study there were 54 illnesses diagnosed as roseola infantum occurring in 54 "outbreaks" in 38 families. Four persons were considered to have had the disease twice. Thus it is apparent that only one case occurred in a family at a time and that there were no secondary cases.

The clinical characteristics of the cases were as follows: The onset was generally sudden, fever and the symptoms usually associated with a febrile illness, such as feverishness, listlessness, anorexia and irritability, being the outstanding features early in the course. In most of the patients the highest temperatures ranged between 102° and 105°F; in only five instances was the highest recorded temperature less than 102°F. Despite the height of the fever, the children appeared, for the most part, to be well or only slightly to moderately ill. Symptoms referable to the respiratory tract, such as sneezing, nasal discharge and obstruction, sore throat and hoarseness, were observed in a few patients. Vomiting occurred in approximately one-fifth of the cases; diarrhea was observed in only two instances. Physical examination generally revealed few abnormalities apart from a rash. Signs that were noted were conjunctivitis, nasal discharge and injection, usually slight, of the nasal mucous membranes, tonsils, palate, and pharynx. In a few

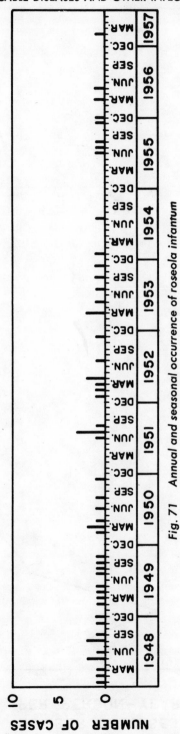

Fig. 71   Annual and seasonal occurrence of roseola infantum

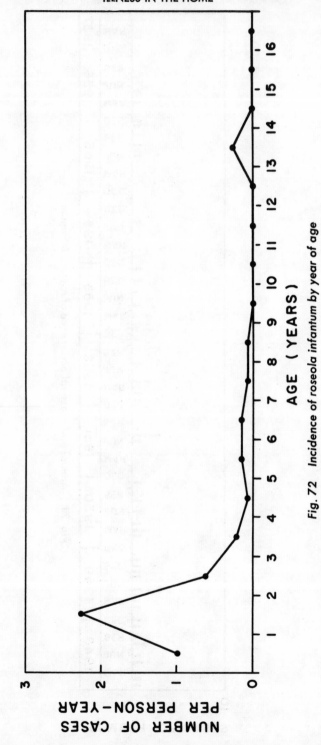

Fig. 72   Incidence of roseola infantum by year of age

instances lymphoid hyperplasia was noted. Slight to moderate anterior and posterior cervical adenopathy was observed in approximately one-third of the cases, but in only two instances were the nodes tender. The interval from the onset of illness to the appearance of the rash varied from 2 to 9 days, but in 49 of the patients the rash appeared on the third, fourth, or fifth day, usually at the time or just before fever subsided. The duration of fever was 4 days or less in 43 patients. There were only two patients who evidenced complications, one having a purulent conjunctivitis which lasted for 3 days and one having a convulsion at the height of the fever. In all instances, recovery was prompt and complete.

ANNUAL AND SEASONAL OCCURRENCE

Cases occurred in every year of the study and ranged in number from 2 to 11 per year (figure 71). There were fewer cases per year as the study progressed, undoubtedly as the result of the aging of the population. The cases occurred throughout the year and showed no seasonal variation although other studies (32, 35) have indicated that there may be two peaks of prevalence, one in the spring and the other in mid-autumn.

FAMILY OUTBREAKS

No information could be obtained regarding the incubation period of roseola since there were no family outbreaks in which more than a single case occurred.

The age distribution of the cases, based on an analysis of children born into the study, is shown in figure 72, which presents the cases per person-year in terms of age. It is apparent that almost all of the illnesses occurred before the age of 3 years and that the oldest case was 13 years of age. There were no cases among parents. Analysis of the cases by sex showed no difference in incidence between males and females.

There were 11 families in which two or more cases occurred: two cases in seven families, three cases in three families, and four cases in one family. The intervals between these cases varied from 133 to 1579 days. The intervals between illnesses in the four individuals who were considered to have had the disease twice varied from 346 to 1252 days. An analysis of the occurrence of roseola among the children born into the study, using a life-table method, showed that 37% of children had had the disease by 33 months of age (figure 73).

In an attempt to detect illnesses which might represent atypical forms of roseola infantum, the illnesses in each family which occurred during the period of 30 days prior to the occurrence of

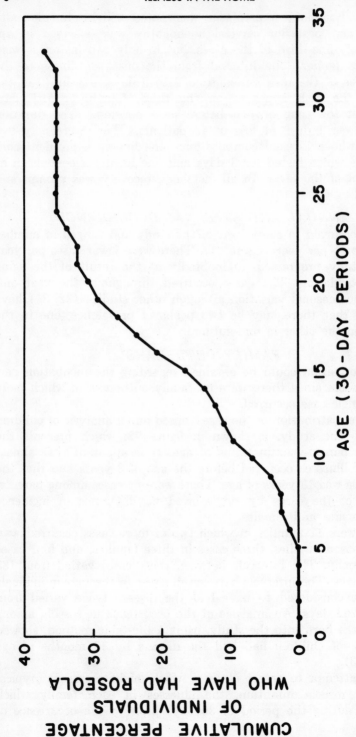

Fig. 73 Cumulative percentage of children born into the study who had had roseola, by age in 30-day periods

the case and 30 days following it were reviewed for the occurrence of fever of unknown origin, adenopathy, and enanthem or exanthem. No cases suggestive of roseola infantum occurred. This finding does not, of course, exclude the occurrence of atypical forms of the disease, but suggests that until the etiological agent is known and specific laboratory tests can be carried out, further information regarding the true occurrence of the disease will be difficult to obtain.

OTHER INFECTIONS

A variety of other infections occurred in this population (table 101 and Appendix 5, table 1). The most frequent of them were conjunctivitis, herpes simplex, furunculosis, and cervical adenitis. Few attempts were made to establish the etiology of these illnesses, so that further comment does not seem warranted.

Chapter XIV
MISCELLANEOUS OBSERVATIONS

A variety of events and illnesses occurred during the study and were recorded but not studied in detail. Since they illustrate the kinds of observations that may be made in "normal" persons and families, however, a survey of them is presented.

LOCAL ABNORMALITIES

A complete list of diagnoses made during the study is given in Appendix 5, table 1. A sample of these is as follows:

Hemorrhoids	Otosclerosis
Rectal polyps	Refractive lens error
Hernia	Muscle imbalance of eye
Appendicitis	Chalazion
Fissure-in-ano	Congenital malformations
Crooked teeth	Localized infections
Duodenal ulcer	Enlarged thymus
Varicose veins	Adenoma of vocal cord
Genitourinary infection	Fractures
Benign prostatic hypertrophy	Bursitis
Renal calculus	Intervertebral disc syndrome
Hydrocele	Ganglion and Baker's cyst
Delayed descent of testis	Moles and hemangiomata
Cervical erosion and cervicitis	Sebaceous cyst
Cervical polyp	Acne
Mass in breast	

The relative infrequency of impetigo and similar skin afflictions, in relation to their occurrence in other studies (100, 125), cannot be explained unless environmental factors were responsible.

MISCELLANEOUS DISEASES

The population selected for study was composed of children and young adults and chronic disorders commonly associated with an older age were not expected to occur. It remains to be seen whether or not recurrent infections, reactions or patterns of behavior represented the initiation of chronic organic disease. Two conditions, rheumatic fever and rheumatoid arthritis, were striking by their absence. Streptococcal infections and the carrier state recurred (Chapter VII). Only time will tell whether or not the appearance of murmurs in childhood were important. The unanticipated diseases that did occur were thyrotoxicosis, diabetes mellitus, chronic glomerulonephritis, gout, and multiple sclerosis.

At age 27 a mother developed thyrotoxicosis which began with marked fatigue, dyspnea on exertion, anorexia, weight loss, night sweats, and a "quivery" feeling. Auricular fibrillation ensued and treatment with propylthiouracil resulted in dramatic improvement. There was no family history of this disorder. During the 4 years prior to the onset of thyrotoxicosis, her thyroid gland had been slightly and diffusely enlarged. A father, aged 44 years, experienced a recurrence of thyrotoxicosis, manifested principally by weight loss and auricular fibrillation. He had had a previous episode 5 years earlier. On both occasions he was treated with propylthiouracil which proved to be effective. Again no family history of this disorder was elicited.

One mother developed diabetes mellitus at age 37 years, and in this instance the family history revealed that her only sibling, a sister, a maternal aunt and a maternal uncle, as well as a first cousin on her mother's side, had diabetes. Her mother was un-affected. There were no obvious precipitating causes and the onset of polyuria and polydipsia was unheralded. At the time of onset she had three children, ages 6, 4, and 1 year, and each child weighed less than 9 pounds at birth; the middle child, however, was born blind. Furthermore, the same child, a boy, was found to have hereditary familial nephritis at the age of 10 years. Further studies on this patient and his family are referred to on p. 117.

Gout occurred in a father at the age of 36 years. The onset was characterized by a tired, uncomfortable feeling in the right ankle which subsequently became swollen and painful. The uric acid level was elevated and the response to colchicine was prompt. No one else in his family to his knowledge had had this disease.

At the age of 26 years a father had an acute respiratory illness which was diagnosed as influenza. Shortly after this illness his feet felt numb. Approximately 10 years later abnormal neurological signs developed, including absence of vibratory sense in the lower extremities, absent abdominal reflexes, difficulty in writing, and a stiff feeling in his legs. The diagnosis of multiple sclerosis was confirmed by several consultants. The disease slowly progressed during the period of the study.

RADIOLOGICAL EXAMINATIONS

During the study 3126 radiographs, principally of the chest, were made of 417 persons, either as part of routine examinations or for specific reasons. These films were all re-examined at the end of the study and any apparent abnormality was reviewed with a radiologist.

Calcified lesions in the lungs were found in 35 of the parents and 3 of the children. Anatomic lesions, either congenital or acquired (such as cervical ribs or healed fractures of the ribs) were noted in 24 adults and 14 children. No relation between these findings and the occurrence, nature or severity of respiratory or other illnesses could be detected, despite detailed analyses. Transient pulmonary infiltrations were detected in 29 cases of respiratory disease in which the physician requested roentgenological examination. Films of the chest were not obtained routinely in all respiratory illnesses, however, so that these data cannot be used to determine frequency of pulmonary involvement.

HYPERSENSITIVITY

Reactions probably due to hypersensitivity were frequent. Many gastrointestinal symptoms were apparently caused by foods and medicines, but the greatest number of allergic responses was seen in the skin and respiratory tract, and in the former more often than in the latter. The most frequent cause of contact dermatitis was a plant, usually poison ivy, while penicillin was responsible for the majority of rashes secondary to medical treatment. The greatest percentage of skin reactions appeared to be endogenous in origin and could not be attributed to any specific cause. They were not due to serious internal disorders such as collagen diseases, systemic fungal infections, metabolic, nutritional or neoplastic processes. There were fewer people with bacterial infections of the skin than with cutaneous allergic reactions. More people had bacterial infections who had experienced an allergic rash at some time, however, than those who had never demonstrated cutaneous hypersensitivity.

In contrast to the skin, the causes of most allergic reactions of the respiratory tract were more specific, such as pollens and molds. Seasonal rhinitis was the most common manifestation and about one-sixth of individuals with seasonal rhinitis experienced bronchial asthma some of the time in conjunction with their nasal allergy. No one in the study had "chronic bronchial asthma." Allergic rhinitis "out of season" was not common and was usually attributed to house dust and animal dander. A small group of individuals complained of chronic nasal congestion with or without nasal discharge and postnasal drip that could be considered as "chronic catarrh" or vasomotor rhinitis. The cause of these symptoms did not appear to be a phenomenon of hypersensitivity to an allergen, but rather secondary to direct irritants such as tobacco smoke. Finally, the association of asthma with respiratory infections was infrequent and the wheezing reported by some mothers often proved to be the result of secretions rather than true bronchospasm.

PSYCHOSOMATIC REACTIONS

Functional disturbances accounted for the highest proportion of noninfectious ailments. A number of complaints recurred so often that they were virtually chronic in nature. Some persons experienced syndromes such as headache, fatigue, and anorexia, while others reported recurrent headaches, fatigability, abdominal pain, constipation, over-eating with weight gain, excessive smoking, insomnia, etc. In a number of parents there was an inverse relationship between smoking and over-eating. As a rule, these symptoms did not interfere with the pursuit of usual activities, but they led to considerable worry in some persons so that they often consulted a physician for a "check-up" or to discuss their problems. Relief from worry rather than prevention of recurrence was usually accomplished by such a visit. In the majority of instances these reactions were accepted for what they were — psychosomatic manifestations — and there was a tendency, once fear of organic disease had been removed, to seek relief by self-medication.

BLOOD PRESSURE

A number of parents had elevated readings at some time although they did not appear to be affected in any specific way. Only two individuals, a mother and a father, age 41 and 40 years, respectively, at the time of entry into the study had a sustained "hypertension", with systolic pressures of 140 or more and diastolic pressures of 90 or more. Both of these people were short and stocky, the so-called "coronary type." The mother was observed for 9 years and the father for 6 years; neither had clinical evidence of heart, kidney or brain injury.

Among the children there were 11 who had a systolic pressure of 130 or more at some time. This particular group of 11 children was interesting when compared with their parents; neither the father nor mother of 1 child had a systolic pressure of 140 or over or a diastolic pressure of 90 or over; 2 children had one parent with a systolic pressure of 140 or over; 4 children had 1 parent with elevation of both systolic and diastolic pressures; 3 children, all siblings, had parents both of whom had an elevation of the systolic pressure and 1 of whom had a diastolic pressure of 90 or over. This sort of observation is far from conclusive, but suggests the need for longitudinal studies of all members of a family.

HEART MURMURS

Interpretation of the importance of heart murmurs has long been debated. Traditionally, murmurs in childhood have been considered as inconsequential as far as the subsequent development of organic heart disease is concerned and there has been a tendency

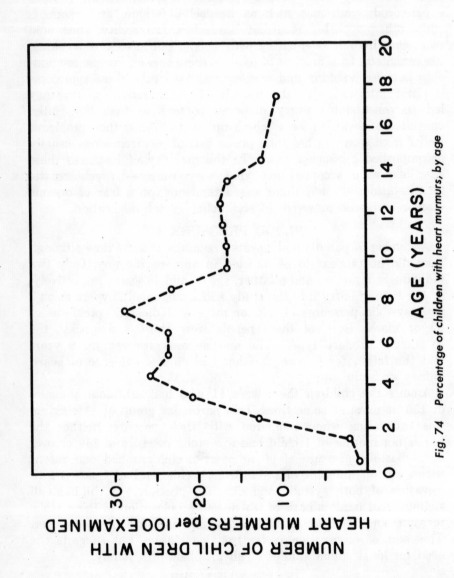

Fig. 74   Percentage of children with heart murmurs, by age

to accept them as a part of the phenomenon of growth. In this study children had systolic murmurs that appeared at one examination and either disappeared at the next, persisted over several years, or vanished only to reappear several years later. In one person, the murmur varied in intensity at different examinations from a soft blowing systolic murmur to a loud, rough murmur. None of the children had frank rheumatic fever or were even suspected of having this disease. Murmurs were most commonly heard in the years from three to nine, with a peak prevalence at 7 years of age (figure 74).

The causes of "functional" murmurs in children are unknown, and may be due to various infections including those that are streptococcal in etiology. For example, one child born during the study had a type 4 streptococcal infection during the month prior to a routine examination and at the latter a systolic murmur was heard for the first time. It was heard again 4 months later and then disappeared for a year only to be heard again 1 month after the child had rubella. Another child born during the study had an influenza-like illness 1 month prior to examination, at which time a murmur was heard for the first time. It was not detected 5 months later. He developed rubella 1 month prior to the next examination and a murmur was heard again; it was still present 5 months later. It was not detected during the 2 succeeding years.

Among the 164 parents in the study, there were seven who had murmurs apparently due to organic heart disease and 29 who had inconstant systolic murmurs most of which could not be explained (table 115). Four had histories of rheumatic fever in childhood; all have developed chronic mitral valvulitis and one had apparent

TABLE 115

Heart murmurs among 164 parents

	Number	Percent
Apparent organic disease:		
Rheumatic heart disease	4	
Suspected congenital septal defect	1	4.3
Suspected organic lesion	2	
Inconstant systolic murmur:		
Without explanation	19	11.6
Associated with hypertension	5	3.0
Associated with pregnancy	5	3.0

involvement of the aortic valve as well. Another had a possible congenital septal defect which had been suspected since infancy; one of her siblings was a "blue baby" who died soon after birth. The remaining two had murmurs which were believed to have organic bases.

OTHER EVENTS

There were three deaths during the study. One (aged 2 years) was due to leukemia, the second (aged 5 weeks) to congenital abnormalities (hydrocephalus and meningo-myelocele), and the third (aged 8 months) was a "sudden death" of a girl whose autopsy (after embalming) revealed widespread bilateral acute and subacute interstitial pneumonitis. She had just recovered from a mild attack of chickenpox and the lesions were incompletely healed. Just prior to her death there was a family episode of an acute respiratory disease which in the father resembled influenza, although this disease was not epidemic at the time. Onset of this illness occurred 3 days prior to her death.

Problems of reproduction were in general minimal. Sterility was not an issue. At least 34 miscarriages* occurred in 27 mothers. There were four stillbirths and seven children had congenital defects, of which four were serious: meningo-myelocele with or without hydrocephalus (three cases), and blindness (one case).

Little can be gained by presenting these episodes in detail. Throughout the study accidents of structure and disorders of function were observed which were probably genetically determined, but the interplay between environment and heredity was so strongly operative that it was impossible to know how significant a role environment actually played in the eventual expression of disease. The relative forces of heredity and environment cannot be easily measured. It is becoming increasingly apparent, however, that the "family unit" is an important entity in itself in the study of disease and serious consideration must be given to the effects of heredity and experience within this unit.

---

*These data are based on special retrospective histories from the mothers and therefore differ from those given in Appendix 5, table 1.

Chapter XV
SIGNIFICANCE OF THE STUDY

This study was originally organized with specific objectives related to factors concerned with the occurrence of illness in families and their individual members over a period of years. By reason of their previous activities, the interests of the staff were primarily in the acute illnesses, especially the acute respiratory diseases. The general plan was that an orderly and scheduled series of observations should be made and recorded at frequent intervals to form the basis for descriptions of these diseases. The type of description which was sought is well illustrated in Chapter VI; it is concerned with both current information and the past experience of individuals and families and how these facts are related to the occurrence and spread of illness.

The choice as to whether a random or selected sample of the population should be studied was considered at length but it was finally decided that a selected sample would be the only one that was practical. The frequency with which observations were to be made restricted the size of the group which could be followed; the desire to observe each family over a period of years required that families be chosen on the basis of factors thought to be related to geographical stability; the degree of intelligent cooperation needed from the subjects dictated selection on the basis of education and intelligence; and the staffing requirements made it necessary to recruit families from an area near the School of Medicine. Finally, a decision was made to confine the study to young married couples with one or more children.

The specific questions asked, then, had to be limited to those that might be answered by observation of a selected sample of the population. Emphasis was placed on the family as an epidemiological unit, and if one objective dominated all others it was to learn something about the role of the family in the spread of common illnesses. Since a family is composed of individual members, however, data were also examined in relationship to individuals; indeed, much of the data included in the present report is of this kind. Similarly, although emphasis was placed on the longitudinal aspects of the study — what happened over time to individuals and to families — many tabulations are presented in the form of incidence rates for specific classes of individuals. In interpreting the latter it must be recognized that the total number of individuals was relatively small and that any one person was included in several classes because age, size of family, and other bases of classification were not constant. Because the size of the group was small, little was learned regarding the non-infectious processes or chronic illnesses.

The absolute levels of incidence rates of illnesses for various classes of individuals or families, then, referred to a selected population and have not been interpreted as measuring the incidence of illness in the general population. On the other hand, relative differences between classes are believed to have a firm basis because the rates for the various classes are to a large, although undescribable, degree based upon the same individuals; therefore, both personal and environmental factors are eliminated to a major degree in such comparisons. Similarly, the longitudinal descriptions, although they refer to a small number of persons and families, have a firm basis, as have the descriptions of intrafamilial events.

While little purpose would be served by repeating in any detail the results reported in the preceding chapters, it does seem pertinent to illustrate by means of specific examples what we consider to be the significance of various parts of the study.

Incidence of illness has been measured in a variety of ways, all of them having limitations. Many of the general issues involved in the counting of clinical illnesses have been discussed in Chapter IV. Problems in diagnosing and properly labeling specific types of illnesses have been discussed in several chapters. Classification of acute respiratory illnesses and infectious gastroenteritis on the basis of symptoms was attempted, but did not prove to be very fruitful. The classification, "Common Respiratory Diseases," was arrived at after ruling out those illnesses that were considered to be etiological entities and is undoubtedly a heterogeneous group. Even if laboratory identification based on present knowledge had been available, making it possible for many of the illnesses to receive specific etiological classification, there would still remain a large group to be placed in the undifferentiated common respiratory disease classification. Similar comments apply to infectious gastroenteritis. In spite of the fact that both of these two major categories of disease are heterogeneous groups, considerable time has been devoted to their study.

In addition to counting clinical illnesses, incidence of infection (due to the adenoviruses, polioviruses, Coxsackie viruses, parainfluenza viruses, and influenza viruses) has been estimated on the basis of serological or virological methods or both. In most of these, identification of infections could not be attempted on an individual case basis, but an index of their incidence was determined through the rate of acquisition of detectable antibodies. This kind of description could only be made by means of a longitudinal study.

Finally, incidence was determined statistically, such as when the frequency of a respiratory-gastrointestinal syndrome and the frequency of undiscriminating symptoms due to poliovirus infection were estimated. The criteria for diagnosing streptococcal illnesses were also confirmed statistically. Again, the longitudinal character of the study made these determinations possible.

For the most part, incidence rates determined by one of these methods and made specific in a variety of ways provided the basis of studying the intrafamilial and the longitudinal factors related to the occurrence of illness.

Determination of the role of the family in the spread of disease was difficult to define and assess. What was being sought was a measurement or series of measurements which could show that members of a family interacted with one another in some way which influenced the incidence of illness. Perhaps the simplest demonstration of this phenomenon is the fact that the average number of respiratory illnesses per individual increased as size of family increased — a reasonable explanation being that there were more individuals to introduce infections into the home, and once in the home a family outbreak occurred.

The fact that infections do spread within families probably needed no demonstration, but was illustrated by the clustering of illnesses in time, as shown by the distribution of incubation periods of the common respiratory diseases and gastrointestinal illnesses, by the family epidemics of clinically diagnosed acute infectious diseases, by the occurrence and spread of streptococci, and by virus isolation and serological studies. These were data which could only be provided by longitudinal observations.

The occurrence of an acute communicable disease in a family and its spread therein seemed to be the simplest model. With these diseases one attack generally induced lasting immunity. What happened within a family depended upon who was susceptible, the degree of intermingling with the population outside the home so that infection might be acquired and brought into the home, and the presence or absence of other susceptible individuals within the home. The past history was a fairly reliable index of susceptibility.

In respect to the less differentiated disease groups the same factors undoubtedly played important roles, although they could be measured only indirectly and with much less precision. Susceptibility to common respiratory disease could only be judged by the occurrence of illness and the level of secondary attack rates, and appeared to be relative rather than absolute. Composition and size of family, school status of family members, and age of children are intrafamilial factors that were shown to be associated with the incidence of these diseases. For example, the attack rates among young children differed according to whether a sibling did or did not attend school, and the differences which occurred were expressed quantitatively for the common respiratory diseases and infectious gastroentertis, as well as for streptococcal infections. Similarly, the fact that secondary attack rates differed according to the age of the primary case was demonstrable. Tabulations of this type led to a description of the introduction and spread of illnesses within the family, and to speculation about frequency of infection from outside the family and levels of immunity. A family group, then, cannot be considered as a combination of average individuals, but as a group of individuals each with his own degree of contact inside and outside of the family and each with his own degree of susceptibility. What was attempted was an assessment of contact and susceptibility of individuals and an integration of these factors into a total for the family. Such assessment showed consistency of a family's behavior with respect to the common respiratory diseases.

The longitudinal character of the study made possible other types of analyses. The high incidence of common respiratory disease upon entering school, yet the apparent lack of immunity as shown both by total incidence and secondary attack rates resulting from this high incidence, illustrates this type of contribution. The consistently high or low incidence rates of the common respiratory diseases which individuals and families as a whole experienced over a period of years, the very considerable variation in number of illnesses experienced per individual, the lack of an effect of tonsillectomy on the incidence of some diseases and on the symptoms of the common respiratory diseases, and the demonstration that influenza incidence within a family was related to past history of influenza in the family, are other longitudinal epidemiological observations.

The orderly collection and recording of data, then, made possible consideration of a variety of questions, not all of which were carefully defined at the start of the study. However, the general areas which were considered in the original planning were those for which the most usable data were collected. The concomitant information, such as data from chest roentgenograms, many items of past history, etc., proved much less usable.

It is quite possible, in fact very likely, that factors other than those considered in this report were important in the occurrence of illness. The principal ones that we recognize as not having been given adequate attention are the psychological factors and other non-physical interpersonal relationships. Efforts were made to evaluate these areas, but adequate methods of description were not available, and we were unable to develop them.

The data that have come from this study do not lend themselves to an interpretation leading to practical methods of prevention or control. In part, this is because etiological determination of most of the illnesses was not possible at the time. The data obtained, however, should be of value in the future when more causative agents are known and identifiable in specific illnesses.

Appendix 1
METHODS OF OBSERVATION

Essentially, there were three broad areas of activity in the study: assemblage of background material, collection of information on current illnesses and other happenings, and conduct of special studies. Intimately related to all of these activities was the maintenance of interest and morale over a long period of time.

Since one of the main purposes of the study was the documentation of illnesses in the families for subsequent analyses, objectivity and uniformity of observation were of prime importance. To this end, forms for recording all the various types of data desired were carefully worked out. But since many different persons (both mothers, and professional staff which changed over the years) were involved in this investigation, the performance of these various individuals in making observations and keeping records was a matter of great concern. A continuing effort was therefore made to maintain consistent procedures and it is believed that the manner of observing and recording data by all concerned was sufficiently uniform to make possible valid analyses.

BACKGROUND MATERIAL

On admission to the study, each family was assigned a number and each individual within the family was identified by a second number. For example, the father of Family 1 was designated 1-1, the mother, 1-2, the oldest child, 1-3, and so on. Basic information about the family was recorded and an inquiry was made concerning the medical history of other relatives. During 1956-57, a more thorough investigation of the family tree was attempted, but the gaps of knowledge about the medical status of relatives and causes of death were so numerous that a sound appraisal of hereditary background could not be made.

A clinical chart was constructed for each individual. This contained records of the initial history and physical examination (including a blood count, urinanalysis and a chest roentgenogram), all subsequent examinations, results of special studies, such as electrocardiograms and blood chemistry, letters to and from other physicians, hospital abstracts, and any other data pertaining to the health of the individual.

At the time of the initial examination a specimen of blood was obtained as a basis of reference for later serological studies. Thereafter blood was collected for the serum library each spring and fall. The parents understood that this material was vital to the aims of the study and this schedule of bleeding was strictly followed over the years. About 10 ml. were collected from the youngest children and a maximum of 30 ml. from the older children and adults. In addition, blood was collected at the end of each trimester of pregnancy and cord blood was obtained at the time of delivery.

Several times each year the school attendance was reviewed and a note made when a child first began to go to school. Not infrequently, this was a nursery school at 4 years of age. Other data, such as dates of immunizations, were gathered from time to time in support of special studies.

COLLECTION OF INFORMATION ON CURRENT ILLNESSES

The bulk of the data in the study came from records that were made by mothers, fieldworkers and physicians as illnesses developed. In each family the mother was primarily responsible for the record-keeping and reporting of illnesses, accidents and miscellaneous symptoms. She was asked to notify the Department of each illness, however minor, in any member of her household (see Appendix 2). When the family went away on a vacation, the mother took the records with her, and if the parents alone went out of town, the person left in charge of the children was instructed about the records and notification of the Department at the time of illness. All tabulations were restricted to the father, the mother and the children. Servants, even though they formed part of the household, were in general too transient to warrant inclusion in the study, as were occasional roomers or relatives.

A telephone call from the mother to the Department was the main line of communication concerning a new illness. The message was either relayed to the staff physician or the mother discussed the illness directly with him. In response to this call, he decided whether to visit the home personally, to send the fieldworker, or simply to make a note in the clinical record. Early in the study practically all illnesses, no matter how minor they seemed, were seen in the home by a staff physician. The mother saw a field-worker regularly each week to go over the events of the preceding week, to report the progress of illnesses, and review her records. Despite her interest, it was recognized from the start that the mother's day would be divided among a number of activities and that it would be natural for her to forget from time to time certain of her obligations to the study. The mothers themselves were the first to admit that constant reminders and checking by the staff in regard to keeping records up to date, reporting at the time of illness and collecting throat cultures routinely were essential and their response to prodding was usually good natured.

The mother's record (Appendix 2, figure 1) for each member of her family was so important that a great deal of effort went into ensuring accurate notations in regard to the presence or absence of symptoms during an illness. For example, it was requested that zeros be included where symptoms were absent during an illness. Each month new record sheets were distributed for each member of the family and the ones of the previous month were collected. During the last 2 years of the study, a few new items, such as anorexia, nausea, and abdominal pain, were added to the mother's record because these symptoms occurred so frequently that it seemed expedient to list them. Also, it seemed worthwhile to try to discover what symptoms appeared to be due to psychosomatic reactions. This was admittedly a difficult project but it was felt that the mothers had had sufficient experience as observers so that the information might be obtained. The mothers were interested but uncertain that they could evaluate these responses. As it turned out, such symptoms as irritability, abdominal pain, listlessness, temper tantrums, feelings of tenseness and nightmares were usually checked in conjunction with the infectious illness, and no reaction patterns, except for headaches and bed-wetting, could be established for any one member of a family by these means.

At this point it is pertinent to examine the adequacy of the information gained from the mothers and their records. Short of an observer living in the home, was this method of collecting information as complete as possible and valid for subsequent analysis? There were 85 mothers in the study so that considerable variation in performance was unavoidable. Over the years, the professional staff became thoroughly familiar with the mothers and knew who might falter, so that more help was given to some than to others. While the objectives of the study were understood by all mothers, and their integrity was beyond question, there was need to check laxity in some and over-zealous recording in others. Written reports were submitted from time to time by the professional staff regarding this matter; it was the composite opinion of staff physicians and fieldworkers that about 20% of the mothers tended to have difficulty in getting information across to the Department. There were a number of different reasons for this, such as forgetfulness in reporting illnesses, failure to keep records up to date, lack of confidence in making observations, and so forth. It was in this area that the efforts of the fieldworkers proved invaluable. They learned to be more watchful of some than others and to anticipate where guidance and discipline were needed.

During the study, two fieldworkers visited all of the families each week in Department-owned cars. In all, 10 women functioned in this capacity: 6 registered nurses, 2 school teachers, 1 student on leave of absence from medical school, and 1 social worker. They made their rounds in the mornings, and the day of the week and the time of morning were arranged by the worker with the mother so that as few appointments as possible were missed. In addition to reviewing the mother's records, the fieldworker collected routine throat cultures and other specimens and made notes of her own. As a rule, the mother took the cultures from each member of the family on the morning of the visit and placed them in the refrigerator until gathered by the fieldworker. Usually this procedure went smoothly but there were times when it was necessary to return for the cultures if they had not been taken on the assigned day. The fieldworker's weekly notes included a statement regarding the presence or absence of illness in each member of the family. She also made note of dates that individuals were away from the family. On returning from her morning rounds, she took the throat cultures to the laboratory and copied her notes concerning illnesses on the reverse side of the physician's clinical record. The date of onset of illness, accident or other symptoms, progress notes, and date of recovery were charted. If, during a routine visit, the fieldworker discovered that a mother had failed to call the Department about a recent illness, she would urge the mother to call and would also confer with the staff physician on returning from her morning visits.

The staff physician, as the result of a telephone call from the mother, or after a conference with the fieldworker, went to the home, obtained facts about the illness, examined that patient, and collected a throat culture and any other specimens required for special studies. The physician's attention was directed not only toward the clinical picture, time of onset, medication, and whether or not the private physician had been called, but also toward the epidemiological aspects of the case such as the likely source of infection, the incubation period of the disease, and the health of other members of the family. The staff physician was primarily an observer, but there were some situations that forced him to urge the parents to call their private physician, for example, the finding of otitis media or rales in the lungs in association with a febrile illness, or exudative pharyngitis in association with group A streptococci that had appeared as a new acquisition. Not infrequently, he called the private physician to learn his impression of the illness or to inform him of any new developments. Subsequent notes on any illness were made by the fieldworker or by the staff physician himself if he saw the patient again. At the end of each month, the mother's records, along with the fieldworker's notes and the clinical records, were reviewed by the staff physician and a diagnosis of each illness was made.

SPECIAL STUDIES

As the study progressed, it was inevitable that new interests and new ideas would emerge from the accumulating data. Despite the special studies that were undertaken, the basic organization and the methods of observation remained the same. Thus any new procedures required by a special study were appended to, but never supplanted, the essential structure of the study. To introduce a special study, a letter was usually written to the parents, followed by individual explanations from the staff physicians and field-workers who expanded on the plans and techniques involved. Most of the special studies pertained to specific infectious diseases such as poliomyelitis, streptococcal infections and influenza. When tissue culture became a practical tool in 1954, certain other respiratory diseases received added attention. Two drugs were studied to evaluate their effectiveness in the prevention and treatment of common respiratory illnesses: antihistamines (22) and oxytetracycline hydrochloride (Terramycin®) (6). A survey was also made of the smoking history of the parents in an effort to determine whether or not there was a relation between smoking and the character and frequency of respiratory illnesses (18).

MAINTENANCE OF INTEREST

The loyalty and cooperation of the families appeared to spring from their estimate of the worthiness of the study's aims, the chance of discovering new knowledge, and the feeling that they themselves were making a significant contribution to the public welfare. Their interest seemed to be an admixture of intellectual stimulation from participation in a scientific investigation and emotional gratification from knowing that they were part of such a venture. The staff was continually alert to the need for maintaining the interest and cooperation of the parents. Letters and instructions to the families not only provided basic information in regard to procedures, but also gave them something to study and think about. Furthermore, each spring a general meeting of the parents was held for which a program of short talks was arranged to acquaint them with different aspects of the investigations being conducted. For example, at the first meeting in 1949 the use of throat cultures, throat washings, bloods and records was discussed and nonbacterial tonsillitis and pharyngitis was described. In subsequent years, the meetings covered a wide range of topics: streptococcal infections and nephritis, antibiotic drugs in common respiratory diseases, viruses and tissue cultures, the role of school and age in the incidence of respiratory diseases, and so forth. At the meeting in 1956, each family was given the results of the tests of their sera for antibodies against all three types of polioviruses; many were surprised to learn that they had had previous infections with these viruses.

In addition, reprints of published reports concerning the study were sent to the families, including an excellent article by one of the mothers which was published in McCall's magazine (95). Moreover, the scientific knowledge of the professional staff was made readily available to the members of the study at all times. This led to discussions on a variety of subjects ranging from the use of glycol vaporizers in one father's business organization to the advisability of immunization with the Asian influenza vaccine. Furthermore, hardly a year went by without a few of the older children making a visit to the Department to obtain material for a school science project.

All in all, a close personal relationship developed over the years between the professional staff and the families in the study. This was a vital factor in maintaining the interest and cooperation of the families. In addition, another factor that contributed greatly to the continuity of the program was the routine nature of the study. The required procedures became a part of the normal lives of the families. Children took the study for granted; they knew they were going to be bled twice a year. The mothers became accustomed to the weekly visits of the fieldworkers and were thoroughly familiar with the items on the records. In fact, cessation of the study left a void in the pattern of their everyday lives to the extent that many of the families expressed the feeling that they missed it.

Appendix 2

INSTRUCTIONS AND FORMS RELATING TO ILLNESS

RECORDS

An example of the records kept by the mothers is shown in figure 1 of this Appendix (1). Detailed forms for the initial history and examination and interim examinations were filled in by the physicians and were of a standard nature.

INSTRUCTIONS TO FAMILIES

NOTIFICATION OF ILLNESS

The general policy of the study is that the Department shall be notified when *any* illness occurs so that the physician may make the necessary observations. Depending on the nature of the illness, the visit by the physician will be made sometime during the first three days of illness.

You should notify the Department of Preventive Medicine as soon as you are sure *that illness of any nature* is present in your family. For example:

1) Whenever one of your family has a temperature which is above normal;
2) Whenever one of your family feels ill enough to go to bed;
3) Whenever a rash appears;
4) Whenever a sore throat is present to such a degree that it hurts to swallow.

These four examples were chosen to illustrate an illness which is clearly present. They should not be taken as the only types of illness in which we are interested. However, it will frequently happen that a minor symptom, such as a dry throat, may be present and the mother will not be sure whether or not a cold is developing. In this case the following rule should be observed:

When a minor symptom is present, but is not severe enough that you are sure the individual is really ill, notify us if the symptom persists for 24 hours. In any case, the symptom should be recorded on the chart and discussed with the physician or nurse at the next visit.

N.B. This 24 hour delay does not apply to the occurrence of definite illness, notification of which should be made promptly.

If any situation arises which is not covered in these instructions, please feel perfectly free to call us.

RECORDING OF ILLNESS

A basic rule in any scientific investigation is that all records should be made as comparable with one another as is humanly possible. A large number of mothers are responsible for the recording of the scientific facts which form the basis of the present investigation. In order that we may have the greatest possible uniformity in our records, the following instructions have been prepared for keeping them. Even if these instructions are carefully observed, there is bound to be individual variation in the way they are interpreted by the various mothers. In order to minimize this, you should feel free to ask the visiting physician or nurse for more detailed explanations whenever you are in doubt as to the meaning of the instructions.

The mother is responsible for recording all departures from normal health within her family. Record forms are provided for this purpose. These records, kept by the mother, may prove to be the most important part of the entire investigation; but unless they are filled out in a comparable manner by every mother, they cannot be properly interpreted by the investigators and much effort may be wasted. Therefore, if the study is to be of true value, the following instructions should be followed:

1) In trying to trace the spread of a disease throughout a family, it must be assumed that all the members of the family are exposed to one another each day. If this is not the case, then this fact must be taken into account. Therefore, if some member of the family is away from home for longer than one day, this fact should be recorded on the form (second line). Upon return, the individual should be questioned as to any symptoms which may have occurred during his absence. If he has forgotten to note symptoms (however minor) which occurred during his absence, this fact should also be recorded.

2) When no member of the family is ill on a particular day, no entry should be made on the record.

3) When *any symptom* is present in any member of the family, *a complete set of entries* should be made for that individual, even though the symptom may not meet the criteria set up for notifying the Department. Accuracy will be improved if entries (both positive and negative) are recorded daily. A complete set of entries includes:

(a) For symptoms other than vomiting, diarrhea, temperature, progress, and restricted activity:

  ∨—for any symptom present;

  0 —for any symptom not present;

  ? —for any symptom which the mother is
    unable to determine because of the age
    of the child, or for other reason.

(b) Vomiting:

  0—if none;

  Number of times—if present.

(c) Diarrhea:

  0—if the bowel habits are normal;

  Number of times—if loose stools are present;

  ? —if no information is available.

(d) Temperature:

  Temperature should be taken on those days when
the mother believes there is a departure from normal
health. Temperatures vary throughout the day. For
this reason, it is preferred that temperatures be taken
at 4:00 p.m. However, all temperatures taken during
an illness are of value and should be recorded in degrees. If temperature is not taken, leave blank.

  If thermometer is used rectally, this should be
noted.

(e) Progress:

  In order to characterize an illness properly, it is
necessary to know its ups and downs. For this reason
a row of spaces is provided for the mother to express
her opinion as to the progress of the disease. Appropriate symbols are given at the bottom of the form.

(f) Restricted activity:

  ∨—stayed home from school or work because
    of illness, or otherwise restricted activ-
    ity because of illness;

  0 —normal activity.

(g) Remarks:

  Any descriptive remarks which the mother can make
regarding the course of events, the severity of symptoms, temperature taken at times other than 4:00 p.m.,
etc., will be of value.

If a space is left blank, the record loses its value because we
have no way of knowing whether the mother neglected to make the

necessary observations or whether the symptom was absent. Since it is necessary to distinguish between these two possibilites, we ask that you make the appropriate entry for each and every symptom. The only space that should ever be left blank is the one for the 4:00 p.m. temperature when the temperature is not taken.

Name ___Johnny D._____ Address ___3517 East Road_____ Number ___10-3___

Dates away from family during month (inclusive dates) _____

Seen by any physician, why? ___Dr. Z. - for cold and cough_____

Month and year ___February, 1950_____

Day of month	4	5	6	7	8	9	10	11	12	13	14
Headache	0	0	0	0	0	0	0	0	0	0	0
Feverish	0	0	✓	✓	0	✓	0	0	0	0	0
Chilly	0	0	0	0	0	0	0	0	0	0	0
Irritable	0	0	✓	0	✓	0	0	0	0	0	0
Listless	0	0	✓	✓	0	0	0	0	0	0	0
Loss of appetite	✓	✓	✓	✓	0	0	0	0	0	0	0
Aches and pains - Describe	✓	✓	✓	✓	0	0	0	0	0	0	0
Sneezing	✓	0	✓	✓	0	0	✓	0	0	0	0
Nasal discharge — Watery	✓	✓	✓	✓	0	0	0	0	0	0	0
Nasal discharge — Thick	0	0	0	0	0	0	✓	✓	✓	✓	0
Obstructed nose	✓	✓	✓	✓	0	0	0	0	0	0	0
Sore throat — Irritated	0	0	✓	✓	✓	0	0	0	0	0	0
Sore throat — Hurts	0	0	✓	✓	0	0	0	0	0	0	0
Hoarse	0	0	✓	✓	✓	0	0	0	0	0	0
Cough — Throat	0	0	✓	✓	✓	✓	✓	✓	✓	✓	0
Cough — Chest	0	0	✓	✓	✓	✓	✓	✓	✓	✓	0
Sputum	✓	✓	✓	✓	✓	✓	✓	✓	✓	✓	0
Other - Explain below (Date)	0	0	0	0	0	0	0	0	0	0	0
Vomiting - No. of times	0	0	0	0	0	0	0	0	0	0	0
Diarrhea - No. of times	0	0	0	0	0	0	0	0	0	0	0
4 p.m. temp. - degrees			99	99¾	99						
Oral or rectal temp.?	O	R	R	R	R	O	O	O	O	O	O
Progress	W	W	S	S	B	B	B	B	B	B	N
Restricted activity	✓	✓	✓	✓	✓	✓	✓	✓	✓	✓	✓

If ill, ✓ each symptom present; 0 if absent (except vomiting, diarrhea, progress, and restricted activity).

Progress: B = Better than yesterday, but not normal;   W = Worse than yesterday;
S = Same as yesterday;   N = Normal.

Oral or rectal temp. - specify which.

Restricted activity: ✓ = stayed home from school or work, etc.; N = normal activity.

REMARKS: 5th - stomach ache
Kept indoors, Feb. 5-15

Please notify Department of each illness.

Rev. 5-15-50
F-4

Appendix 2 Fig. 1   Form used by mother for daily recording of symptoms

Appendix 3
LABORATORY METHODS

The procedures used for the collection and examination of specimens are detailed in the publications to which reference has been made. In general, standard or conventional methods were used for the isolation and identification of bacteria and viruses, and in the performance of serological tests. A brief description of these methods is appended here for orientation and completeness.

BACTERIOLOGICAL METHODS

Paired cotton-tipped swabs were used to sample pharyngeal flora both routinely once a week and at the time of illness. Early in the study when pneumococci were sought routinely, the swabs were placed in tryptose phosphate broth to prevent drying during the delay in transportation (127). Material from dry swabs, swabs held in non-selective broth, or swabs held in media selective for streptococci (106) was inoculated on sheep blood agar plates for the isolation of pneumococci, streptococci, and staphylococci, and on Fildes' medium for isolation of influenza bacilli. During the period of January, 1948, to May, 1950, pneumococci were sought by injecting swab cultures intraperitoneally in mice; this procedure was reinstituted during the study of Asian (A2) influenza in 1957. Pneumococci were identified by bile solubility and quellung reaction. Streptococci were grouped and typed by the methods of Lancefield et al. (92, 129). Typing sera for 33 types were employed.* Staphylococci and influenza bacilli were identified by colonial morphology and gram stain; few influenza bacilli could be typed with specific antisera.

Stool emulsions and material from rectal swabs were cultured on Endo agar and desoxycholate plates, and inoculated into selenite broth for isolation of *Shigella* and *Salmonella* organisms.

VIROLOGICAL METHODS

Throat washings (garglings) of sterile skim milk or pharyngeal swabs placed immediately in one of several fluids (variously Hank's balanced salt solution (BSS), tryptose phosphate broth, veal infusion broth, beef-heart infusion broth) were collected for isolation of viruses. Penicillin and streptomycin were added to supress bacterial growth. The majority of the specimens were sealed in glass ampules, rapidly frozen and stored at -70° C. Pharyngeal and stool

---

*Antisera for the following types were available: 1-6, 12-15, 17-19, 22-26, 28-33, 36-44, 46 and 47.

specimens for poliovirus study were stored at -20° C. Stool specimens were collected in cardboard containers and transported to
the laboratory within 5 hours; samples were stored in lusteroid
screw-cap containers.

Pharyngeal specimens were tested without further treatment by
inoculating 0.1 ml. into each of 6 eggs or 3 to 6 tissue culture tubes.
Influenza viruses were sought by amniotic passage in 9 to 11-day
old embryonated chicken eggs. During the period 1950-1953, broth
from individual swabs was initially tested by pooling 0.25 ml. of
fluid from each of five swabs to make a single inoculum. Following
definite identification of viruses, the individual swabs of the pool
were examined singly. In 1957, all specimens were tested individually. After 3-4 days' incubation at 35°C. or 37°C., the amniotic
fluids were harvested and tested for their capacity to agglutinate
both chicken and either guinea-pig or human erythrocytes. Adenoviruses, polioviruses, and other agents were sought by inoculation
of tube cultures of continuous cell lines, usually HeLa or DMB.
The cells were grown on glass in 32-oz. prescription bottles in nutri-
ent fluid; for the majority of the studies, this fluid consisted of
40% pooled human serum and 60% Hanks' BBS. Cells were dis-
pensed into culture tubes in numbers sufficient to produce a sheet
of cells within 24 hours. After washing, maintenance medium (0.9
ml.) and inoculum (0.1 ml.) were added For most of the studies,
the maintenance medium was composed of 67.5% Scherer's solution,
12% tryptose phosphate broth, and 7.5% chicken serum (66). Tubes
were incubated in stationary racks at 36-37°C. for 12 to 14 days,
with the medium being changed two to three times.

Stool specimens were processed in several ways. In general, 10 or
20% suspensions were made in distilled water, BSS, or maintenance
solution. The crude suspensions were centrifuged at 1000 to 2000
R.P.M. for 10 to 20 minutes; the supernate was then centrifuged at
12,000 R.P.M. for 30 to 45 minutes. Final concentrations of antibiotics ranged from 0.5 to 10 mg. per ml. for streptomycin, and from
400 to 2000 units per ml., for penicillin. For poliovirus studies, 0.2
ml. was inoculated into each of three tubes of HeLa cells, and incubated at 36°C. in a stationary position. If atypical degeneration
occurred within 24 hours, presumably due to toxicity of the stool,
0.2 ml. of culture fluid was transferred to fresh cell culture tubes.
Frequently the isolation attempt was repeated using an 0.1 ml.
inoculum, replacing the maintenance fluid after 2 to 3 hours with
fresh medium, adding a second 0.1 ml. of stool supernate, and
changing fluid again after another 2 to 3 hours.

SEROLOGICAL PROCEDURES

Influenza viruses were typed by specific antisera in a standard hemagglutination-inhibition test (47). Cytopathic viruses were identified by tissue culture neutralization tests.

Influenza studies utilized standard complement-fixation and hemagglutination-inhibition tests (82), the sera for the latter test being pretreated with either periodate or *Vibrio cholerae* filtrate (RDE). Titers were expressed as the highest initial dilution of serum producing 3+ to 4+ fixation of complement or complete inhibition of hemagglutination. All serum specimens from an individual, and usually from a family, were examined in the same test. In addition to the widely used PR8 (A), FM1 (A1), Japan 305 (A2), and Lee (B) strains, two others were used as antigens. A/FW1/53 was isolated from a specimen collected at Francis E. Warren Air Force Base, Wyoming; B/WRU/53/50 was isolated from an individual in the family study (83). A 4-fold or greater rise in titer was considered as indicative of infection by influenza virus during the time period spanned by the serum specimens. Because the sera were tested at different times, different lots of antigen were used. Initially, sera collected from the time of an individual's entrance into the study through the spring of 1952 were tested with PR8, FM1, Lee, and B/WRU/53/50 antigens. Following the occurrence of influenza A1 infections in 1953, the specimens collected in the spring of 1952 were re-examined along with subsequent sera through the fall of 1953. These were tested with FM1, A/FW1/53 and B/WRU/50/53 antigens. Specific chicken immune sera were included in each day's test, each serum being run against all virus antigens. In 1957, a pool of eleventh and twelfth egg passages of an egg-animal line of A/Japan/305 supplied by Jensen (48) was used as antigen for both hemagglutination-inhibition and complement-fixation tests (17).

Complement-fixing antibody titers for measles* and mumps viruses were determined with the micromethod of Fulton and Dumbell (64). Measles virus antigen was prepared with the Edmonston strain grown in human amnion cells. Mumps virus antigen was allantoic fluid from infected chick embryos.

For tissue culture neutralization tests, virus infectivity was measured by preparing serial 1:3.2 ($10^{-0.5}$) dilutions in Hanks' BSS and inoculating 0.1 ml. of each dilution into each of two tubes. The appropriate amount of virus was added to each serum dilution under test and the mixture held, usually for 30 to 60 minutes at room temperature, before the inoculation of culture tubes (65). Tubes

---

*We are indebted to Dr. Frederick C. Robbins for confirming some of these titers.

were incubated at 37°C. in stationary racks. Cell lines and tissue culture doses used with different viruses were as follows: adenoviruses, Coxsackie viruses, and polioviruses, DMB or HeLa, 50-100 TCD_{50}; parainfluenza 1, primary monkey kidney, 100 TDC_{50}; parainfluenza 2, primary human amnion, 100 TCD_{50}; parainfluenza 3, HeLa, 100-200 TCD_{50}. Titers were expressed as the reciprocal of the final dilution of serum which protected 50% or more of the cells from cytopathic damage.

SERUM STORAGE

Sera were stored at -20°C. in a walk-in freezer. Aliquots were inactivated at 56°C. for 30 minutes prior to testing.

Appendix 4

APPENDIX 4, TABLE 1

Number of person-days, number of family-days, and number of families according to size of family

Family size	Total number person-days	Total number family-days	Number of families	Average number of person-days per family	Median number of person-days per family
3	38,991	12,997	20	1,950	1,181
4	269,604	67,401	61	4,420	2,876
5	399,450	79,890	57	7,008	5,580
6	201,396	33,566	26	7,746	8,430
7	36,491	5,213	8	4,561	3,560
8	31,104	3,888	3	10,368	8,856

APPENDIX 4, TABLE 2

Distribution of parents according to their education at time of entry into study

Highest education attained	Number of husbands	Number of wives
High school	1	9
High school + special training	1	4
Junior college	1	11
College	56	48
College + postgraduate training	23	10
Total	82*	82*

*Excludes the families of three staff members and includes family 35 only once.

APPENDIX 4, TABLE 3

Distribution of husbands according to their occupation at time of entry into study

Occupation	Number of families
Professional	31
Managerial	37
Sales	14
Total	82*

*Excludes the families of three staff members and includes family 35 only once.

APPENDIX 4, TABLE 4

Distribution of families according to income at time of entry into study

Annual income	Number of families
$3,000-3,999	1
$4,000-4,999	12
$5,000-7,499	18
$7,500-9,999	13
$10,000+	35
Unknown	3
Total	82*

*Excludes the families of three staff members and includes family 35 only once.

APPENDIX 4, TABLE 5

Distribution of families according to home ownership at time of entry into study

Class of home ownership	Number of families
Own	73
Rent	7
Unknown	2
Total	82*

*Excludes the families of three staff members and includes family 35 only once.

Appendix 5
PERIOD OF ILLNESS

None of the analyses of our data have been concerned with periods of ill health. In fact, it became evident very early that the records were quite unsatisfactory for this purpose, primarily because of the nature of the record form in use (Appendix 2). This form required mothers to check the presence or absence of each of several listed symptoms; space was provided for daily checks and covered the period of a calendar month. New forms were distributed on the first day of the month and old ones were collected. The general pattern of recording seemed to be that during the acute phases of illness the records were quite complete, even though the illness extended into the next month; however, if only one or two symptoms of a relatively chronic nature (e.g., cough) remained from an acute illness, then, as judged by the records, illnesses tended to end on the last day of the month. Because the interests of the study did not include the determination of how long such symptoms persisted, no attempt was made to overcome this deficiency. However, if one were interested in counting, or describing, periods of ill health, this could not be done with any accuracy from our records; the artificial termination of a period of illness on the last day of the month would make it possible for a new period of illness to start at any time after the second day of the following month when, in truth, the old symptoms might still be present. This factor would not be operating, at least to the same intensity, at other times during the month.

APPENDIX 5, TABLE 1
Total number of illnesses by clinical diagnosis

Diagnosis	Number of cases	Total	1	2	3	4	5	6	7	8	9	10	11	12	13	14	15	16+	No. of operations	No. of individuals
Common respiratory diseases	14,990	See Appendix 5, Table 2																		
Specific respiratory diseases:																				
Streptococcal tonsillitis and pharyngitis	437	220	116	54	18	11	14	5	1	1										
Non-bacterial tonsillitis and pharyngitis	219	150	105	26	16	1	2													
Primary atypical pneumonia	42	37	33	3	1															
Pneumococcal pneumonia	6	6	6																	
Undiagnosed pneumonia	15	14	13	1																
Influenza (laboratory diagnosis)	74	73	72	1																
Gastrointestinal infections:																				
Gastroenteritis	2,139	397	58	64	46	34	41	34	21	22	21	13	6	11	3	4	7	12		
Gastroenteritis, epidemiological	1,169	324	98	53	51	33	19	19	18	10	7	2	3	4	1	4	1	1		
Gastroenteritis, probable	749	290	112	65	45	24	21	5	8	5	5									
"Other" infections:																				
Chickenpox	165	163	161	2																
Measles	156	150	144	6																
Mumps	114	113	112	1																
German measles	66	63	60	3																
Roseola infantum	54	50	46	4																
Erythema infectiosum	5	5	5																	
Fever of unknown origin	259	155	94	38	13	4	4	1		1										
Other constitutional symptoms, etiology unknown	110	88	72	12	2	2														
Conjunctivitis, etiology unknown	188	141	109	25	2	4														
Miscellaneous infection of the eye	30	25	21	3	1				1											
Herpes simplex	172	50	30	1	3	2	1	5		2	2			1	1	1	1			
Herpes zoster	2	2	2																	
Stomatitis of unknown etiology	9	9	9																	
Furunculosis	186	76	48	17	4	2	1	1		2									2	2
Poststreptococcal illness, nonsuppurative complication	67	57	48	8	1															

(Continued on following page)

APPENDIX 5, TABLE 1 (Continued)
Total number of illnesses by clinical diagnosis

Diagnosis	Number of cases	Total	_____ Number of individuals _____																Operations	
			_____ Number of illnesses _____																	No. of operations	No. of individuals
			1	2	3	4	5	6	7	8	9	10	11	12	13	14	15	16+		
Primary otitis media	77	46	26	13	4	2	1													
Obscure infection of the ear	19	17	15	2																
Cervical adenitis, etiology unknown	55	46	38	7	1														26	24
Infected tooth and extraction	43	37	32	4	1															
Gingivitis	5	5	5																	
Fungus infection of the skin	25	23	21	2															1	1
Thrush	1	1	1																	
Miscellaneous skin lesion, infected blister, etc.	68	51	39	10	1			1											3	3
Impetigo	25	22	19	3																
Warts	27	25	23	2															18	18
Acne	5	3	1	2																
Intestinal worms	28	15	10	3	1	1														
Trichinosis	4	4	4																	
Pityriasis rosea	5	5	5																	
Pleurodynia	5	5	5																	
Erysipelas	4	3	2	1																
Infectious Mononucleosis	2	2	2																	
Pulmonary tuberculosis	2	2	2																	
Infectious hepatitis	1	1	1																	
Malaria	1	1	1																	
Poliomyelitis	1	1	1																	
Other illnesses:																				
Hay fever, allergic rhinitis	321	88	25	18	10	10	5	5	3	6	2	2	1					1		
Asthma	21	10	5	1	3		1													
Asthma and hay fever (combined)	6	5	4	1																
Allergic conjunctivitis	9	6	4	1	1															
Urticaria	84	60	45	9	3	3														
Contact dermatitis	45	35	30	3	1			1												
Eczema	42	28	20	4	3		1													
Purpura, nonthrombocytopenic	1	1	1																	
Abrasion, contusion, cut, etc.	240	146	90	38	6	8	2		2										1	1
Dislocation, sprain	57	47	51	11	3	8	2													

Diagnosis									
Fracture	23	21	39	6	2				
Animal bite or scratch	18	18	20		1				
Burn	18	18	18						
Concussion	82	65	18						
Miscellaneous trauma	39	35	31	4					
Gastrointestinal symptoms, dietary causes	120	90	68	15	6	1			
Infant diarrhea	8	8	8						
Condition leading to tonsillectomy, adenoidectomy, or both	63	63	63					63	63
Condition leading to appendectomy	12	12	12					12	12
Miscellaneous operations	35	32	29	3				35	32
Reactions to vaccine, drug, etc.	115	89	70	12	7				
Noninfectious dermatitis	148	93	60	19	8	5	1		
Live birth	83	56	33	19	4				
Miscarriage	8	8	8						
Condition related to pregnancy	17	12	7	5					
Miscellaneous disease of the female genital tract	30	20	14	4	1	1		8	7
Pyelitis, pyelonephritis, kidney infection	20	14	11	2	1				
Cystitis	17	12	10		1	1			
Urinary frequency, dysuria, burning	7	7	7	1					
Albuminuria	3	2	1	1					
Renal calculus	2	2	2					2	2
Varicocele and hydrocele	5	4	3	1					
Orchitis	2	2	2						
Prostatic disease	2	2	2						
Miscellaneous gastrointestinal disorder	22	19	16	3				5	5
Anemia	8	7	6	1				7	7
Leukemia	1	1	1					7	7
Disorder of bone, joint and related structures	59	41	29	7	4	1		1	1
Hemorrhoids, varicosity, phlebitis	22	18	15	2	1		1		
Epistaxis	77	43	27	8	2	3	2	1	
Headaches, including migraine	488	119	49	28	13	8	2	5	2
Localized aches and pains	273	125	74	24	11	3	3	3	1
Otalgia	121	70	50	9	5	1	1		
Functional symptoms	396	164	87	27	19	6	4	2	3
Miscellaneous illnesses and disorders	214	135	88	31	10	3	2	1	1
Total	25,155								

APPENDIX 5, TABLE 2

Number of individuals with indicated number of common respiratory diseases (CRD)

Number of CRD	Number of individuals	Number of CRD	Number of individuals	Number of CRD	Number of individuals	Number of CRD	Number of individuals
0	3	26	8	52	5	88	1
1	6	27	7	53	6	90	3
2	4	28	6	54	5	91	2
3	5	29	6	55	3	92	2
4	8	30	11	57	1	94	1
5	3	31	10	58	4	96	2
6	7	32	8	59	1	99	1
7	5	33	5	61	3	105	1
8	5	34	9	62	3	114	1
9	10	35	5	63	4	Totals:	
10	10	36	6	64	5	14,990	439
11	5	37	6	65	2		
12	8	38	6	66	2		
13	8	39	5	67	8		
14	6	40	13	69	3		
15	7	41	7	70	3		
16	14	42	5	71	5		
17	10	43	5	73	2		
18	8	44	7	74	1		
19	5	45	2	75	1		
20	4	46	6	77	2		
21	9	47	7	78	1		
22	12	48	2	79	1		
23	8	49	7	80	1		
24	7	50	2	81	2		
25	3	51	7	83	3		

APPENDIX 6, TABLE 1

Incidence of specific respiratory diseases by year

Diagnosis	1948		1949		1950		1951		1952	
	Number cases	Cases per person-year	Number cases	Cases per person-year	Number cases	Cases per person-year	Number cases	Cases per person-year	Number cases	Cases per person-year
Streptococcal tonsillitis & pharyngitis	14	.08	40	.16	53	.21	62	.23	67	.20
Nonbacterial tonsillitis & pharyngitis	40	.24	6	.02	26	.10	26	.10	52	.16
Primary atypical pneumonia	7	.04	13	.05	9	.04	2	.01	3	.01
Pneumococcal pneumonia	2	.01	0	....	1	.00	2	.01	1	.00
Undiagnosed pneumonia	0	....	0	....	0	....	2	.01	1	.00
Influenza (laboratory diag.)	0	....	1	.00	16	.06	30	.11	1	.00
Total	63	.38	60	.24	105	.41	124	.46	125	.38

Diagnosis	1953		1954		1955		1956		1957	
	Number cases	Cases per person-year	Number cases	Cases per person-year	Number cases	Cases per person-year	Number cases	Cases per person-year	Number cases	Cases per person-year
Streptococcal tonsillitis & pharyngitis	70	.22	59	.18	30	.09	33	.11	9	.07
Nonbacterial tonsillitis & pharyngitis	14	.04	15	.05	30	.09	8	.03	2	.02
Primary atypical pneumonia	1	.00	4	.01	1	.00	1	.00	1	.01
Pneumococcal pneumonia	0	....	0	....	0	....	0	....	0	....
Undiagnosed pneumonia	0	....	3	.01	2	.01	4	.01	3	.02
Influenza (laboratory diag.)	22	.07	0	....	0	....	4	.01	0	....
Total	107	.33	81	.25	63	.20	50	.16	15	.12

APPENDIX 6, TABLE 2

Incidence of illnesses by age and by broad diagnostic groups

Age	Common respiratory diseases	Infectious gastroenteritis	All other illnesses	Total illnesses
<1	6.72	1.00	1.85	9.57
1	8.28	1.92	2.65	12.84
2	8.07	1.89	2.24	12.20
3	7.84	1.90	2.42	12.16
4	7.62	1.89	2.61	12.13
5	7.42	2.11	2.99	12.51
6	6.16	2.01	3.01	11.19
7	6.12	2.17	2.99	11.28
8	5.99	2.05	2.59	10.63
9	5.34	1.71	2.74	9.79
10	5.70	1.84	2.47	10.01
11	5.09	1.60	2.45	9.14
12	5.00	0.98	2.07	8.05
13	4.58	1.03	1.69	7.30
14	4.73	0.95	1.53	7.21
15	4.76	0.58	1.80	7.14
16	5.54	0.74	3.08	9.36
17	3.83	1.74	2.26	7.84
18	0.00	1.72	3.45	5.17
22 - 24	4.09	1.02	2.16	7.27
25 - 29	4.82	1.12	2.02	7.96
30 - 34	4.45	1.08	1.75	7.28
35 - 39	3.83	1.21	1.93	6.97
40 - 44	3.68	1.14	2.01	6.83
45 - 49	3.97	0.75	2.26	6.99
50 - 51	3.62	0.23	0.90	4.75

APPENDIX 6, TABLE 3

Percentage distribution of illnesses by broad diagnostic groups according to age

Age	Common respiratory diseases	Infectious gastroenteritis	All other illnesses
<1	70.2	10.4	19.4
1	64.5	14.9	20.6
2	66.1	15.5	18.4
3	64.5	15.6	19.9
4	62.9	15.6	21.6
5	59.3	16.8	23.9
6	55.1	18.0	26.9
7	54.2	19.3	26.5
8	56.3	19.3	24.4
9	54.5	17.5	28.0
10	57.0	18.4	24.7
11	55.7	17.5	26.8
12	62.1	12.2	25.7
13	62.7	14.1	23.2
14	65.6	13.2	21.2
15	66.7	8.1	25.2
16	59.2	7.9	32.9
17	48.9	22.2	28.9
18	0.0	33.3	66.7
22 - 24	56.2	14.1	29.7
25 - 29	60.6	14.1	25.3
30 - 34	61.1	14.9	24.0
35 - 39	54.9	17.4	27.7
40 - 44	53.9	16.7	29.5
45 - 49	56.8	10.8	32.4
50 - 51	76.2	4.8	19.0

Appendix 7

ILLNESS DURING THE FIRST YEAR OF LIFE

TOTAL ILLNESS

The analysis of total illness was based on 107 infants who were under 1 year of age. Total illness included all maladies that were reported by the mothers in their records. Most of the infectious diseases were seen and diagnosed by the staff physicians. A number of the minor complaints such as diaper rash, colic, reactions to immunizations, and so forth, were included on the basis of the mother's description which may or may not have been confirmed by the fieldworker, family pediatrician or a staff physician. Appendix 7, table 1, shows a progressive rise in total illness from 3.4 cases per person-year under 30 days of age to a maximum of 12.1 cases per person-

APPENDIX 7, TABLE 1

Incidence of total illnesses and of common respiratory diseases in 107 children less than one year of age, by periods of 30 days of age

30-day period number	Number person-days	Total number illnesses	Total illnesses per person-year	Number common respiratory diseases	Common respiratory diseases per person-year
1	2,490	23	3.37	13	1.91
2	2,483	45	6.61	30	4.41
3	2,572	50	7.10	40	5.68
4	2,583	60	8.48	45	6.36
5	2,633	76	10.54	51	7.07
6	2,688	71	9.64	58	7.88
7	2,752	91	12.07	71	9.42
8	2,823	84	10.86	57	7.37
9	2,852	94	12.03	63	8.06
10	2,868	86	10.94	60	7.64
11	2,837	82	10.55	57	7.33
12	2,871	92	11.70	61	7.76
13*	500	15	10.95	7	5.11
Total	32,952	869	9.63	613	6.79

*This is not a complete 30-day period; it consists of the interval from the 361st day to the end of the first year.

year during the seventh month of age. Thereafter, total illness by month of age ranged from 10.6 to 12.0 cases per person-year. It is apparent that the shape of the curve of total illness (figure 8) was directly affected by the incidence of common respiratory disease. Appendix 7, table 2, shows the ratio of common respiratory disease to total illness during each month of age. For the entire first year of life it remained fairly constant by month of age, and on the average, 71% of total illnesses were due to the common respiratory diseases (figure 9).

COMMON RESPIRATORY DISEASES

The occurrence of the common respiratory diseases during the first year of life is discussed in Chapters V and VI.

APPENDIX 7, TABLE 2

Ratio of common respiratory diseases to total illnesses in 107 children less than one year of age, by periods of 30 days of age

30-day period number	Number of common respiratory diseases	Number of other illnesses	Total number of illnesses	Common respiratory diseases, percent of total illnesses
1	13	10	23	57
2	30	15	45	67
3	40	10	50	80
4	45	15	60	75
5	51	25	76	67
6	58	13	71	82
7	71	20	91	78
8	57	27	84	68
9	63	31	94	67
10	60	26	86	70
11	57	25	82	70
12	61	31	92	66
13*	7	8	15	47
Total	613	256	869	71

*See footnote, Appendix 7, table 1.

ILLNESSES OTHER THAN COMMON RESPIRATORY DISEASES

Illnesses other than the common respiratory diseases accounted for 29% of the total illnesses. There was a gradual increase in incidence with age to a maximum of four cases per person-year or one-third illness per person per month. Two-thirds of these illnesses were infectious diseases, foremost among them being gastroenteritis (91 cases). The rest of the infections (Appendix 7, table 3) formed a heterogeneous group of illnesses, including 17 cases of primary conjunctivitis, 11 cases of chickenpox, 9 cases of roseola infantum, 7 instances of bacterial skin infection, 2 cases each of primary atypical pneumonia and laboratory-proved influenza, and 3 cases of rubeola. There were isolated instances of rubella, mumps, thrush, pinworms, etc. Rashes of noninfectious origin were recorded 22 times. Many of them could not be readily classified but were believed to be allergic in nature. Reactions to immunizations were recorded 17 times and usually were associated with fever and irritability. Without exception, each infant received the recommended schedule of vaccination against smallpox and immunization against diphtheria, pertussis and tetanus. Fever of unknown origin occurred 10 times.

APPENDIX 7, TABLE 3

Percentage distribution of illnesses other than common respiratory diseases in 107 infants during the first year of life

Illnesses	Number of cases	% of total
Infections	159	62.1
Infectious gastroenteritis	91	
Primary conjunctivitis	17	
Chickenpox	11	
Roseola infantum	9	
Bacterial skin infection	7	
Other infections	24	
Noninfectious dermatitis	22	8.6
Reactions to immunizations	17	6.6
Fevers of unknown origin	10	3.9
Miscellaneous diseases	44	17.2
Accidents	4	1.6
Total	256	100.0

Except for one boy with congenital dislocation of the hip and a girl with meningomyelocele who subsequently died after surgery, miscellaneous diseases consisted of minor disorders. There were four accidents, two burns, one animal bite, and one fractured skull (when the mother fell with the baby).

Appendix 8
TREND OF INCIDENCE OF THE COMMON
RESPIRATORY DISEASES IN TIME

Examination of figure 3 gave the impression that the downward trend in incidence of the common respiratory diseases occurred primarily during the months of high incidence. Graphs for each calendar month (Appendix 8, figure 1) bear out this impression in that each of the months from September through April showed quite marked decreases in incidence, while only slight decreases were noted for May through August. Appendix 8, figure 2 summarizes the data for these two groups of months and shows the downward trend for the months of high incidence and the slight drop for May through August. These data were examined by age, and the downward trend in incidence during the September through April periods was present at all ages. Contrariwise, there was little evidence of a downward trend for any age group for the months of May through August.

In summary, the evidence was quite consistent that there was a decreased incidence of the common respiratory diseases recorded as the study progressed and that this decrease was most evident in the months of high incidence (September through April), and was consistent for each age group. There was little if any decrease during the summer months.

The decrease in the crude incidence rates for the common respiratory diseases, however, might have been due to the shift in the age of the childhood population. For example, during 1948-1949, 60% of the individuals in the study were less than 5 years old and were subjected to the highest incidence rates, while in 1956-1957, only 20% were in this group. The effects of this are illustrated by the age-adjusted rates shown in Appendix 8, figure 3.

Each age-adjusted rate was computed by applying the age-specific rates for the period in question to a standard population. For example, the age-adjusted rates for ages 0 to 18, September through April (the upper left graph in Appendix 8, figure 3) were computed as follows:

1) The total person-years of family study experience for the nine September-through-April periods was taken as the standard population. These numbers are shown in the second column of Appendix 8, table 1.

2) The age-specific rates (the remaining columns of Appendix 8, table 1) which were observed in a given year were applied to the standard population. Thus the age-specific rate for infants in 1948-

320

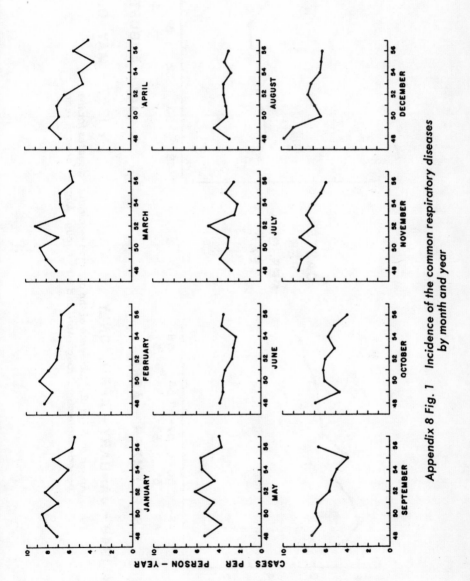

Appendix 8 Fig. 1   Incidence of the common respiratory diseases
by month and year

22

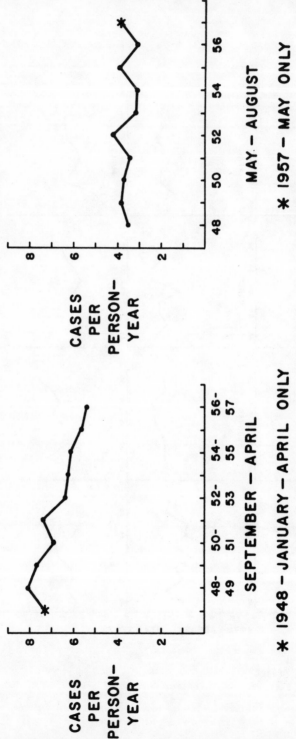

Appendix 8 Fig. 2   Incidence of the common respiratory diseases for the periods September through April and May through August, for each year

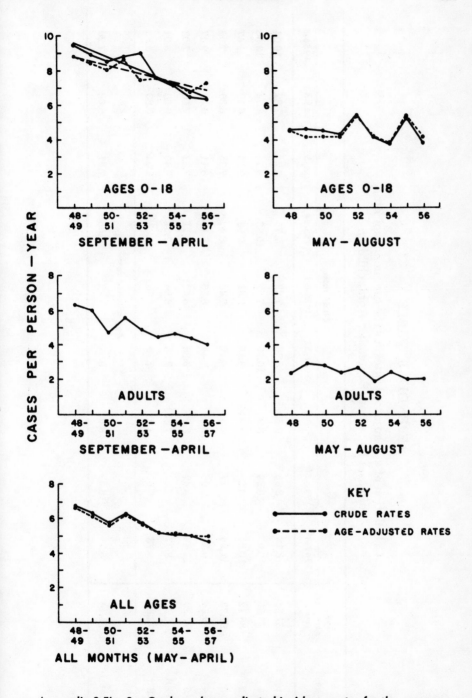

Appendix 8 Fig. 3   Crude and age-adjusted incidence rates for the common
respiratory diseases for the periods September through April and
May though August, for each year

APPENDIX 8, TABLE 1

Calculation of age-adjusted rates for the common respiratory diseases by season, September-April: children

Age	Total person-years	Crude rates								
		1948-49	1949-50	1950-51	1951-52	1952-53	1953-54	1954-55	1955-56	1956-57
Under 1	61.35	8.18	8.96	9.39	8.96	7.62	7.75	6.24	7.82	10.04
1	77.96	10.05	10.33	8.93	10.76	7.52	10.53	8.76	8.74	12.36
2	88.12	10.81	9.61	9.93	9.75	9.81	9.66	9.16	6.19	7.47
3	91.78	11.94	10.17	9.63	9.12	7.43	8.67	7.35	8.30	7.06
4	99.34	9.21	9.06	10.09	9.44	8.36	8.45	8.11	6.50	9.47
5	97.29	11.48	8.42	8.96	9.88	8.52	8.11	7.82	7.06	7.03
6 - 8	262.92	8.77	7.87	7.35	7.85	6.94	7.31	6.40	6.22	5.91
9 +	272.38	5.73	6.87	5.82	7.19	6.30	5.33	6.54	5.83	5.53
						Age-adjusted rates				
Total	1051.14	8.78	8.37	8.01	8.57	7.42	7.56	7.21	6.68	7.20

1949 (8.18 cases per person-year) was multiplied by 61.35 person-years to determine the number of cases (502) which would have occurred among children under 1 in the standard population if this population of 61.35 children suffered the 1948-1949 incidence rates. This procedure was done for each age as follows:

Age	Cases per person-year	Standard population	Expected number of cases
Under 1	8.18	61.35	501.8
1	10.05	77.96	783.5
2	10.81	88.12	952.6
3	11.94	91.78	1095.9
4	9.21	99.34	914.9
5	11.48	97.29	1116.9
6-8	8.77	262.92	2305.8
9+	5.73	272.38	1560.7
Total		1051.14	9232.1

$$\text{Age adjusted rate} = \frac{9232.1 \text{ cases}}{1051.14 \text{ person-years}} = 8.78 \text{ cases per person-year}$$

In this way it was determined that if the age-specific rates for 1948-1949 were occurring in the standard population, a total of 9232 cases would be recorded. The total rate would be 8.78 cases per person-year.

The age-adjusted rates were computed in this way for each year (Appendix 8, table 1). These adjusted rates showed what the incidence would have been if the age distribution of the population had remained constant. The adjusted rates, together with the total (crude) rates for this group of children, are shown in Appendix 8, figure 3 (upper left diagram). The average decrease per year in these rates was computed by fitting straight lines by the method of least squares to each of these two groups of data.

The trend line for the observed rates showed an average annual decrease in incidence of 0.392 cases per person-year. The average decrease for the age-adjusted rates was 0.233 cases per person-year. The difference between these two slopes represents the change which can be attributed to the aging of the population. It is estimated, then, that $\frac{0.392-0.233}{0.392}$ or 40% of the drop was due to the aging of the population, while 60% was due to some other unknown factor or factors.

The data just presented refer to children aged 0-18 years during the September-April periods. Calculations were performed for children during the May-August periods and trend lines (not shown in Appendix 8, figure 3) were fitted. Neither line showed a significant change in incidence during the study. Age-adjusted rates were not determined for adults.

In computing the age-adjusted rates for the total experience, adults were taken to represent one age group. On the basis of the computed trend lines the observed (crude) rates showed an average annual decline of 0.253 case per person-year. The average annual decline of the age-adjusted rates was 0.197 cases per person-year. So it may be estimated that $\frac{0.056}{0.253}$ or 22% of the drop in the total incidence rate was due to the change in the age distribution of the population in the study, and 78% was due to some other factor or factors which could not be determined.

It must be recognized that this analysis provides only an estimate, and the use of other standard populations would lead to other estimates.

Appendix 9

APPENDIX 9, TABLE 1

Incidence of the common respiratory diseases, by age

Age (years)	Person-days	Number of illnesses	Illnesses per person-year
Under 1	33,317	613	6.7
1	42,196	957	8.3
2	48,183	1,065	8.1
3	50,131	1,077	7.8
4	53,891	1,125	7.6
5	53,176	1,081	7.4
6	51,485	869	6.2
7	48,209	808	6.1
8	43,322	711	6.0
9	36,853	539	5.3
10	30,999	484	5.7
11	25,759	359	5.1
12	20,085	275	5.0
13	13,796	173	4.6
14	9,569	124	4.7
15	5,677	74	4.8
16 +	5,270	67	4.6
Fathers	202,163	1,912	3.5
Mothers	202,955	2,677	4.8
Totals	977,036	14,990	5.6

APPENDIX 9, TABLE 2

Incidence of the common respiratory diseases in male children, by age

Age (years)	Person-days	Number of illnesses	Illnesses per person-year
Under 1	18,002	341	6.9
1	22,414	510	8.3
2	25,397	580	8.3
3	26,431	577	8.0
4	27,649	586	7.7
5	27,335	584	7.8
6	25,101	435	6.3
7	23,589	408	6.3
8	21,653	361	6.1
9	18,180	280	5.6
10	15,629	266	6.2
11	14,061	217	5.6
12	10,459	151	5.3
13	7,457	101	4.9
14	5,151	68	4.8
15	2,792	43	5.6
16	1,433	26	6.6
17	1,077	12	4.1
18	156	0	0.0
Totals	293,966	5,546	6.9

APPENDIX 9, TABLE 3

Incidence of the common respiratory diseases
in female children, by age

Age (years)	Person-days	Number of illnesses	Illnesses per person-year
Under 1	15,315	272	6.5
1	19,782	447	8.2
2	22,786	485	7.8
3	23,700	500	7.7
4	26,242	539	7.5
5	25,841	497	7.0
6	26,384	434	6.0
7	24,620	400	5.9
8	21,669	350	5.9
9	18,673	259	5.1
10	15,370	218	5.2
11	11,698	142	4.4
12	9,626	124	4.7
13	6,339	72	4.1
14	4,418	56	4.6
15	2,885	31	3.9
16	1,530	19	4.5
17	1,019	10	3.6
18	55	0	0.0
Totals	277,952	4,855	6.4

APPENDIX 9, TABLE 4

Incidence of the common respiratory diseases
in parents by sex, according to age

Age group in years	Number of illnesses	Number of person-days	Cases per person-year
A. Males			
22 - 31	267	26,722	3.65
32 - 41	1,357	146,177	3.39
42 - 51	288	29,264	3.59
B. Females			
22 - 31	900	62,935	5.22
32 - 41	1,611	125,678	4.68
42 - 51	166	14,342	4.22
C. Total			
22 - 31	1,167	89,657	4.75
32 - 41	2,968	271,855	3.98
42 - 51	454	43,606	3.80

Appendix 10

INTRODUCTION OF COMMON RESPIRATORY DISEASES INTO THE HOME

The relative rates with which various classes of family members introduced common respiratory diseases into the home were determined for five categories of individuals: fathers (F), mothers (M), preschool children (P), school children less than 6 years of age (S<6) and school children 6 years of age and older (S6+).

The methods of determining the rates may be illustrated first in terms of the simplest type of family in the study: that consisting of a father, mother, and one preschool child. In families of this composition there were 177 index cases: 40 were among the fathers, 45 among the mothers, and 92 among the preschool children. Mothers, then, introduced 45/40=1.13 as many infections as did the fathers, while preschool children introduced 92/40=2.30 as many. These ratios are considered to mean that in families of this composition the relative risk of contracting an infection outside the home was 1.13 times as great for the mothers as for the fathers, and was 2.30 times as great for the preschool children as for the fathers. It is this ratio, the number of introductions by each class of individual divided by the number of introductions by the fathers in the same families, that is employed here to indicate the relative risk of each class.

In the example cited above, determination of the relative number of introductions for the three classes of persons—father, mother, and preschool child—is simple because each family considered had only one member of each class. When the analyses are extended to include all episodes in all families, the relationship of mothers to fathers is readily determined because each family had one of each. This ratio, which is taken to be the best measure of the relative risk for mothers, was $\frac{833 \text{ index cases among mothers}}{620 \text{ index cases among fathers}} = 1.34$ to 1.

The analyses became much more complicated when expanded to include the data for all families containing more than one child. The problem is illustrated in Appendix 10, table 1, which shows the number of index cases in three types of families, containing respectively one, two, and three school children 6 years of age or older. In those families with one such child, on the average those children were index cases 2.58 times as often as were the fathers. The ratio increased with the number of children, to 5.13 in families with three such children. The obvious explanation is that there were

APPENDIX 10, TABLE 1

Number and relative number of index cases of common respiratory disease among various classes of individuals in 3 types of families

Class of individual	Number of index cases		
	F M S6+	F M S6+ S6+	F M S6+ S6+ S6+
Father (F)	12	64	53
Mother (M)	15	75	67
School child 6+ (S6+)	31	307	272

$$\frac{\text{Index cases among school children } 6+}{\text{Index cases among fathers}} : \text{F M S6}+ : \frac{31}{12} = \frac{2.58}{1}$$

$$\text{F M S6}+ \text{ S6}+ : \frac{307}{64} = \frac{4.80}{1}$$

$$\text{F M S6}+ \text{ S6}+ \text{ S6}+ : \frac{272}{53} = \frac{5.13}{1}$$

three times as many children to accomplish these introductions in the latter type of family than in the former. If one is interested in the average relative risk per individual, the ratio 4.80 (families with two school children 6 years of age or older) is twice as great as it should be and that of 5.13 is three times as large. Appendix 10, table 2, shows the method of computing the relative risk per person for school children 6 years of age or older in these three types of families.

There were, of course, many variants of families containing school children 6 years of age or older. There were altogether 42 types of families at the onset of episodes, of which 31 contained children of the type S6+. Appendix 10, table 3, shows the steps followed in order to arrive at a figure describing the relative introduction ratio for this type of child based on the total experience of these 31 types of families:

1) The index cases among fathers in the 10 types of families containing one S6+ child were determined to be 133.

2) The index cases among S6+ children in these same families were found to be 395.

3) These 528 index cases occurred in only 516 episodes, for in some episodes there was more than one index case.

4) The ratio 395/133=2.97 was determined.

5) Similar accumulations were made for families containing two, three, four, and five children S6+, respectively. The ratios were of the type derived in Appendix 10, table 2: the relative number of index cases per person.

APPENDIX 10, TABLE 2

Adjusted number and relative number of index cases of common respiratory disease among various classes of individuals in 3 types of families

Class of individual	Adjusted number of index cases		
	F M S6+	F M S6+ S6+	F M S6+ S6+ S6+
Father (F)	12	64	53
Mother (M)	15	75	67
School child 6+ (S6+)	31	153.5	90.67

$$\frac{\text{Adjusted number of index cases}}{\text{Index cases among fathers}} : \text{F M S6+} : \frac{31}{12} = \frac{2.58}{1}$$

$$\text{F M S6+ S6+} : \frac{153.5}{64} = \frac{2.40}{1}$$

$$\text{F M S6+ S6+ S6+} : \frac{90.67}{53} = \frac{1.70}{1}$$

6) A weighted average of these ratios was computed to be 2.20. In this process each ratio was weighted according to the number of episodes in which either the father or a school child (S6+) or both were involved as an index case. This method of weighting is somewhat different from that used in previously published papers.

Similar computations were made for preschool children and school children under 6 years of age (Appendix 10, table 3). These ratios indicate the relative frequency with which each class of person introduced common respiratory disease into the home. Another and somewhat different interpretation is that they measure the relative risk of having been infected in the community outside the home.

The basic assumption in the ratios used here was that when a family became eligible for the development of an index case, each member of the family was automatically at risk of becoming an index case; in computing the ratio, each class of individual was weighted according to the frequency with which such persons were present in families when episodes started.

Theoretically a more direct approach to measuring these relative risks would be to determine the absolute rate of acquiring infections in the community for each class of individual. Such incidence rates would, of course, imply a measure not only of the number of infections acquired, but also a measure of the time during which one was exposed to the risk of acquiring infection. It was not pos-

APPENDIX 10, TABLE 3

Summary table showing relative introduction ratios of the common respiratory diseases for mothers and 3 classes of children

	Number of index cases		No. of episodes	Ratio	Ratio x no. episodes	Relative introduction ratio
A. Mothers	Fathers	Mothers				
	620	833	1432	$\dfrac{833}{620} = 1.34$		1.34
B. No. Preschool children in family	Fathers	Preschool children				
1	242	642	865	$\dfrac{642}{242} = 2.65$	2292	
2	130	713	758	$\dfrac{356.5}{130} = 2.74$	2077	
3	23	174	166 ⎫	$\dfrac{59.75}{23} = 2.60$	450	
4	.....	7	7 ⎭			
			1796		4819	$\dfrac{4819}{1796} = 2.68$

C. No. school children <6 in family	Fathers	School children <6				
1	195	633	811	$\frac{633}{195} = 3.25$	2636	
2	15	99	105	$\frac{49.5}{15} = 3.30$	346	
			916		2982	$\frac{2982}{916} = 3.26$

D. No. school children 6+ in family	Fathers	School children 6+				
1	133	395	516	$\frac{395}{133} = 2.97$	1533	
2	196	727	878	$\frac{363.5}{196} = 1.85$	1624	
3	81	536	586	$\frac{178.7}{81} = 2.21$	1295	
4	20	125	133	$\frac{31.25}{20} = 1.56$	207	
5	1	6	7	$\frac{1.20}{1} = 1.20$	8	
			2120		4667	$\frac{4667}{2120} = 2.20$

sible to determine for many of the illnesses whether they were acquired outside or inside the home and, therefore, proper incidence rates for infections acquired outside the home could not be computed. It might be possible to determine for each individual the period when he was at risk of becoming an index case, and to compute the following ratio for each class of individual:

$$\frac{\text{Number of index cases}}{\text{Person-days eligible to become an index case}}$$

The denominators of such ratios, however, would be extremely difficult to determine. More importantly, they represent a residue of time after eliminating other periods of time which have very complex descriptions (see definition of episode and some of the exclusions described in Chapter VI, pages 40 and 41). The periods excluded are not random periods of time, but are selected because complex events were occurring in the family. It would be difficult indeed to argue that such a ratio represented the true rate of incidence of infection acquired outside the home. The measure which was used does not eliminate these objections. It is one which was easier to compute and which possibly contains no more distortions than the alternative just described.

Appendix 11

APPENDIX 11, TABLE 1

Secondary attack rates from the common respiratory diseases, by age

Age of contact (years)	Number of times exposed	Number of illnesses	Illnesses per exposure
Under 1	660	243	.37
1	707	345	.49
2	804	378	.47
3	810	325	.40
4	910	345	.38
5	875	272	.31
6	912	243	.27
7	860	212	.25
8	846	205	.24
9	712	156	.22
10	602	154	.26
11	480	109	.23
12	362	69	.19
13	280	45	.16
14	184	33	.18
15	121	20	.17
16	76	22	.29
17	48	6	.13
18	4	0	.00
Fathers	4331	602	.14
Mothers	4118	954	.23
Totals	18,702	4738	.25

Note: Includes all episodes regardless of number of index cases.

APPENDIX 11, TABLE 2

Secondary attack rates from the common respiratory diseases, by family size

Size of family	Number of illnesses	Number of times exposed	Illnesses per exposure
3	132	500	.26
4	1189	4492	.26
5	1902	7741	.25
6	1116	4346	.26
7	218	899	.24
8	180	729	.25
Totals	4737	18,707	.25

APPENDIX 11, TABLE 3

Observed and expected secondary attack rates for the common respiratory diseases among children 1 year of age and older, according to length of time since last common respiratory illness

Days since last illness	Number of contacts	Number of secondary cases		Secondary attack rates %	
		Observed	Expected	Observed	Expected
10-12	184	55	66.3	29.9	36.0
13-15	231	70	82.8	30.3	35.8
16-19	398	122	149.8	30.7	37.6
20-24	571	205	207.1	35.9	36.3
25-29	545	218	192.6	40.0	35.3
30-34	466	190	169.3	40.8	36.3
35-39	405	155	146.0	38.3	36.0
40-49	668	230	233.6	34.4	35.0
50-59	538	204	190.0	37.9	35.3
60-69	430	152	141.7	35.3	33.0
70-99	744	238	236.7	32.0	31.8
100-129	440	129	129.9	29.3	29.5
130-159	261	65	72.4	24.9	27.7
160-199	188	52	50.5	27.7	26.9
200-365	281	53	65.2	18.9	23.2
366-730	43	5	8.3	11.6	19.3
731+	7	1	1.7	14.3	24.3
Totals	6400	2144	2144.0	33.5	33.5

APPENDIX 11, TABLE 4

Observed and expected secondary attack rates for the common respiratory diseases in adults, according to length of time since last common respiratory illness

Days since last illness	Number of contacts	Number of secondary cases		Secondary attack rates %	
		Observed	Expected	Observed	Expected
10-12	107	20	25.6	18.7	23.9
13-15	113	26	25.6	23.0	22.7
16-19	198	40	44.3	20.2	22.4
20-24	294	67	67.5	22.8	23.0
25-29	281	51	63.1	18.1	22.5
30-34	256	52	57.6	20.3	22.5
35-39	262	54	57.4	20.6	21.9
40-49	471	102	104.4	21.7	22.2
50-59	425	82	94.6	19.3	22.3
60-69	342	65	70.7	19.0	20.7
70-99	797	179	159.5	22.5	20.0
100-129	501	107	96.4	21.4	19.2
130-159	332	70	58.6	21.1	17.7
160-199	342	66	58.8	19.3	17.2
200-365	555	95	81.3	17.1	14.6
366-730	168	9	17.6	5.4	10.5
731+	50	2	4.0	4.0	8.0
Totals	5494	1087	1087.0	19.8	19.8

Appendix 12

DESCRIPTION OF THE EPISODES WHICH WERE ELIMINATED FROM THE STUDY OF SUSCEPTIBILITY TO REPEATED ATTACKS OF THE COMMON RESPIRATORY DISEASES

In the tabulations presented in the text (Chapter VI) which relate secondary attack rates to the interval since an individual was last ill, certain of the family episodes of common respiratory disease were omitted:

1. Not infrequently a decision had to be made as to whether an exacerbation of previously existing symptoms, or the appearance of new symptoms superimposed on those already present, reflected a new illness or the progression of an old one. These decisions were made on the basis of clinical judgment (see Chapter IV) and most of the rates included in the present monograph are based on cases so judged. In the present study the correctness of such decisions assumes major importance, for they were required most frequently during the period of time undergoing special scrutiny, that is, soon after the onset of the last respiratory illness in an individual. For these tabulations, therefore, family contacts were excluded if either the index case or the contact had respiratory symptoms at any time during the 3 days prior to the onset of the episode. For similar reasons, contacts were excluded if a concurrent illness, such as measles, was present which might have caused confusion in establishing whether or not a common respiratory illness was present.

2. Another practice used in most of the tabulations was to ignore temporary absences from home. The reason for this has been stated (page 41). In the present tabulations, a contact was excluded if he or the index case was away from home for 1 day or more during the episode.

3. There were many instances where the interval from the preceding illness to the present episode was unknown. With few exceptions, these were exposures which occurred to persons before their first respiratory illnesses after entering the study. These were of necessity omitted.

4. For reasons mentioned in the text, children under 1 year of age were omitted as contacts.

Appendix 12, table 1, compares the secondary attack rates in these selected episodes with the secondary attack rates in the total study (see Appendix 11, table 1). The similarity of these two sets of rates implies that the clinical criteria used for diagnosis and the ignoring of temporary absences from home were justified.

APPENDIX 12, TABLE 1

Comparison of secondary attack rates for the common respiratory diseases in all episodes with those in the selected episodes

		All episodes	Selected episodes
Adults	Number of times exposed	8,449	5,494
	Number of secondary cases	1,556	1,087
	Secondary attack rates (%)	18.4	19.8
Children 1 year of age and older	Number of times exposed	9,593	6,400
	Number of secondary cases	2,939	2,144
	Secondary attack rates (%)	30.6	33.5

Appendix 13

APPENDIX 13, TABLE 1

Number of common respiratory illnesses in which the specific symptoms were present, by age

Symptoms	Age					
	Under 1	1-5	6-18	Fathers	Mothers	Total
Coryza	489	3748	2258	1186	1555	9236
Sore throat	25	615	980	892	1323	3835
Hoarseness	48	755	469	319	585	2176
Cough	262	2304	1209	621	917	5313
No. of cases	512	4088	2610	1455	1898	10,563

APPENDIX 13, TABLE 2

Number of common respiratory illnesses in which specific combinations of symptoms were present, by age

| Symptoms* | | | | Age | | | | | |
Coryza	Sore throat	Hoarseness	Cough	Under 1	1-5	6-18	Fathers	Mothers	Total
x	x	x	x	4	153	147	170	346	820
x	x	x	o	1	26	63	47	88	225
x	x	o	x	7	194	269	206	265	941
x	x	o	o	8	124	279	251	346	1008
x	o	x	x	35	394	136	42	60	667
x	o	x	o	6	99	62	19	27	213
x	o	o	x	201	1345	501	123	140	2310
x	o	o	o	227	1413	801	328	283	3052
o	x	x	x	0	16	17	24	26	83
o	x	x	o	0	13	20	10	20	63
o	x	o	x	2	16	30	29	38	115
o	x	o	o	3	73	155	155	194	580
o	o	x	x	1	30	13	3	10	57
o	o	x	o	1	24	11	4	8	48
o	o	o	x	12	156	96	24	32	320
o	o	o	o	4	12	10	20	15	61
Totals				512	4088	2610	1455	1898	10,563

*x = Present; o = Absent

APPENDIX 13, TABLE 3

Number of cases of common respiratory diseases by age according to presence or absence of specific pairs of symptoms

Age	Symptom	Number of cases	Sore throat		Hoarseness		Cough	
			Present	%	Present	%	Present	%
Under 1	Coryza	489	20	4.1	46	9.4	247	50.5
	No coryza	23	5	21.7	2	8.7	15	65.2
	Total	512	25	4.9	48	9.4	262	51.2
1-5	Coryza	3748	497	13.3	672	17.9	2086	55.7
	No coryza	340	118	34.7	83	24.4	218	64.1
	Total	4088	615	15.0	755	18.5	2304	56.4
6-18	Coryza	2258	758	33.6	408	18.1	1053	46.6
	No coryza	352	222	63.1	61	17.3	156	44.3
	Total	2610	980	37.5	469	18.0	1209	46.3
Fathers	Coryza	1186	674	56.8	278	23.4	541	45.6
	No coryza	269	218	81.0	41	15.2	80	29.7
	Total	1455	892	61.3	319	21.9	621	42.7
Mothers	Coryza	1555	1045	67.2	521	33.5	811	52.2
	No coryza	343	278	81.0	64	18.7	106	30.9
	Total	1898	1323	69.7	585	30.8	917	48.3
Under 1	Sore throat	25			5	20.0	13	52.0
	No sore throat	487			43	8.8	249	51.1
	Total	512			48	9.4	262	51.2
1-5	Sore throat	615			208	33.8	379	61.6
	No sore throat	3473			547	15.8	1925	55.4
	Total	4088			755	18.5	2304	56.4

APPENDIX 13, TABLE 3 (cont.)

Age	Symptom	Number of cases	Sore throat		Hoarseness		Cough	
			Present	%	Present	%	Present	%
6-18	Sore throat	980			247	25.2	463	47.2
	No sore throat	1630			222	13.6	746	45.8
	Total	2610			469	18.0	1209	46.3
Fathers	Sore throat	892			251	28.1	429	48.1
	No sore throat	563			68	12.1	192	34.1
	Total	1455			319	21.9	621	42.7
Mothers	Sore throat	1323			480	36.3	675	51.0
	No sore throat	575			105	18.3	242	42.1
	Total	1898			585	30.8	917	48.3
Under 1	Hoarseness	48					40	83.3
	No hoarseness	464					222	47.8
	Total	512					262	51.2
1-5	Hoarseness	755					593	78.5
	No hoarseness	3333					1711	51.3
	Total	4088					2304	56.4
6-18	Hoarseness	469					313	66.7
	No hoarseness	2141					896	41.8
	Total	2610					1209	46.3
Fathers	Hoarseness	319					239	74.9
	No hoarseness	1136					382	33.6
	Total	1455					621	42.7
Mothers	Hoarseness	585					442	75.6
	No hoarseness	1313					475	36.2
	Total	1898					917	48.3

APPENDIX 13, TABLE 4

Percentage of cases* of the common respiratory diseases in which fever was present, by year of age

Age	Number of cases	Fever present	
		Number	%
Under 1	547	105	19.2
1	835	164	19.6
2	896	191	21.3
3	857	173	20.2
4	917	197	21.5
5	857	175	20.4
6	648	130	20.1
7	538	89	16.5
8	459	69	15.0
9	343	48	14.0
10	265	34	12.8
11	186	20	10.8
12	126	11	8.7
13	75	12	16.0
14	36	1	2.8
15	21	1	4.8
16	14	1	7.1
17	6	0	0.0
Fathers	1495	99	6.6
Mothers	2013	102	5.1
Totals	11,134	1622	14.6

*This table is based on all cases (11,134) of common respiratory diseases occurring during the period 1948 through 1954; it was not necessary to exclude for this purpose the 571 cases for which there was some question regarding the localizing symptoms.

APPENDIX 13, TABLE 5

Occurrence of complications in persons with the common respiratory diseases*

Complication	Number	% with complication
Mastoiditis	1	0.01
Herpes simplex	6	0.05
Cervical adenitis	22	0.20
Earache	48	0.43
Sinusitis	53	0.48
Asthma	76	0.68
Conjunctivitis	108	0.97
Otitis media	213	1.91

*This table is based on all cases (11,134) of common respiratory diseases occurring during the period 1948 through 1954; it was not necessary to exclude for this purpose the 571 cases for which there was some question regarding the localizing symptoms.

Appendix 14

APPENDIX 14, TABLE 1

Incidence of streptococcal tonsillitis and pharyngitis, by age

Age in years	Person-days	Number of cases	Number of cases per 1000 person-days
0	33,317	0	0.00
1	42,196	15	0.36
2	48,333	20	0.41
3	49,981	24	0.48
4	53,891	37	0.69
5	53,176	58	1.09
6	51,485	52	1.01
7	48,209	54	1.12
8	43,322	31	0.72
9	36,853	27	0.73
10	30,999	15	0.48
11	25,759	15	0.58
12	20,085	12	0.60
13	13,796	4	0.29
14	9,569	3	0.31
15	5,677	1	0.18
16	2,963	1	0.34
17	2,096	0	0.00
18	211	0	0.00
Parents	405,118	68	0.17

APPENDIX 14, TABLE 2

Secondary carrier rates for typable group A streptococci when index
carrier had streptococcal illness, by age

Age	No. of exposures	No. of carriers	%
Under 1 yr.	10	0	0
1 - 2 yrs.	18	6	33
3 - 4 yrs.	26	14	54
5+ yrs.	38	15	39
Fathers	47	1	2
Mothers	44	10	23
Totals	183	46	25

APPENDIX 14, TABLE 3

Secondary carrier rates for typable group A streptococci when index
carrier did not have streptococcal illness, by age

Age	No. of exposures	No. of carriers	%
Under 1 yr.	14	1	7
1 - 2 yrs.	33	2	6
3 - 4 yrs.	34	6	18
5+ yrs.	73	8	11
Fathers	65	3	5
Mothers	72	6	8
Totals	291	26	9

APPENDIX 14, TABLE 4

Secondary carrier rates for group A streptococci
by class of family member

Class of index case	Fathers			Mothers			School children			Preschool children		
	No. of exposures	No. of carriers	%	No. of exposures	No. of carriers	%	No. of exposures	No. of carriers	%	No. of exposures	No. of carriers	%
Father	....	....	....	9	1	11	15	1	7	6	0	0
Mother	9	0	0	....	....	....	15	4	27	8	0	0
School child	81	3	4	84	13	15	71	16	23	96	23	24
Preschool child	22	1	5	23	2	9	22	6	27	13	2	15
Multiple	5	0	0	4	1	25	5	1	20	3	2	67
Total	117	4	3	120	17	14	128	28	22	126	27	21

APPENDIX 14, TABLE 5

Frequency with which a recurrence of symptoms was diagnosed as "post-streptococcal illness"*

Year	No. of cases of streptococcal tonsillitis and pharyngitis	Cases with recurrence of acute symptoms	
		No.	%
1948	14	3	21
1949	40	7	18
1950	53	7	13
1951	62	14	23
1952	66	18	27
1953	69	7	10
1954	56	6	11
1955	30	3	10
1956	33	0	0
1957	9	0	0
Total	432	65	15

*In this table the five instances mentioned in the text are included as "post-streptococcal illness" although initially they had been diagnosed as cases of streptococcal tonsillitis and pharyngitis. Therefore there are five less cases of streptococcal tonsillitis and pharyngitis than are included elsewhere and 65 cases of the type described in the title of this table.

Appendix 15

SPECIAL STUDY OF POST-STREPTOCOCCAL COMPLICATIONS

During a short period an intensive attempt was made to discover any evidence of post-streptococcal complications following the acquisition of a group A streptococcus. A control group consisted of individuals who acquired a non-group A streptococcus during the same interval of time. In three instances acquisitions of *alpha*-hemolytic streptococci were included as controls because on the initial culture they were mistakenly considered to be *beta*-hemolytic streptococci. A total of 58 individuals was studied, 38 of whom had acquired group A streptococci and 20 of whom had acquired non-group A streptococci.

As soon as possible after acquisition was known, observations were made as follows: nose and throat cultures were obtained, an acute-phase blood for the antistreptolysin test was drawn, clinical observations of any illness were made and an electrocardiogram was taken. This tracing included the three standard limb leads, the augmented unipolar leads, and the six chest leads. At weekly intervals for 3 weeks after acquisition, clinical observations, throat cultures by both the method of Pike and streaking on a blood agar plate, and electrocardiograms were repeated. On the fourteenth day following acquisition the urine was examined microscopically and tested for albumin. The period of observation terminated on about the twenty-first day following acquisition. On this occasion, another

APPENDIX 15, TABLE 1

Results of cultures taken at weekly intervals from 38 individuals acquiring group A streptococci who received antibiotic treatment

Time of culture	No. of individuals harboring streptococci by	
	Pike method	Blood agar plate
When acquisition first detected (routine culture)	26	23
As soon as possible after acquisition	10	8
1 week after acquisition	12	11
2 weeks after acquisition	10	10
3 weeks after acquisition	12	10

blood was drawn for erythrocyte sedimentation rate. An antistreptolysin test was later performed on this blood and on the
acute-phase blood specimen. Detailed information regarding the
choice of therapy, the quantity administered, and the duration of
treatment was obtained from the mother and family doctor or
pediatrician.

Appendix 15, table 1 presents the results of cultures taken from
38 individuals who acquired group A streptococci. All of these patients received antibiotic treament, the therapy consisting of varying
doses of sulfonamides, penicillin, aureomycin, chloramphenicol, ter-
ramycin alone or in combination, for 1-7 days. Only one individual
received treatment for a week. The majority received treatment for
about 3 days. It can be pointed out from these data that the treat-
ments administered were inadequate to eradicate streptococci.
Analysis of the antistreptolysin data indicated that the therapy
administered failed to suppress antibody formation, since at least
one-half of the individuals showed a significant rise in titer. This
result would be expected if no treatment had been given. Thus,
one may conclude that the therapy administered should not have
materially interfered with any post-streptococcal complications that
might have occurred.

A search for such post-streptococcal complications was, however,
barren, with the possible exception of T wave changes in the electrocardiograms. Only one urine was positive for protein. This urine
did not show cells on careful microscopic examination. On repeated
urinalysis no abnormality was detected. In Appendix 15, table 2,

APPENDIX 15, TABLE 2

Erythrocyte sedimentation rates 21 days after acquisition
of streptococci

Corrected sedimentation rate (mm./hr.)	Individuals with group A streptococci	Individuals with non-group A streptococci
<10	2	4
10-14	8	3
15-19	12	2
20-24	4	0
25-29	0	1
30+	4	2
Total	30	12

a comparison of the erythrocyte sedimentation rates is given. Although the average difference in the level of the sedimentation rate between individuals who acquired group A streptococci and those who acquired non-group A streptococci was not significant, the comparison is based on small numbers. The difference which was found is in the direction one might expect—an elevated rate in cases of group A infections.

In analyzing the electrocardiograms, five P-R intervals in lead II in each record were measured and averaged. Differences between the P-R interval in the initial control record and subsequent exam-

APPENDIX 15, TABLE 3

Average change in P-R interval (seconds) after acquisition
of hemolytic streptococci

Group of streptococci	Days after acquisition		
	7	14	21
A	−.00071	−.00226	−.00250
Non-A	−.00312	−.00167	−.00278

inations at 7, 14 and 21 days were determined. Appendix 15, table 3 shows the average difference for each of these times. The average change in P-R interval was very small and was no greater among those acquiring a group A streptococcus than among those acquiring a non-group A streptococcus.

Changes in T waves between the two groups were also compared at 7, 14, and 21 days. The only difference occurred among children

APPENDIX 15, TABLE 4

Distribution of children according to number of leads
showing T wave changes at 14 days

Group of streptococci	Number of leads showing T wave changes		Total	% with 2 or more
	0 or 1	2 or more		
A	9	15	24	62.5
Non-A	10	1	11	9.1
Total	19	16	35	

14 days after acquisition. Appendix 15, table 4 shows that 62.5% of the children harboring group A streptococci had T wave changes in two or more leads, as compared with 9.1% of the children harboring streptococci other than group A. This difference, while impressive, is difficult to interpret. Changes in T waves were observed largely in leads III, AVR, V3, and V4. In these leads, non-specific T wave changes are known to occur frequently. No T wave changes occurred in standard leads I and II. No definite evidence of post-streptococcal activity indicative of rheumatic fever was observed.

Appendix 16

APPENDIX 16, TABLE 1

Age-specific incidence rates of several diagnostic groups of illnesses in children according to status with respect to tonsillectomy

	Tonsillec-tomy	Age group (years)			
		3-5	6-7	8-9	10+
Number of person-days	Yes	18,121	29,916	35,110	67,268
	No	139,077	69,778	45,065	43,887
Common respiratory diseases:					
Number of cases	Yes	421	580	607	933
	No	2,862	1,097	643	623
Cases per 1000 person-days	Yes	23.2	19.4	17.3	13.9
	No	20.6	15.7	14.3	14.2
Nonbacterial tonsillitis and pharyngitis:					
Number of cases	Yes	8	14	3	10
	No	77	23	19	11
Cases per 1000 person-days	Yes	0.44	0.47	0.09	0.15
	No	0.55	0.33	0.42	0.25
Streptococcal tonsillitis and pharyngitis:					
Number of cases	Yes	7	11	14	19
	No	112	95	44	32
Cases per 1000 person-days	Yes	0.39	0.37	0.40	0.28
	No	0.81	1.36	0.98	0.73

Fevers of unknown origin:					
Number of cases	Yes	8	7	8	11
	No	68	37	13	9
Cases per 1000 person-days	Yes	0.44	0.23	0.23	0.16
	No	0.49	0.53	0.29	0.21
Infectious gastroenteritis:					
Number of cases	Yes	104	186	188	233
	No	743	385	228	180
Cases per 1000 person-days	Yes	5.74	6.22	5.35	3.46
	No	5.34	5.52	5.06	4.10

APPENDIX 16, TABLE 2

Secondary attack rates for the common respiratory diseases in persons who had not had tonsillectomy, by age and sex

Age (years)	Males			Females		
	No. times ill	No. times exposed	Illnesses per exposure	No. times ill	No. times exposed	Illnesses per exposure
Under 1	127	364	.35	116	296	.39
1	194	396	.49	151	311	.49
2	202	422	.48	175	379	.46
3	169	440	.38	147	345	.43
4	144	414	.35	163	388	.42
5	103	354	.29	113	353	.32
6	76	301	.25	85	351	.24
7	61	265	.23	74	313	.24
8	61	261	.23	53	247	.21
9	42	185	.23	36	185	.19
10	41	149	.28	33	141	.23
11	40	138	.29	12	75	.16
12	19	68	.28	6	69	.09
13	14	64	.22	2	19	.11
14	12	30	.40	2	12	.17
15	7	26	.27	1	8	.13
16	6	17	.35	2	7	.29
17	2	16	.13	....	....	....
18	....	....	....	....	....	....
Parents	80	610	.13	271	1103	.25

APPENDIX 16, TABLE 3

Secondary attack rates for the common respiratory diseases in persons who had had tonsillectomy according to age and sex

Age (years)	Males			Females		
	No. times ill	No. times exposed	Illnesses per exposure	No. times ill	No. times exposed	Illnesses per exposure
Under 1	....	....	....	....	....	....
1	....	....	....	....	....	....
2	1	3	.33	....	....	....
3	8	17	.47	1	6	.17
4	21	65	.32	17	37	.46
5	31	93	.33	24	69	.35
6	40	134	.30	43	121	.36
7	37	135	.27	40	142	.28
8	46	165	.28	44	165	.27
9	32	154	.21	44	181	.24
10	37	145	.26	42	160	.26
11	25	127	.20	32	133	.24
12	17	118	.14	27	105	.26
13	16	90	.18	12	106	.11
14	7	68	.10	12	74	.16
15	2	29	.07	10	58	.17
16	6	21	.29	8	31	.26
17	1	9	.11	3	23	.13
18	0	3	.00	0	1	.00
Parents	503	3617	.14	683	3015	.23

APPENDIX 16, TABLE 4

Observed and expected attack rates for the common respiratory
diseases in 59 children according to time before and
after tonsillectomy

Period before or after operation	Person-days	Number of cases		Rates per 1000 person-days	
		Expected*	Observed	Expected*	Observed
Before operation:					
7th year or earlier	3,324	66	55	19.9	16.5
6th year	3,377	71	75	21.0	22.2
5th year	5,171	101	122	19.5	23.6
4th year	7,554	149	168	19.7	22.2
3rd year	10,982	222	227	20.2	20.7
2nd year	14,740	292	314	19.8	21.3
1st year	19,699	383	431	19.4	21.9
Year of operation	10,647	226	264	21.2	24.8
After operation:					
Year of operation	10,330	167	179	16.2	17.3
1st year	17,342	310	363	17.9	20.9
2nd year	14,140	243	295	17.2	20.9
3rd year	11,679	189	221	16.2	18.9
4th year	7,861	124	152	15.8	19.3
5th year	5,856	89	112	15.2	19.1
6th year	4,198	61	64	14.5	15.2
7th year or later	2,277	34	26	14.9	11.4

*Expected numbers are based on age-specific and season-specific rates for the entire child-
hood population. Since 17 of the 59 tonsillectomies were performed during May and June,
it was necessary to consider seasonal variation in arriving at these expected numbers.
Since the rates for the common respiratory diseases are fairly constant between September
and April and lower between May and August, the seasonal adjustment was based on these
two groups of months.

APPENDIX 16, TABLE 5

Observed and expected attack rates for streptococcal tonsillitis and pharyngitis in 59 children according to time before and after tonsillectomy

Period before or after operation	Person- days	Number of cases		Rates per 1000 person-days	
		Expected*	Observed	Expected*	Observed
Before operation:					
7th year or earlier	3,044	0.85	0	0.28	0.00
6th year	3,588	1.49	4	0.42	1.11
5th year	5,656	3.01	3	0.53	0.53
4th year	7,980	4.34	5	0.54	0.63
3rd year	11,475	6.65	14	0.58	1.22
2nd year	15,007	9.20	13	0.61	0.87
1st year	20,175	14.71	19	0.73	0.94
Year of operation	8,569	8.16	21	0.95	2.45
After operation:					
Year of operation	12,070	8.81	1	0.73	0.08
1st year	16,888	14.81	4	0.88	0.24
2nd year	14,258	12.63	5	0.89	0.35
3rd year	11,285	9.49	2	0.84	0.18
4th year	7,889	6.18	4	0.78	0.51
5th year	5,614	3.47	1	0.62	0.18
6th year	3,833	2.36	2	0.62	0.52
7th year or later	1,850	0.84	0	0.46	0.00

*Expected numbers are based on age-specific and season-specific rates for the entire childhood population. The year was divided into four groups of months for this purpose, based on similarity of incidence rates within these months.

Appendix 17

METHOD OF TABULATION OF ANTIBODY ACQUISITION DATA FOR ADENOVIRUSES AND TYPE 3 PARAINFLUENZA VIRUS

Figures 43 and 44 are based on antibody studies of serial sera obtained from children born into the study. Sera were collected from the mother during the third trimester of pregnancy or at term, from the umbilical cord at birth, and from the child at intervals of approximately 6 months thereafter. For a variety of reasons, few children had a complete set of sera. Sera were tested for neutralizing antibodies in a final dilution of 1:8 and all sera from a single person were tested simultaneously.

The following rules were applied in the tabulation of the adenovirus results to take advantage of longitudinal observation of the same subject:

Antibody present: On and after the time of appearance of antibody until the last serum tested (except in two cases subsequently noted).

Antibody absent: Up to the last negative serum before the first positive, including the interval between two negative specimens.

Antibody status unknown: Between the last negative and the first positive serum.

The method is shown in Appendix 17, table 1. No serum specimens were available from this child at 1, 3, 3½, and 4½ years. At 1 year the status of type 2 antibody was classified as "unknown." After its demonstration at 1½ years, type 2 antibody was tabulated as "present" at 3, 3½, and 4½ years as well as at the periods actually tested. The status of type 1 antibody was classified as "absent" at 1 year, "unknown" at 3 and 3½ years, and "present" at 4½ years. Antibodies for the other types were tabulated as being "absent" at all periods. It is believed that these tabulation rules were justified because of the infrequent disappearance of antibody once it had been detected. Neutralizing antibody, once present, disappeared only three times from the subsequent sera of two subjects. In one case, type 5 antibody was measured in the serum collected at 1 year of age, but was not detected at 18 months or thereafter. The same child had type 2 antibody in all serum specimens from 6 months to 5 years. In the other child, type 2 antibody was present from 18 months to 3 years, absent from 3½ to 4½ years, and present again at 5 years; type 7 antibody appeared at 3 years, was still present at 4½ years, but was absent at 5 years. In the same

APPENDIX 17, TABLE 1

Adenovirus neutralizing antibodies in serial serum specimens
from one individual

Serum date	Approximate age (years)	Antibodies* to adenovirus type					
		1	2	3	5	6	7
3-10-48	Mother	o	x	x	o	o	x
4- 1-48	Cord - 0.0	o	x	x	o	o	x
11-15-48	0.5	o	o	o	o	o	o
—	1.0						
12-16-49	1.5	o	x	o	o	o	o
5-29-50	2.0	o	x	o	o	o	o
10-26-50	2.5	o	x	o	o	o	o
—	3.0						
—	3.5						
10-13-52	4.0	x	x	o	o	o	o
—	4.5						
3-31-53	5.0	x	x	o	o	o	o

*Tested at 1:8 final dilution: o=absent; x=present.

child, type 6 antibody appeared at 3½ years and persisted; there
was no indication that the sera had been mislabeled.

For the work with the parainfluenza virus, type 3, the following
rules of tabulation were employed:

Antibody present: At the time of the demonstration of
antibody, including the intervals between positive sera.
(For an exception, see "antibody status unknown").

Antibody absent: At the time of the demonstration of
the absence of antibody including the intervals between
negative sera.

Antibody status unknown: The interval between a negative and a positive serum or between a positive and a negative serum. In addition, because it was not known how long
maternal antibody persisted in the sera of the child, and
because antibody to parainfluenza virus is apparently developed quite early in life in some instances, the antibody
status after the cord blood was obtained was classified as
"unknown" until the presence or absence of antibody was
demonstrated in the next available serum.

It is believed that these tabulation rules were justified because in only four instances were sera found to be negative for antibody to parainfluenza virus 3 after demonstration of antibody in an earlier serum. In one case antibody developed at 3 years, persisted until 4½ years, and was absent at 5 years. In another case, antibody was present at 3½ and 4 years, but absent at 4½ years; the status at 5 years was unknown. In still another case, antibody was present at 3 years, absent at 4 years, and present again at 5 years. It is of interest that a serum from this patient at the age of 9 years, tested in another study, showed the absence of antibody. The fourth case showed antibody at 2½ years and no antibody at 3½ years; the antibody status at later periods was unknown.

The two somewhat different criteria for analyzing the data dealing with adenoviruses and parainfluenza viruses were adopted because of the more frequent disappearance of antibody for the parainfluenza viruses in an individual in whom this antibody had once appeared.

Appendix 18

ISOLATION OF INFLUENZA VIRUSES

In general, specific attempts to isolate influenza viruses were made when an unusual occurrence of "influenza-like" illness was noted in the study group, or when influenza was known to be occurring in the community or the country. Specimens examined for this purpose were of two types: a) those obtained from persons with symptoms of respiratory infections and b) routine pharyngeal swabs collected weekly from the entire population (Appendix 18, table 1).

VIRUS ISOLATIONS, 1950

In 1950, the illness specimens were inoculated into embryonated eggs on the day they were taken; specimens collected from each individual routinely at weekly intervals were stored at -70°C. and examined 3 to 6 months later.

Throat washings.—Sixteen throat washings that were collected from individuals with acute respiratory illnesses between October 17, 1949, and January 1, 1950, did not yield virus. Fourteen additional washings were collected between January 27 and May 6, 1950; virus was isolated from two of these—one collected in March and one in April.

Illness swabs.—During a period of 7 months (November 1, 1949 to May 26, 1950) 1017 swabs in broth were collected from individuals with respiratory symptoms, multiple swabs being collected from some patients. The swabs were first examined in 241 pools. Following definite or questionable identification of viruses, 237 swabs from 52 pools were tested singly. Virus was not isolated from the single components of 14 positive pools. Nineteen strains of virus were isolated from 17 individuals, including the 2 with positive throat washings ill between February 25 and May 13.

Routine swabs.—During a period of 4 months, January 30 to May 22, 1950, encompassing the pre-epidemic and most of the epidemic period, 2361 swabs in broth were collected at the time of routine weekly home visits. These swabs were tested initially in 472 pools, then 63 individual swabs from 13 pools were examined. Virus was not isolated from the individual components of three positive pools. Viruses were isolated from only two individuals whose specimens were collected in mid-March. The two persons, mother and maid, were members of the same household, but influenza virus A1 was isolated from the specimens collected from one and influenza virus B from the other. No respiratory illnesses were occurring in the family; one of the children developed gastroenter-

APPENDIX 18, TABLE 1

Detection of type A1 influenza virus

| Year | Reason for collection of specimen | | | | | | Total number individuals with type A1 virus |
| | Respiratory symptoms | | | Routine weekly | | | |
	Collection period	Number tested	No. persons with virus	Collection period	Number tested	No. persons with virus	
1949-50	10/17/49-5/26/50 (7 months)	1047	17	1/30-5/22 (4 months)	2361	1	18
1951	1/17-4/26 (3 months)	244	31	2/20-3/12 (3 weeks)	555	3*	31
1953	1/14-3/7 (2 months)	235	22	None			22
Total		1526	70		2916	4	71

*These persons were ill at time of routine weekly culture; virus also isolated from illness specimens.

itis with fever the day after the swabs were collected. The B viruses detected in this year were isolated from swabs collected in April.

Total for 1950.—Forty-eight strains of influenza virus A1 were isolated from pools, individual swabs, and throat washings. In three instances, two strains were isolated from the same individuals; these specimens had been obtained at intervals of 2, 5, and 9 days, and the strains isolated were antigenically similar. The net result was the identification of influenza virus A1 in specimens from 18 persons.

VIRUS ISOLATIONS, 1951

In 1951, instead of examining illness swabs on a current basis and storing positive harvests for later passage, any positive or doubtful amniotic fluids were passed until virus was obtained in high titer.

Throat washings.—Twenty-seven washings were collected from individuals ill between February 10 and April 26, 1951. Virus was isolated from 16 of these specimens.

Illness swabs.—Seventy-eight swabs were collected from individuals ill between January 17 and February 3, 1951. Because of the experience in the previous year, swabs from six persons with febrile illnesses during this period were tested; virus was not isolated. Between February 20 and April 14, 1951, 211 illness swabs were collected; 23 swabs, collected simultaneously with washings, were tested separately as described below; the rest were examined in 38 pools. Virus was not isolated when the individual components of three positive pools were tested. Viruses were isolated from 26 individuals, including 11 with positive washings, ill between February 21 and March 23, 1951.

Routine swabs.—During the period January 17 to March 31, 1951, 1770 swabs in broth were collected routinely at weekly intervals. Only those collected during the 3 weeks (February 20-March 12) when illness specimens yielded the greatest number of isolations, were examined. These 555 routine swabs were tested in 112 pools. Virus was obtained from one swab for each of the three positive pools. Viruses were also isolated from illness swabs collected from these three persons. From one, the routine swab had been collected 1 day before onset and from another on the second day of an influenza-like illness. The situation in the third instance was as follows: Two of the children in the family had influenza-like illnesses beginning on February 26 and February 27. The mother had a headache, but no other symptoms, on February 27 when a routine swab was obtained. The father had an influenza-like illness on March 15. On March 26 the mother developed typical influenza and an illness swab was collected the following day. Influenza viruses, both A1 strains, were isolated from swabs collected from the mother on February 27 and March 22, an interval of 24 days.

Total for 1951.—Fifty-nine A1 strains were isolated from pools, individual swabs and throat washings. Two strains were isolated from 2 different specimens from each of 12 individuals; 3 strains were isolated from 1 individual. The net result was the identification of virus in specimens from 31 persons.

Comparison of throat washing and swab in broth.—In 1951, swabs and washings were collected simultaneously from 23 individuals. These swabs were tested separately, but to make the dilution factor correspond to that which obtained when swabs were tested in pools of five, 0.2 ml. of each specimen was added to 0.8 ml. of sterile broth prior to the addition of antibiotics. If the results

APPENDIX 18, TABLE 2

Comparison of throat washings and swabs as sources of
influenza virus

Isolations		Throat washings		
		Positive	Negative	Total
Swab in broth	Positive	12	4	16
	Negative	4	14	18
	Total	16	18	34

from 1950 are added, the comparison shown in Appendix 18, table 2, is obtained, indicating that the swab in broth is comparable to the throat washing as a source of influenza virus.

VIRUS ISOLATIONS, 1952

During a period of 20 days (March 11 to March 31, 1952) 48 swabs in broth were collected from individuals with respiratory symptoms. Influenza virus B was isolated from one pool and a single swab of this pool. Difficulty was experienced in obtaining these B strains, as well as a similar one isolated from a hospitalized patient, in high titer.

VIRUS ISOLATIONS, 1953

Throat washings.—Virus was isolated from a single washing collected on January 14, 1953.

Illness swabs.—During a period of 6 weeks, from January 27 to March 7, 235 swabs in broth were collected from individuals with respiratory symptoms. These were tested in 47 pools; no virus was isolated from the individual components of 3 of 17 positive pools. Viruses were isolated from 21 individuals ill between January 31 and February 24.

Total for 1953.—Thirty-nine A1 strains were isolated from pools, individual swabs and a throat washing in the 7-week period from January 14 to February 24. The net result was the identification of virus in specimens from 22 persons.

SENSITIVITY OF HEMAGGLUTINATION-INHIBITION TEST

Because of the interval between the serum specimens, some indication of the sensitivity of the serological method was sought by examining the responses of those individuals from whom virus had been isolated (Appendix 18, table 3). Sera that immediately spanned

APPENDIX 18, TABLE 3

The frequency of increases in titer of antibodies to influenza A antigens in individuals from whom virus was isolated in corresponding year

Individuals	Year		
	1950	1951	1953
Number with virus isolated	18	31	22
Number with properly spaced sera	14	25	13
Number with 4-fold or > increase in titer	9	23	11
Percent with increase in titer	64	92	85

the period of isolation were available from 52 of the 71 persons with A viruses isolated in 1950, 1951 or 1953. Of individuals from whom virus was isolated in 1950, only 64% showed four-fold or greater rises in titer, in contrast to such rises in 92% of persons with virus in 1951 and 85% of those with virus in 1953. One explanation for this difference could be that some of the strains isolated in 1950 represented laboratory contamination, yet three of the five persons who did not show significant increases in titer had influenza-like illnesses. Alternate interpretations could be that there was a more rapid decline of antibody level in some individuals or that measurement of the frequency of occurrence of influenza by such antibody studies provides an estimate slightly below the actual value.

Appendix 19

THE IDENTIFICATION AND CLASSIFICATION OF GASTROINTESTINAL ILLNESSES

Complete characterization of gastrointestinal illnesses in man will not be possible until methods are available to identify the responsible agent or agents. Lacking such methods, attempts to describe these illnesses epidemiologically or clinically must use a somewhat arbitrary and inexact approach. Which cases to include in these descriptions is a matter of definition and judgment. The purpose of this section is to present the definitions that were used and the considerations upon which judgments were based in selecting the cases of gastrointestinal illness included in Chapter XI. The results presented were based on two somewhat different methods of classifying gastrointestinal illness; both methods are discussed here.

Regardless of the method used to identify and classify gastrointestinal illnesses, the basic source of information was the monthly check sheet of symptoms kept by the mothers. For the first 8 years of the study this sheet listed two gastrointestinal symptoms: vomiting and diarrhea (Appendix 2, figure 1). Abdominal pain, when present, was indicated by checking "aches and pains" and describing them in a footnote. During the final 2 years, nausea and stomachache were added to the list of signs and symptoms whose presence or absence was to be noted by the mothers.

ROUTINE CLASSIFICATION OF GASTROINTESTINAL SYMPTOMS, 1948-1957

In the routine procedure for diagnosing illnesses used over the entire 10-year period, the check sheet of symptoms for each individual was reviewed at regular intervals by a member of the departmental staff. Gastrointestinal symptoms encountered in this review were judged to be 1) the result of primary gastrointestinal disease, 2) secondary to another diagnosed illness or to some cause other than illness, or 3) too minor to warrant being considered a true symptom. There were no specific rules governing which occurrences of gastrointestinal symptoms should be attributed to other causes and which should be considered gastrointestinal illness, nor as to what constituted the beginning of a new illness rather than the continuation of an old one. Symptoms assigned to categories 2) and 3) were dismissed from further consideration. Those placed in the first category were further classified as being of infectious or noninfectious origin. Included in the latter group were gastroin-

testinal symptoms due to dietary causes (120 cases), infant diarrhea (8 cases), functional gastrointestinal symptoms such as constipation, globus hystericus, and the like (192 cases), and miscellaneous gastrointestinal disorders including gastrointestinal symptoms attributed to peptic ulcer, diverticulitis, ulcerative colitis, etc.
(22 cases). The remaining gastrointestinal illnesses were presumed
to be infectious in nature. The clinical and epidemiological evidence
for this presumption varied from case to case, however, and three
categories of presumably infectious gastrointestinal illness were distinguished on the basis of clinical and epidemiological characteristics:

Infectious gastroenteritis. This category included all gastrointestinal illnesses, with the exception of those classified as being in
one of the various noninfectious diagnostic groups, during which
two or more of the following occurred: vomiting, abdominal pain,
diarrhea, and fever (2139 cases).

Infectious gastroenteritis-epidemiological. Cases placed in this
group were less distinct gastrointestinal illnesses during which one
of the above major symptoms (vomiting, abdominal pain, diarrhea,
and fever) or minor symptoms (nausea, anorexia, etc.) occurred,
provided the illness began within 10 days of another case of infectious gastroenteritis or infectious gastroenteritis-epidemiological in
the same family (1169 cases).

Probable infectious gastroenteritis. These cases had the same
clinical characteristics as infectious gastroenteritis-epidemiological
but were not associated, within 10 days, with the onset of another
case of infectious gastroenteritis in the same family (749 cases).

The 4057 cases included in the above categories form the basis
for the description of the incidence of infectious gastroenteritis presented in Chapter V and the first part of Chapter XI.

DETAILED STUDY OF GASTROINTESTINAL ILLNESSES,
1948-1950

A separate study of all gastrointestinal symptoms during 1948-1950
was also carried out. The purposes of this study are discussed in
Chapter XI. To identify gastrointestinal illnesses, the check sheets
kept by the mothers were examined for any entry of vomiting,
diarrhea, or abdominal pain. Every occurrence of one or more of
these three symptoms in an individual who had been free of all
of them for at least 5 days was listed for further study. There were
1466 instances that fulfilled these criteria.

The record sheets, including footnotes made by mothers, fieldworkers and physicians, were then examined further for accompanying events or causes that might explain the occurrence of gastrointestinal symptoms. A number of possible explanations were offered

and all were considered in detail. Those that seemed to explain the gastrointestinal symptoms adequately were combined to form a list of acceptable explanatory circumstances. The purpose of this list was to provide a describable set of criteria by which to decide, in a consistent manner, whether or not each occurrence of gastrointestinal symptoms could be attributable to some recognizable cause. If one of the listed explanatory circumstances was recorded as accompanying an occurrence of gastrointestinal symptoms, it was considered to have caused the symptoms. Gastrointestinal symptoms occurring in the absence of acceptable explanatory circumstances were considered, for want of better diagnostic criteria, to represent cases of infectious gastroenteritis.

Of the 1466 occurrences of gastrointestinal symptoms during 1948-1950, 362 seemed to be reasonably attributable to causes other than infectious gastroenteritis. In some cases the cause was a specific gastrointestinal disorder, e.g., dietary indiscretion, peptic ulcer, or diverticulitis, while in other cases the primary cause was considered to be outside the gastrointestinal tract. The explana-

APPENDIX 19, TABLE 1

Circumstances accepted as explaining gastrointestinal symptoms

Explanatory circumstance	Number of cases
Acute infectious diseases	116
Dietary indiscretion	63
Coughing, gagging, etc.	59
Medication	45
Emotional causes	18
Other	61
Total	362

tions accepted are summarized in Appendix 19, table 1. Although these circumstances comprise many categories, approximately 80% of the 362 instances included in this table were attributed entirely or in part to five different causes: a) acute infectious diseases, most often streptococcal infections or one of the common diseases of childhood such as measles or chickenpox, b) dietary indiscretions, c) coughing, including gagging on mucus, d) antibiotics or other medications given on the day before or the day of onset of the gastrointestinal symptoms, and e) emotional causes such as nervousness and excitement.

In general, all reasonable explanations offered by mothers, field-workers, or visiting physicians were accepted. The major exception was the occurrence of a common respiratory disease in an individual at the time of onset of gastrointestinal symptoms. In the routine diagnosing of illness, gastrointestinal symptoms were sometimes attributed to a concurrent respiratory disease *per se*, and it seems reasonable to expect that respiratory infections, like other acute infectious diseases, may at times give rise to gastrointestinal symptoms. Since both infectious gastroenteritis and the common respiratory diseases occurred with considerable frequency in this population, it also seems reasonable to expect a certain number of individuals to be affected by both concurrently but independently. It was not possible to separate these two situations on the basis of the clinical records. Since it was felt that a considerable error would be introduced by attributing gastrointestinal symptoms to common respiratory disease whenever an individual was afflicted by both at the same time, the concurrence of these two sets of symptoms was analyzed in different ways in Chapter XI depending on the purpose of the analysis.

Appendix 20

METHODS OF RECORDING AND ANALYZING GASTROINTESTINAL SYMPTOMS

PRESENCE OR ABSENCE OF GASTROINTESTINAL SYMPTOMS

The accuracy and completeness of the records cannot be determined precisely. In less than 1% of the gastrointestinal illnesses was there doubt as to whether or not diarrhea and vomiting were present. In slightly less than 10% there was some question as to the presence of abdominal pain; this question arose either because pain was recorded as present but was not described (3.5%) or because there was neither a " √ " nor "0" entry for aches and pains. In analyzing the results, a symptom was considered to have been absent if the record left its presence in doubt. In the light of intimate knowledge regarding the recording habits of the participants, this procedure is thought to have led to only minor errors.

DEFINITION OF ONSET AND DURATION OF ILLNESS AND OF INDIVIDUAL SYMPTOMS

Onset of an illness.—The onset of an illness was the first day on which vomiting, diarrhea or abdominal pain occurred in an individual who had been free from all three symptoms for at least 5 days; the onset was not dated from the occurrence of any nonspecific prodromal symptom, such as anorexia or malaise, which may have been present.

Presence of a symptom.—A symptom other than vomiting, diarrhea and abdominal pain was considered to be present only if it began on or before the third day of the gastrointestinal illness. Fever was considered to be present if a temperature, either oral or rectal, of 100°F. or higher was recorded.

Duration of illness and of individual symptoms.—The duration of an illness included the period from the first day on which vomiting, diarrhea or abdominal pain occurred through the last day in that illness on which any of these symptoms occurred. All intervening days were included as part of the illness even though the individual may have been free from all symptoms for one or more of these days. Only when an individual had been free from all three major gastrointestinal symptoms for more than 5 days did the reappearance of a symptom constitute a new illness. Similarly, the duration of individual symptoms included the period from the first day on which the symptom occurred through the last day on which it occurred in that illness, even though the symptom may have been absent on one or more of the intervening days.

374

Appendix 21

METHODS USED TO COMPUTE INCIDENCE OF INFECTIOUS GASTROENTERITIS AT INTERVALS FROM COMMON RESPIRATORY DISEASES

During the 3-year period, 1948-1950, there were 130 cases of infectious gastroenteritis that began on the day that a common respiratory disease was diagnosed in the same individual. Since, during this same period, there were 4200 cases diagnosed as common respiratory diseases, it follows that there were 4200 person-

APPENDIX 21, TABLE 1

Experience of a hypothetical individual for a month illustrating the method used to classify infectious gastroenteritis and person-days according to the interval to the nearest common respiratory disease

Day of month	Onset of illness*	Days from onset of nearest common respiratory disease**	Day of month	Onset of illness*	Days from onset of nearest common respiratory disease**
1		−1	16		+1
2	CRD	0	17		+2
3		+1	18		+3
4	GE	+2	19		+4
5		+3	20		+5
6		+4	21		−5
7		+5	22		−4
8		+6	23		−3
9		−6	24		−2
10		−5	25		−1
11		−4	26	CRD	0
12		−3	27		+1
13		−2	28		+2
14		−1	29		+3
15	CRD & GE	0	30		+4

*CRD=Onset of common respiratory disease in this individual.
 GE=Onset of infectious gastroenteritis in this individual.

**A minus sign indicates that the day preceded, and a plus sign that it followed, the diagnosed onset of the nearest common respiratory disease.

days on which common respiratory diseases began. The incidence of infectious gastroenteritis on the days of onset of common respiratory diseases was $\frac{130}{4200} = .031$ cases per person-day, or 3.1 cases per 100 person-days. The method by which the data necessary for rates of this kind were obtained is illustrated in Appendix 21, tables 1 and 2. The hypothetical individual whose experience is shown suffered three respiratory illnesses and two gastroenteric illnesses during the month. The first gastroenteric illness was classified as beginning on a +2 day, since it began 2 days after the onset of the nearest common respiratory disease. The second was classified as beginning on a zero day, since it began on the day of onset of a common respiratory disease. This illness would be one of the 130 cases forming the numerator of the incidence rate shown above.

APPENDIX 21, TABLE 2

Number of cases of infectious gastroenteritis according to the interval from the nearest common respiratory disease in the same individual (1948-1950)

Days from onset of nearest common respiratory disease	Number of cases of infectious gastroenteritis	
	According to original method of diagnosing	According to modified method of diagnosing
−5	9	11
−4	15	16
−3	11	12
−2	17	26
−1	10	24
0	130	145
+1	48	52
+2	45	45
+3	31	32
+4	28	28
+5	25	24
Total in this period	369	415*

*This includes: 369 cases of the preceding column, 45 cases reclassified according to the method described in text, and one case originally classified by mistake as more than 5 days from the onset of respiratory disease.

The gastroenteric illness starting 2 days after the nearest respiratory illness would be included as a case in the numerator of another incidence rate, that referring to the +2 day. In order to determine denominators for these rates, it was necessary to classify each person-day on the same scale, as shown in the third column of Appendix 21, table 1. The denominator of the rate for the zero day was obtained by counting the number of person-days classified as 0; the denominator for the +1 day, by counting the number of person-days classified as +1, etc. Those days that could not be classified on this basis and the corresponding cases were omitted from the tabulations.

Compilation of the person-days of observation showed that there were 4200 zero person-days corresponding to the 4200 diagnosed onsets of common respiratory disease. There were 3279 and 3259 person-days of experience, respectively, 10 days after and 10 days before the nearest common respiratory disease. This trend continued so that there were 1946 person-days that were 20 days after and 1937 person-days that were 20 days before the nearest common respiratory disease. Such decrease was due to the fact that respiratory infections often occurred at rather short intervals.

The methods used in arriving at the data presented in figure 58 were described in a previous publication (12). As explained therein, the analyses brought to light a few inconsistencies in the specification of diagnosis and the dating of onsets of illnesses in which gastrointestinal and respiratory symptoms occurred more or less simultaneously. The frequency of such inconsistencies was too small to warrant re-analysis of the data for the purpose of making minor corrections, and figure 58 is based on data uncorrected for these errors. Other data and calculations presented in Chapter XI were made after the inconsistencies had been recognized and eliminated. The results of these corrections were: 1) to increase the total number of diagnosed onsets of common respiratory diseases (and, therefore, the number of person-days on which a common respiratory disease began) from 4200 to 4245 and 2) to alter the number of cases of infectious gastroenteritis at various intervals from a common respiratory disease as shown in Appendix 21, table 2. Figure 58 is based on column 2 of this table; all subsequent calculations are based on column 3.

Appendix 22

METHOD OF ESTIMATING SYMPTOMATOLOGY OF "RESPIRATORY-GASTROINTESTINAL" SYNDROME

The method used to estimate the gastrointestinal symptoms present in the 216 cases of "respiratory-gastrointestinal" syndrome was as follows:

1. An examination was made of the records of the 683 instances of gastrointestinal symptoms which were not associated with respiratory disease and which were not otherwise explained. The relative frequency of each symptom in these cases of infectious gastroenteritis was presented in table 79. For example, vomiting was noted in 53% of the cases.

2. The records of the entire 326 cases of infectious gastroenteritis that started on one of the first 6 days of respiratory disease were examined to determine in how many of them each particular symptom was present. For example, vomiting was recorded for 149 of the cases.

3. It was assumed that the 110 expected cases of infectious gastroenteritis were the same type of disease as those whose records were examined in step 1, and that they would have the same percentage distribution of symptoms. Thus, 53% (58 cases) of them would be expected to have had vomiting.

4. The remaining instances of each particular gastrointestinal symptom among the 326 cases were considered to have occurred as part of the 216 cases of "respiratory-gastrointestinal" syndrome. Thus, vomiting was attributed to 91 (149 minus 58) cases of "respiratory-gastrointestinal" syndrome, or 42% of the 216 cases.

An estimate was also made of the proportion of cases of "respiratory-gastrointestinal" syndrome manifesting one, two, and all three of the major gastrointestinal symptoms: vomiting, diarrhea and abdominal pain. The method used was the same as that just described. Calculations were based on data shown in table 78.

Data were not available to estimate the occurrence of such symptoms as nausea, flatulence, constipation and dizziness, which may also be part of the syndrome.

A similar process of calculation was carried out with regard to respiratory symptoms. The relative frequency of each symptom was determined for common respiratory illnesses occurring during 1948-1950 whose onsets were at least 6 days removed from the nearest onset of infectious gastroenteritis. These data are shown in Appen-

APPENDIX 22, TABLE 1

Symptoms present in cases of the common respiratory diseases that
started 6 or more days from the onset of infectious
gastroenteritis (1948-1950)

Symptoms	No. of cases for which adequate information was available*	No. of cases with symptom present	% of cases with symptom present
Sneezing	3,574	2,223	62.2
Watery nasal discharge	3,553	2,393	67.4
Thick nasal discharge	3,537	1,663	47.0
Obstructed nose	3,534	1,922	54.4
Sore or irritated throat	3,575	1,223	34.2
Hoarseness	3,568	815	22.8
Cough	3,494	1,784	51.1
Fever or feverishness	3,581	828	23.1

*The variation in the numbers of this column is chiefly due to the persistence of a symptom from a previous illness, or the chronic presence of a symptom in a person, so that it could not be determined whether or not the symptom was present during the illness in question.

dix 22, table 1. With the exception of that referring to fever or feverishness, these percentages were taken as the relative frequencies with which respiratory symptoms occurred in the 110 cases of coincident but unrelated gastroenteritis and respiratory disease.

The evaluation of fever or feverishness in the "respiratory-gastrointestinal" syndrome required a modification of this method of analysis because fever or feverishness may be present both in gastrointestinal illnesses not associated in time with respiratory symptoms and in respiratory illnesses unassociated with gastrointestinal symptoms. Thus, the fever or feverishness of the 110 cases of simultaneous but otherwise unrelated instances of gastroenteritis and common respiratory disease might have come from either one or both of these infections.

Of the 683 cases of infectious gastroenteritis, 25.3% had accompanying fever or feverishness, while 23.1% of the cases of common respiratory disease described in Appendix 22, table 1, were accompanied by this finding. If, as was assumed throughout this analysis, there were 110 cases of coincident but causally unrelated gastroenteritis and common respiratory disease, the proportion of these 110 cases which would have been expected to show fever or feverishness is $0.253 + 0.231 \, (1 - 0.253)$ or 0.426.

APPENDIX 22, TABLE 2

Symptoms present in 326 cases of concurrent infectious gastroenteritis and common respiratory disease

Symptoms	No. of cases for which adequate information was available	No. of cases with symptom or indicated number of symptoms present	% of cases with symptom or indicated number of symptoms present
Sneezing	321	195	60.7
Watery nasal discharge	322	205	63.7
Thick nasal discharge	313	134	42.8
Obstructed nose	312	168	53.8
Sore or irritated throat	323	117	36.2
Hoarseness	321	90	28.0
Cough	311	184	59.2
Fever or feverishness	323	180	55.7
Vomiting	326	149	45.7
Diarrhea	326	173	53.1
Abdominal pain	326	115	35.3
Number of gastrointestinal symptoms*: 1	326	235	72.1
2	326	71	21.8
3	326	20	6.1

*Includes vomiting, diarrhea and abdominal pain

The symptoms recorded for the 326 instances of coincident respiratory and gastrointestinal symptoms are shown in Appendix 22, table 2. It will be seen that some of the data could not be included in this analysis. In three cases, the record of respiratory symptoms was too meager to warrant inclusion; in others the persistence of symptoms from a previous illness, or the chronicity of some symptoms, was the reason for exclusion from the tabulation.

Appendix 23

APPENDIX 23, TABLE 1

Maximum temperature per illness in four groups of cases

Maximum temperature, °F.	Poliovirus isolated in 1952		No evidence of infection in 1952	
	1952 illnesses Group I	1951 illnesses Group II	1952 illnesses Group III	1951 illnesses Group IV
Normal	0	11	5	16
99	3	5	1	2
100	4	0	1	3
101	9	2	4	0
102	3	1	1	1
103	11	2	0	1
104	2	0	2	1
Feverish, temperature not taken	6	2	1	1
Not feverish, temperature not taken	1	18	24	15
Unknown	1			
Total illnesses	40	41	39	40

See text (Chapter XII, page 224) for descriptions of groups.

APPENDIX 23, TABLE 2

Duration of illness in four groups of cases

Duration of illness (days)	Poliovirus isolated in 1952		No evidence of infection in 1952	
	1952 illnesses Group I	1951 illnesses Group II	1952 illnesses Group III	1951 illnesses Group IV
1	6	4	6	11
2	8	3	6	3
3	11	4	2	2
4	4	4	2	2
5	2	4	3	3
6	2	2	3	—
7	1	2	2	1
8	—	3	—	2
9	—	5	1	—
10	1	1	3	1
11	—	2	1	2
12	—	1	1	2
13	—	3	1	2
14	1	—	1	1
15+	3	1	4	5
Unknown	1	2	3	3
Total illnesses	40	41	39	40

APPENDIX 23, TABLE 3

Physical findings in four groups of cases

Finding	Poliovirus isolated in 1952		No evidence of infection in 1952	
	1952 illnesses Group I	1951 illnesses Group II	1952 illnesses Group III	1951 illnesses Group IV
Appearance: Moderately ill	6	0	1	2
Injection of nose or throat	18	9	4	10
Pharyngeal exudate	5	1	1	1
Vesicles on palate or pharyngeal wall	5	0	2	0
Cervical adenopathy	9	6	2	4
Nuchal rigidity	2	0	0	0
Other findings*	0	6	6	6
Unknown	10	17	25	18
Total illnesses	40	41	39	40

*Minor injury, allergic reactions, acute exanthems, furunculosis, conjunctivitis, otitis media, abdominal tenderness.

APPENDIX 23, TABLE 4

Isolation of poliovirus from 40 persons in relation to their post-epidemic neutralizing antibody titers

Type of poliovirus	Virus isolated	Antibody titer*				Total
		100 or <	280-400	512-768	1024 or >	
1	Yes	0	3	0	2	5
	No	1	1	2	0	4
2	Yes	5	8	3	7	23
	No	2	3	1	1	7
3	Yes	0	1	0	0	1
	No	0	0	0	0	0
Total	Yes	5	12	3	9	29
	No	3	4	3	1	11

*Expressed as reciprocal of dilution end-point.

APPENDIX 24, TABLE 1

The relationship of a history of mumps and pre-outbreak antibody status to the occurrence of mumps and antibody response among children exposed to mumps within the home

History of Mumps	Pre-outbreak antibody status*	Post-outbreak antibody status**						Total
		Clinical mumps			No clinical mumps			
		Rise	No rise	Unk.	Rise	No rise	Unk.	
Yes	Present	0	0	0	0	16	1	17
	Absent	0	0	0	1	1	0	2
No	Present	3	1	0	3	9	0	16
	Absent	26	0	2	12	19	4	63
	Unknown	0	0	6	0	4	5	15
Unknown	Absent	0	0	0	0	1	0	1
Total								114

*A complement-fixing titer of 8 or greater, using either viral or soluble antigens, was considered to indicate the presence of antibodies.

**A rise indicates a fourfold or greater increase in antibody titer.

APPENDIX 24, TABLE 2

The relationship of a history of mumps and pre-outbreak antibody status to the occurrence of mumps and antibody response among parents exposed to mumps within the home*

History of Mumps	Pre-outbreak antibody status	Clinical mumps			No clinical mumps			Total
		Post-outbreak antibody status			Post-outbreak antibody status			
		Rise	No rise	Unk.	Rise	No rise	Unk.	
Yes	Present	0	0	0	6	61	6	73
	Absent	0	0	0	4	2	1	7
	Unknown	0	0	0	0	0	7	7
No	Present	0	0	1	8	19	2	30
	Absent	5	1	0	1	0	0	7
Unknown	Present	0	0	0	1	1	1	3
	Absent	0	0	0	0	0	1	1
Total								128

*See Appendix 24, Table 1 for legends.

REFERENCES

Note: References 1-26 comprise a complete list of papers based upon this study up to April 1, 1964. Most of them are referred to in the text.

References 1-21 comprise a numbered series with the general title "A Study of Illness in a Group of Cleveland Families."

1. Dingle, J. H., Badger, G. F., Feller, A. E., Hodges, R. G., Jordan, W. S., Jr. and Rammelkamp, C. H., Jr. I. Plan of study and certain general observations. Am. J. Hyg., 58:16-30, 1953

2. Badger, G. F., Dingle, J. H., Feller, A. E., Hodges, R. G., Jordan, W. S., Jr. and Rammelkamp, C. H., Jr. II. Incidence of the common respiratory diseases. Am. J. Hyg., 58:31-40, 1953

3. Badger, G. F., Dingle, J. H., Feller, A. E., Hodges, R. G., Jordan, W. S., Jr. and Rammelkamp, C. H., Jr. III. Introduction of respiratory infections into families. Am. J. Hyg., 58:41-46, 1953

4. Badger, G. F., Dingle, J. H., Feller, A. E., Hodges, R. G., Jordan, W. S., Jr. and Rammelkamp, C. H., Jr. IV. The spread of respiratory infections within the home. Am. J. Hyg., 58:174-178, 1953

5. Badger, G. F., Dingle, J. H., Feller, A. E., Hodges, R. G., Jordan, W. S., Jr. and Rammelkamp, C. H., Jr. V. Introductions and secondary attack rates as indices of exposure to common respiratory diseases in the community. Am. J. Hyg., 58:179-182, 1953

6. Katz, S., Badger, G. F., Jordan, W. S., Jr., Rosenbaum, H. B. and Dingle, J. H. VI. Controlled study of reactions to oxytetracycline hydrochloride. New Eng. J. Med., 251:508-513, 1954

7. Jordan, W. S., Jr., Gordon, I. and Dorrance, W. R. VII. Transmission of acute non-bacterial gastroenteritis to volunteers: evidence for two different etiologic agents. J. Exper. Med., 98:461-475, 1953

8. McCorkle, L. P., Hodges, R. G., Badger, G. F., Dingle, J. H. and Jordan, W. S., Jr. VIII. Relation of tonsillectomy to incidence of common respiratory diseases in children. New Eng. J. Med., 252:1066-1069, 1955

9. Jordan, W. S., Jr., Stevens, D., Katz, S. and Dingle, J. H. IX. Recognition of family epidemics of poliomyelitis and pleurodynia during a search for respiratory-disease viruses. New Eng. J. Med., 254.687-691, 1956

10. Jordan, W. S. Jr., Badger, G. F. Curtiss, C., Dingle, J. H., Ginsberg, H. S. and Gold, E. X. The occurrence of adenovirus infections. Am. J. Hyg., 64:336-348, 1956

11. Hodges, R. G., McCorkle, L. P., Badger, G. F., Curtiss, C., Dingle, J. H. and Jordan, W. S., Jr. XI. The occurrence of gastrointestinal symptoms. Am. J. Hyg., 64:349-356, 1956

12. McCorkle, L. P., Badger, G. F., Curtiss, C., Dingle, J. H., Hodges, R. G. and Jordan, W. S., Jr. XII. The association of respiratory and gastrointestinal symptoms; an estimation of the magnitude and time relations of the association. Am. J. Hyg., 64:357-367, 1956

13. Dingle, J. H., McCorkle, L. P., Badger, G. F., Curtiss, C., Hodges, R. G. and Jordan, W. S., Jr. XIII. Clinical description of acute nonbacterial gastroenteritis. Am. J. Hgy., 64:368-375, 1956

14. Badger, G. F., McCorkle, L. P., Curtiss, C., Dingle, J. H., Hodges, R. G. and Jordan, W. S., Jr. XIV. The association of respiratory and gastrointestinal symptoms; an estimation of the specific symptomatology. Am. J. Hyg., 64:376-382, 1956

15. Jordan, W. S. Jr., Badger, G. F. and Dingle, J. H. XV. Acquisition of type-specific adenovirus antibodies in the first five years of life—Implications for the use of adenovirus vaccine. New Eng. J. Med., 258:1041-1044, 1958

16. Jordan, W. S., Jr., Badger, G. F. and Dingle, J. H. XVI. The epidemiology of influenza, 1948-1953. Am. J. Hyg., 68:169-189, 1958

17. Jordan, W. S., Jr., Denny, F. W., Jr., Badger, G. F., Curtiss, C., Dingle, J. H., Oseasohn, R. and Stevens, D. A. XVII. The occurrence of Asian influenza. Am. J. Hyg., 68:190-212, 1958

18. Boake, W. C. XVIII. Tobacco smoking and respiratory infections. New Eng. J. Med., 259:1245-1249, 1958

19. James, W. E. S., Badger, G. F. and Dingle, J. H. XIX. The epidemiology of the acquisition of group A streptococci and of associated illnesses. New Eng. J. Med., 262:687-694, 1960

20. McCorkle, L. P. XX. Blood groups O and A and the occurrence of certain minor illnesses. Am. J. Hyg., 75:33-43, 1962

21. Miller, I. XXI. The tendency of members of a given family to have a similar number of common respiratory diseases. Am. J. Hyg., 79:207-217, 1964

22-26 Other articles based in part, at least, on the present study.

22. Feller, A. E., Badger, G. F., Hodges, R. G., Jordan, W. S., Jr., Rammelkamp, C. H., Jr. and Dingle, J. H. The failure of antihistaminic drugs to prevent or cure the common cold and undifferentiated respiratory diseases. New Eng. J. Med., 242:737-744, 1950

23. Ginsberg, H. S., Gold, E., Jordan, W. S., Jr., Katz, S., Badger, G. F. and Dingle, J. H. Relation of the new respiratory agents to acute respiratory diseases. Am. J. Pub. Health, 45:915-922, 1955

24. Dingle, J. H. Studies of respiratory and other illnesses in Cleveland (Ohio) families (Summary). Proc. Royal Soc. Med., 49:259-260, 1956

25. Jordan, W. S., Jr. Occurrence of adenovirus infections in civilian populations. A.M.A. Arch. Int. Med., 101:54-59, 1958

26. Dingle, J. H. An epidemiological study of illness in families. The Harvey Lectures, 1957-1958. Academic Press, New York, 1959, 1-24.

27-139 Other References

27. Anderson, S. G. Experimental rubella in human volunteers. J. Immunol., 62:29-40, 1949

28. Andrewes, C. H. The viruses of the common cold. Scientific American, 203: 88-102, 1960

29. Annual Reports of City of Cleveland, Department of Public Health and Welfare, Cleveland's Health, 1948-1957.

30. Bell, J. A., Rowe, W. P., Engler, J. I., Parrott, R. H. and Huebner, R. J. Pharyngoconjunctival fever. Epidemiological studies of a recently recognized disease entity. J.A.M.A. 157:1083-1092, 1955

31. Bell, S. D., Rota, T. R. and McComb, D. E. Adenoviruses isolated from Saudi Arabia. III. Six new serotypes. Amer. J. Trop. Med. and Hyg., 9:523-526, 1960

32. Berenberg, W., Wright, S. and Janeway, C. A. Roseola infantum (exanthem subitum). New Eng. J. Med., 241:253-259, 1949

33. Bhatt, P. N., Brooks, M. and Fox, J. P. Extent of infection with poliomyelitis virus in household associates of clinical cases as determined serologically and by virus isolation using tissue culture methods. Am. J. Hyg., 61:287-301, 1955

34. Bodian, D. and Paffenbarger, R. S. Poliomyelitis infection in households: Frequency of viremia and specific antibody response. Am. J. Hyg., 60: 83-98, 1954

35. Breese, B. B., Jr. Roseola infantum (exanthem subitum). New York State J. Med., 41:1854-1859, 1941

36. Brimblecombe, F. S. W., Cruickshank, R., Masters, P. L., Reid, D. D. and Stewart, M. D. Family studies of respiratory infections. Brit. Med. J., 1:119-128, 1958

37. Brown, G. C., Francis, T., Jr. and Pearson, H. E. Rapid development of carrier state and detection of poliomyelitis virus. J. A. M. A., 129:121-123, 1945

38. Brown, G. C., Rabson, A. S. and Schieble, J. H. The effect of gamma globulin on subclinical infection in familial associates of poliomyelitis cases. I. Quantitative estimation of fecal virus. J. Immunol., 73:54-61, 1954

39. Brown, G. C., Rabson, A. S. and Schieble, J. H. The effect of gamma globulin on subclinical infection in familial associates of poliomyelitis cases. II. Serological studies and virus isolations from pharyngeal secretions. J. Immunol., 74:71-80, 1955

40. Buck, Carol. Acute upper respiratory infections in families. Am. J. Hyg., 63:1-12, 1956

41. Casey, A. E., Fishbein, W. I., Schabel, F. M., Jr., Smith, H. T. and Bundesen, H. N. Epidemiologic implication of poliomyelitis virus in the throat. South. Med. J., 42:427-429, 1949

42. Chamovitz, R., Rammelkamp, C. H., Jr., Wannamaker, L. W. and Denny, F. W., Jr. The effect of tonsillectomy on the incidence of streptococcal respiratory disease and its complications. Pediatrics, 26:355-367, 1960

43. Collins, S. D., Phillips, R. F. and Oliver, D. S. Age incidence of specific causes of illness found in monthly canvasses of families. Pub. Health Rep., 66:1227-1245, 1951

44. Commission on Acute Respiratory Diseases. Experimental transmission of minor respiratory illness to human volunteers by filter-passing agents. II. Immunity on reinoculation with agents from the two types of minor respiratory illness and from primary atypical pneumonia. J. Clin. Invest., 26:974-982, 1947

45. Commission on Acute Respiratory Diseases. Exudative tonsillitis and pharyngitis of unknown cause. J. A. M. A., 133:588-593, 1947

46. Commission on Chronic Illness. Chronic illness in the United States. Vol. 1, Chapter 2, Promotion of health, 8-15. The Commonwealth Fund, Cambridge, Mass., Harvard University Press, 1957

47. Committee on Standard Serological Procedures in Influenza Studies. An agglutination-inhibition test proposed as a standard of reference in influenza diagnostic studies. J. Immunol., 65:347-353, 1950

48. Communicable Disease Center influenza report, U. S. Dept. of Health, Education, and Welfare, No. 8:4, 1957

49. Cramblett, H. G., Rosen, L., Parrott, R. H., Bell, J. A., Huebner, R. J. and McCullough, N. B. Respiratory illness in six infants infected with a newly recognized ECHO virus. Pediatrics, 21:168-177, 1958

50. Dingle, J. H., Ginsberg, H. S., Badger, G. F., Jordan, W. S., Jr. and Katz, S. Evidence for the specific etiology of acute respiratory disease (ARD). Trans. Assn. Amer. Phys., 67:149-154, 1954

51. Dingle, J. H., Ginsberg, H. S., Gold, E., Jordan, W. S., Jr., Katz, S. and Badger, G. F. Relationship of certain characteristics of the new respiratory viruses to the clinical and epidemiological behavior of non-bacterial pharyngitis. Trans. Assn. Amer. Phys., 68:73-77, 1955

52. Dorn, H. F. A classification system for morbidity concepts. Pub. Health Rep., 72:1043-1048, 1957

53. Downes, J. Change with age in susceptibilty to minor respiratory illness. Milbank Mem. Fund Quart., 30:211-223, 1952

54. Downes, J. Control of acute respiratory illness by ultra-violet lights. Am. J. Pub. Health, 40:1512-1520, 1950

55. Downes, J. and Mertz, J. C. Effect of frequency of family visiting upon the reporting of minor illnesses. Milbank Mem. Fund Quart., 31:371-390, 1953

56. Drachman, R. H., Hochbaum, G. M. and Rosenstock, I. M. Chapter II., A seroepidemiologic study in two cities. In: The impact of Asian influenza on community life. Pub. Health Ser. Pub. No. 766, U. S. Government Printing Office, 1960, 27-54

57. Dungal, N. Convalescent serum against measles. J. A. M. A., 125:20-22, 1944

58. Dunn, F. L. Pandemic influenza in 1957. Review of international spread of new Asian strain. J. A. M. A., 166:1140-1148, 1958

59. Eichenwald, H. F., Ababio, A., Arky, A. M. and Hartman, A. P. Epidemic diarrhea in premature and older infants caused by ECHO virus type 18. J. A. M. A., 166:1563-1566, 1958

60. Enders, J. F., Weller, T. H. and Robbins, F. C. Cultivation of Lansing strain of poliomyelitis virus in cultures of various human embryonic tissues. Science, 109:85-87, 1949

61. Evans, A. S. Adenovirus infections in children and young adults, with comments on vaccination. New Eng. J. Med., 259:464-468, 1958

62. Fox, J. P., Gelfand, H. M., LeBlanc, D. R. and Conwell, D. P. A continuing study of the acquisition of natural immunity to poliomyelitis in representative Louisiana households. Am. J. Pub. Health, 46:282-294, 1956

63. Frost, W. H. and Gover, M. The incidence and time distribution of common colds in several groups kept under continuous observation. Pub. Health Rep., 47:1815-1841, 1932

64. Fulton, F. and Dumbell, K. R. The serological comparison of strains of influenza virus. J. Gen. Microbiol., 3:97-111, 1949

65. Ginsberg, H. S., Badger, G. F., Dingle, J. H., Jordan, W. S., Jr. and Katz, S. Etiologic relationship of the RI-67 agent to acute respiratory disease (ARD). J. Clin. Invest., 34:820-831, 1955

66. Ginsberg, H. S., Gold, E. and Jordan, W. S., Jr. Tryptose phosphate broth as supplementary factor for maintenance of HeLa cell tissue cultures. Proc. Soc. Exper. Biol. and Med., 89:66-71, 1955

67. Gordon, I. The nonamebic nonbacillary diarrheal disorders. Am. J. Trop. Med. and Hyg., 4:739, 1955

68. Gordon, I., Ingraham, H. S. and Korns, R. F. Transmission of epidemic gastroenteritis to human volunteers by oral administration of fecal filtrates. J. Exper. Med., 86:409-422, 1947

69. Hammon, W. McD., Ludwig, E. H., Sather, G. E. and Schrack, W. D., Jr. A longitudinal study of infection with poliomyelitis viruses in American families on a Philippine military base during interepidemic period. Ann. N. Y. Acad. Sci., 61:979-988, 1955

70. Heinbecker, P. and Irvine-Jones, E. I. M. Susceptibility of Eskimos to the common cold and a study of their natural immunity to diphtheria, scarlet fever and bacterial filtrates. J. Immunol., 15:395-406, 1928

71. Hilleman, M. R., Werner, J. H., Dascomb, H. E. and Butler, R. L. Epidemiologic investigations with respiratory disease virus RI-67. Am. J. Pub. Health, 45:203-210, 1955

72. Hilleman, M. R., Werner, J. H., Adair, C. V. and Dreisbach, A. R. Outbreak of acute respiratory illness caused by RI-67 and influenza A viruses, Fort Leonard Wood, 1952-1953. Am. J. Hyg., 61:163-173, 1955

73. Hilleman, M. R. and Werner, J. H. Recovery of new agents from patients with acute respiratory illness. Proc. Soc. Exper. Biol. and Med., 85:183-188, 1954

74. Howe, H. A., Bodian, D. and Wenner, H. A. Further observations on the presence of poliomyelitis virus in the human oropharynx. Bull. Johns Hopkins Hosp., 76:19-24, 1945

75. Huebner, R. J., Rowe, W. P., Ward, T. G., Parrott, R. H. and Bell, J. A. Adenoidal-pharyngeal-conjunctival agents: a newly recognized group of common viruses of the respiratory system. New Eng. J. Med., 251:1077-1086, 1954

76. Ingalls, T. H., Babbott, F. L., Hampson, K. W. and Gordon, J. E. Rubella: Its epidemiology and teratology. Am. J. Med. Sci., 239:363-383, 1960

77. Isacson, P., Melnick, J. L. and Walton, M. Environmental studies of endemic enteric virus infection. II. Poliovirus infections in household units. Am. J. Hyg., 65:29-42, 1957

78. Jackson, G. G., Dowling, H. F. and Anderson, T. O. Neutralization of common cold agents in volunteers by pooled human globulin. Science, 128:27-28, 1958

79. Jackson, G. G. and Dowling, H. F. Transmission of the common cold to volunteers under controlled conditions. IV. Specific immunity to the common cold. J. Clin. Invest., 38:762-769, 1959

80. Jackson, G. G., Dowling, H. F., Spiesman, I. G. and Boand, A. V. Transmission of the common cold to volunteers under controlled conditions. A.M.A. Arch. Int. Med., 101:267-278, 1958

81. Jaffe, N. B. Epidemic gastroenteritis. Amer. J. Digest. Dis., 15:131-134, 1948

82. Jensen, K. E. Influenza. In: Diagnostic Procedures for Virus and Rickettsial Diseases. American Public Health Association, New York, 1956, 241-262

83. Jordan, W. S., Jr. and Gaylin, S. G. The antigenic variation of influenza B viruses. Demonstration of an antigenic spectrum by use of titer ratios. J. Immunol., 70:393-399, 1953

84. Jordan, W. S., Jr. The mechanism of spread of Asian influenza. Amer. Rev. Resp. Dis., 83:29-35, 1961

85. Jordan, W. S., Jr. and Oseasohn, R. O. The use of RDE to improve the sensitivity of the hemagglutination-inhibition test for the serologic diagnosis of influenza. J. Immunol., 72:229-235, 1954

86. Kaiser, A. D. Results of tonsillectomy: Comparative study of 2200 tonsillectomized children with equal number of controls 3 and 10 years after operation. J.A.M.A., 95:837-842, 1930

87. Kaiser, A. D. Significance of tonsils in development of child. J.A.M.A., 115:1151-1156, 1940

88. Kessel, J. F. and Moore, F. J. The occurrence of poliomyelitis virus in tonsils and stools of noncontacts during an interepidemic period. Am. J. Hyg., 41:25-29, 1945

89. Klein, J. O., Lenner, A. M. and Finland, M. Acute gastroenteritis associated with ECHO virus, Type II. Am. J. Med. Sci., 240:749-753, 1960

90. Kojima, S., Fukumi, H., Kusama, H., Yamamoto, S., Suzuki, S., Uchida, T., Ishimaru T., Oka, T., Kuretani, K., Ohmura, K., Nishikawa, F., Fujimoto, S., Fujita, K., Nakano, A. and Sunakawa, S. Studies on the causative agent of the infectious diarrhea. Records of the experiments on human volunteers. Japan Med. J., *1*:467-476, 1948

91. Krugman, S., Ward, R., Jacobs, K. G. and Lazar, M. Studies on rubella immunization. I. Demonstration of rubella without rash. J.A.M.A., *151*:285-288, 1953

92. Lancefield, R. C. Studies on antigenic composition of group A hemolytic streptococci. I. Effects of proteolytic enzymes on streptococcal cells. J. Exper. Med., *78*:465-476, 1943

93. Lidwell, O. M. and Sommerville, T. Observations on the incidence and distribution of the common cold in a rural community during 1948 and 1949. J. Hygiene, *49*:365-381, 1951

94. McLean, D. M., McNaughton, G. A. and Wyllie, J. C. Infantile gastroenteritis: Further viral investigations. Canad. Med. Assn. J., *85*:496-497, 1961

95. Marshall, M. O. We are a family of guinea pigs. McCall's, *77*:26-36, 1949

96. Medical Research Council. Epidemics in schools: An analysis of the data collected during the first five years of a statistical inquiry. Med. Res. Council Spec. Rep. Series No. 227, 1938

97. Melnick, J. L., Horstmann, D. M. and Ward, R. The isolation of poliomyelitis virus from human extra-neural sources. II. Comparison of virus content of blood, oral pharyngeal washings, and stools of contacts. J. Clin. Invest., *25*:275-277, 1946

98. Melnick, J. L., Walton, M., Isacson, P. and Cardwell, W. Environmental studies of endemic enteric virus infections. I. Community seroimmune patterns and poliovirus infection rates. Am. J. Hyg., *65*:1-28, 1957

99. Mertz, J. C. Tonsillectomy and respiratory illness in populations of two communities in New York State. Milbank Mem. Fund Quart., *32*:5-21, 1954

100. Miller, F. J. W., Court, S. D. M., Walton, W. S. and Knox, E. G. Growing Up in Newcastle upon Tyne. Oxford University Press, London, 1960, 1-369

101. Murray, E. S., Chang, R. S., Bell, S. D., Tarizzo, M. L. and Snyder, J. C. Agents recovered from acute conjunctivitis cases in Saudi Arabia. Am. J. Ophth., *43*:32, Part II, April 1957

102. Neter, E. Enteritis due to enteropathogenic Escherichia coli. Present day status and unsolved problems. J. Pediat., *55*:223-239, 1959

103. Oseasohn, R., Adelson, L. and Kaji, M. Clinicopathologic study of 33 fatal cases of Asian influenza. New Eng. J. Med., *260*:509-518, 1959

104. Patton, J. H. P. Tonsil-adenoid operation in relation to health of group of schoolgirls. Quart. J. Med., *12*:119-128, 1943

105. Paul, J. H. and Freese, H. L. An epidemiological and bacteriological study of the common cold in an isolated arctic community (Spitzbergen). Am. J. Hyg., *17*:517-535, 1933

106. Pike, R. M. Isolation of hemolytic streptococci from throat swabs. Experiments with sodium azide and crystal violet enrichment broth. Am. J. Hyg., *41*:211, 1945

107. Rammelkamp, C. H., Jr. and Weaver, R. S. Acute glomerulonephritis. The significance of the variations in the incidence of the disease. J. Clin. Invest., *32*:345-358, 1953

108. Ramos-Alvarez, M. and Sabin, A. B. Enteropathogenic viruses and bacteria: Role in summer diarrheal diseases of infancy and early childhood. J.A.M.A., *167*:147-156, 1958

109. Reimann, H. A. Viral and bacillary dysentery: A dual epidemic. J.A.M.A., *149*:1619-1623, 1952

110. Reimann, H. A. Viral infections of the respiratory tract: Their treatment and prevention. J.A.M.A., *132*:487-493, 1946

111. Rosen, L., Hovis, J. F., Mastrota, F. M., Bell, J. A. and Huebner, R. J. Observations on a newly recognized virus (Abney) of the reovirus family. Am. J. Hyg., *71*:258-265, 1960

112. Rosen, L., Baron, S. and Bell, J. A. Four newly recognized adenoviruses. Proc. Soc. Exper. Biol. and Med., *107*:434-437, 1961

113. Rowe, W. P., Huebner, R. J., Gilmore, L. K., Parrott, R. H. and Ward, T. G. Isolation of cytopathogenic agents from human adenoid undergoing spontaneous degeneration in tissue culture. Proc. Soc. Exper. Biol. and Med., *84*:570-573, 1953

114. Rowe, W. P., Hartley, J. W. and Huebner, R. J. Serotype composition of adenovirus group. Proc. Soc. Exper. Biol. and Med., *97*:465-470, 1958

115. Sabin, A. B. Personal communication.

116. Sabin, A. B. Reoviruses. Science, *130*:1387-1389, 1959

117. Sabin, A. B. and Steigman, A. J. Poliomyelitis virus of low virulence in patients with epidemic summer grippe or sore throat. Am. J. Hyg.,*49*: 176-193, 1949

118. Sanford, J. P. and Sulkin, S. E. Clinical spectrum of ECHO-virus infections. New Eng. J. Med., *261*:1113-1122, 1959

119. Sartwell, P. E. The distribution of incubation periods of infectious disease. Am. J. Hyg., *51*:310-318, 1950

120. Schabel, F. M., Jr., Casey, A. E., Fishbein, W. I. and Smith, H. T. Isolation of the virus of poliomyelitis from the stools, oropharynx and nose of contacts. J. Inf. Dis., *87*:152-157, 1950

121. Scherer, W. F., Syverton, J. T. and Gey, G. O. Studies on propagation *in vitro* of poliomyelitis viruses. IV. Viral multiplication in a stable strain of human malignant epithelial cells (strain HeLa) derived from epidermoid carcinoma of cervix. J. Exper. Med., *97*:695-710, 1953

122. Shope, R. E. Influenza: History, epidemiology, and speculation. Pub. Health Rep., *73*:165-178, 1958

123. Sickles, G. M., Feorino, P. and Plager, H. Isolation and type determinations of Coxsackie virus, group B, in tissue culture. Proc. Soc. Exper. Biol. and Med., *88*:22-24, 1955

124. Siegel, A. C., Rammelkamp, C. H., Jr. and Griffeath, H. I. Epidemic nephritis in a school population. The relation of hematuria to group A streptococci. Pediatrics, *15*:33-44, 1955

125. Spence, J., Walton, W. S., Miller, F. J. W. and Court, S. D. M. A. Thousand Families in Newcastle upon Tyne. Oxford University Press, London, 1954, 1-217

126. Stallones, R. A., Hilleman, M. R., Gauld, R. L., Warfield, M. S. and Anderson, S. A. Adenovirus (RI-APC-ARD) vaccine for prevention of acute respiratory illness. 2. Field evalution. J.A.M.A., *163*:9-15, 1957

127. Stevens, D. A. Studies on the technique of transporting throat swabs to the laboratory for the isolation of pneumococci. J. Lab. and Clin. Med., *39*:437-439, 1952

128. Sommerville, R. G. Enteroviruses and diarrhoea in young persons. Lancet, *2*:1347-1349, 1958

129. Swift, H. F., Wilson, A. T. and Lancefield, R. C. Typing group A hemolytic streptococci by M precipitin reactions in capillary pipettes. J. Exper. Med., *78*:125-133, 1943

130. Sydenstricker, E. A study of illness in a general population. Hagerstown morbidity studies No. 1: The method of study and general results. Pub. Health Rep., *41*:2069-2088, 1926

131. Tateno, I., Suzuki, S., Kagawa, S., Naito, H. and Goto, T. On an ECHO-like agent constantly recoverable from volunteers given Niigata strain of acute epidemic gastroenteritis. Japan. J. Exper. Med., *26*:125-138, 1956

132. Trotter, Y., Dunn., F. L., Drachman, R. H., Henderson, D. A., Pizzi, M. and Langmuir, A. D. Asian influenza in the United States, 1957-1958. Am. J. Hyg., *70*:34-50, 1959

133. Tyrell, D. A. J. Personal communication containing data analyzed by J. W. Field and A. T. Roden, some of which appeared in: Roden, A. T. Variations in the clinical patterns of experimentally induced colds. J. Hyg., *61*:231-246, 1963

134. U.S. Bureau of the Census, 1950 Census of the Population. Alphabetical Index of Occupations and Industries (revised edition). U.S. Government Printing Office, Washington, D. C., 1950

135. Vignec, A. J., Paul, J. R. and Trask, J. D. Recovery of viruses of poliomyelitis from extra-neural sources in man, with survey of literature. Yale J. Biol. and Med., *11*:15-31, 1938

136. Wehrle, R. F., Hammon, W. McD., Coriell, L. L. and McAllister, R. M. Spread of poliovirus infection during an epidemic of unusual activity, Woodbury County, Iowa, and Dakota County, Nebraska, 1952. Am. J. Hyg., *65*:386-403, 1957

137. Weil, W. B., Jr., Rammelkamp, C. H., Jr. and Bolande, R. P. Unpublished data.

138. Wenner, H. A. and Tamm, W. A. Poliomyelitis in families attacked by disease. I. Distribution of virus in stool and oropharynx of members of household. Am. J. Med. Sci., *216*:258-269, 1948

139. Zaintek, A. R. The rapid infection of a family after introduction of poliomyelitis virus. Am. J. Hyg., *46*:248-253, 1947

INDEX

Adenoviruses. *See* Common respiratory diseases *and* Tonsillitis and pharyngitis (non-bacterial)

Blood pressure, 283

Cervical adenitis, 279

Chickenpox, 241-246
annual and seasonal occurrence, 241
family outbreaks, 244-246
incubation periods, 244
secondary attack rates, 244-245

Cold, common. *See* Common respiratory diseases

Common respiratory diseases, 33-96
clinical aspects
attempts to classify by symptomatology, 66-80
definition of, 19, 162
episodes in families
definition, 41
intervals between index and secondary cases, 47
inverse correlation between intervals and secondary attack rates, 48-49
possible role of immunity, 49
etiology, 129-161
adenoviruses, 129-148
antibodies, occurrence and distribution of, 129-140
laboratory properties in relation to epidemic spread, 146
occurrence of illness due to, 136-148
Coxsackie viruses, 153-157
parainfluenza viruses, 157-161
polioviruses, 148-153
first year of life, 80-96
clinical characteristics, 80-86
complications, 85-86
epidemiological aspects, 89-96
incidence by month of age, 89
incidence by season of birth, 91
relationship of respiratory infection in mother during pregnancy to onset of first illness in infant, 94-96
secondary attack rates by month of age, 93-94
incidence
age, 33
age at which child first attended school, 38-39
cumulative, 26
family composition, 42-43
school attendance, 35-37
sex, 35
size of family, 39-40
total, 33
variation in individuals and families, 56-66
indices of exposure within the community, 49-52
introduction and spread in the family, 40-52
role of various family members, 41-42
secondary attack rates
age, 45-46
age of contact and age of index case, 46
size of family, 46-47
spread within the family, 43-52
role of immunity, 55-56
susceptibility to repeated attacks, 52-56
tonsillectomy, relation to symptoms and incidence, 118-124

Communicable diseases, 240-279
occurrence in Cleveland, 240
occurrence in study population, 241
See also specific diseases

Conjunctivitis, 279

Coxsackie viruses
isolation at time of respiratory symptoms, 141
See also Common respiratory diseases

Deaths, 7, 286

Diseases
miscellaneous, 280-286

Exanthem subitum, 274-279
See also Roseola infantum

Families
accuracy of recorded data, 12-13
age of individuals, 8
economic status, 9
education of parents, 9
methods of observation, 4-6
number of individuals studied, 7
number studied, 7
occupation of parents, 9
selection of, 2, 4, 287
size of, 8

396